W0227826

HIGH RISK
PREGNANCY
AND CHILD

HIGH RISK PREGNANCY AND CHILD

Z. Štembera, M. D.,
K. Znamenáček, M. D.,
K. Poláček, M. D.

Institute for the Care of Mother and Child, Prague

MARTINUS NIJHOFF / MEDICAL DIVISION
THE HAGUE 1976

ISBN-13:978-94-010-1422-9   e-ISBN-13:978-94-010-1420-5
DOI: 10.1007/978-94-010-1420-5

Copyright 1976 by Martinus Nijhoff b. v., P.O. Box 269, The Hague
The Netherlands
© Translation: M. Schierlová
Softcover reprint of the hardcover 1st edition 1976

This book is published with the arrangement of AVICENUM,

Czechoslovak Medical Press, Prague.

All rights reserved.
No part of this book may be reproduced by print, photoprint, or any other
means without written permission of the publishers.

CO-WORKERS

V. Čiperová, M.D.
J. Dittrichová, Ph.D.
J. Dolanský, M.D.
K. Hodr, M.D.
M. Janovský, M.D.
M. Kittrich, M.D.
J. Koch, Ph.D.
J. Kučera, M.D.
R. Lodinová, M.D.
V. Melichar, M.D.
J. Tomanová, Ph.D.
B. Vedra, M.D.
V. Vlach, M.D.
J. Zezuláková, M.D.
J. Židovský, M.D.
A. Zwinger, M.D.

CONTENTS

7

INTRODUCTION TO ENGLISH EDITION

This book, written in 1971, was first published in Czech, in 1972. In the four years which have elapsed since then, perinatal medicine has made rapid progress, and new findings have been made in prevention, diagnosis and therapy. This meant that some chapters have had to be supplemented, corrected or revised. Since Dr. K. Znamenáček, the author of several of the paediatric chapters and editor of the paediatric part of the book, died in 1973, his work as corrector and editor was taken over by Dr. K. Poláček, DrSc. In its main outlines, the English version is the same as the Czech, the only difference being the omission of parts specifically concerning Czechoslovak perinatological problems. We hope that the reception given to the English edition of this book will be as favourable as that received by its Czech counterpart.

INTRODUCTION TO CZECH EDITION

It is customary for the introductory chapter of a book to explain what the book is about or to give a concise idea of its contents. In our case, we thought it better to make a break with tradition and state what we did **not** wish this book to be − a scientific monograph, a symposial bibliographic review, a textbook of modern obstetrics and paediatrics, a survey of the latest research results or a doctrine (the only one correctly embracing, describing and explaining perinatal medicine).

All the above negatives severely limited our positive possibilities, but even so we found it difficult to say exactly what we wanted our book to be. Perhaps the formulation "A perinatological compendium", or "A guide to perinatology" would best express our aims, since perinatology is still not recognized as a separate branch of medicine, although the European Perinatological

Society has been in existence for several years and has already held four European congresses.

This book is intended primarily for those who have the most to do with perinatology, that is to say, for obstetricians and neonatologist paediatricians, i.e. specialists in their own field. It must thus presuppose that each of these possesses the necessary basic knowledge of his own specialization. On the other hand, how much can he be expected to know of the other's field? It would, however, be entirely contrary to our aims if the obstetrician were to read only the first part of the book, and the paediatrician only the second part, and both were to ignore the last, i.e. the psychological and neurological, part. The situation is still more difficult for other specialists in contiguous fields, whose work is even more remote from obstetrics and paediatrics, but for whom it is still necessary to read the whole of this book. In our opinion, reciprocal acquaintance with the problems and difficulties encountered in each of these branches of medicine ought, in principle, to abolish the under-estimation and superficial criticism of other people's work which we still encounter from time to time, and replace them by full appreciation and understanding. Precisely perinatology, as an interdisciplinary branch of medicine, is a typical example of how further progress is impossible without the closest cooperation. In fact, it is this repeatedly demonstrated fact which makes perinatology a branch of medicine in its own right.

The stormy development of perinatology during the past 10 years and the hundreds of papers published on this subject (only a few of which are available to the majority of workers) make it hard to decide on the best way to proceed in daily practice. As a result, some workers prefer to keep to the old, well-worn diagnostic and therapeutic paths. Not all of the newly proposed tech-niques have been adequately verified; some, painted in glowing colours, have failed to live up to expectations, while others, less intensively propagated, have proved to be of very real value. Some, although proven and tried, will not be able to be used on a large scale, because the expensive and exacting apparatus required puts them beyond the reach of small institutions. It is necessary for every worker concerned with perinatology to be acquainted with the true present situation as objectively as possible, however. On the other hand, is it within the power of a single individual or a small team to give such objective information? After describing the contemporary situation, we consequently sometimes leave the last word with the reader, who is a spe-cialist, like the authors.

Only methods whose use in practical perinatology can really be recommen-ded are included in the book. Some readers will no doubt feel that other, more modern methods are lacking — and in some cases they will probably be right. Others will imagine that some of the methods described are unnecessary fantasies of the future because at the moment they cannot be used in normal practice. Where is the golden mean between these two views? If these parts of the book were to produce predominantly one or the other reaction, it would be a mark of failure. On the contrary, the purpose of these chapters is to stimulate the reader to increase his efforts to improve the equipment of his own workplace, so that some of the methods recommended can be introduced there. He may often find a lack of comprehension and encounter obstacles, but progress can never be achieved without overcoming them.

This book is the collective product of the workers of one institute and its closest external consultants. It is the outcome of their own daily experiences in antenatal clinics, in hospital wards, in the delivery theatre and the intensive care unit and in some cases of the results of research work. Although the authors have many years' experience in perinatology, because they work in a research institute where, for two decades, it has formed the essence of their clinical and research work, they cannot, and have no desire to, claim that the views expressed in this book are the only right ones. Perinatology is developing so rapidly that by the time this book reaches the reader's hand, some parts of it will probably already be out of date.

The decision as to whether we shall be able to keep up with this stormy development does not rest with the perinatologists alone, but also with those who are responsible for providing them with the necessary conditions, that is to say with the administrative and executive authorities at all levels, from the director of the hospital to the district and regional authorities, right up to government level. Some of the chapters of this book are therefore intended form them also. Today, medicine (and perinatology in particular) is no longer a "non-productive" profession. On the contrary, its influence on the national economy is extremely marked and it is up to all of us to see to it that its influence is as positive as is humanly possible.

THE PRESENT STATE, MISSION AND SOCIAL SIGNIFICANCE OF PERINATAL MEDICINE

Questions associated with human reproduction are being studied with mounting interest all over the world. The most discussed and the most serious problem is the population explosion in the underdeveloped countries, but reproduction problems (though of a different type) also occur in the more advanced countries. Here, more and more interest is being focussed on the care of mother and child, with special reference to the quality of the offspring. This type of very exacting care requires close cooperation not only between the obstetrician and the paediatrician, but also with specialists in other, related fields (the geneticist, children's neurologist, psychologist, sociologist, pedadogue, etc). Successful team-work presupposes at least partial knowledge, by each member of the team, of the work of the others, however. On the other hand, diagnostics and therapeutic techniques (intensive antenatal and postnatal care) have progressed so rapidly during the past decade, owing to the development of medical electronics and modern biochemistry, that the obstetrician and the paediatrician, who previously concerned themselves with the whole of their subject, can hardly keep pace and, by a natural process, this development has of necessity given rise to a new interdisciplinary branch — perinatal medicine.

PERINATAL MORTALITY

Perinatal mortality is an internationally acknowledged index of the quality of care of the pregnant woman and the newborn infant. Its marked drop in Czechoslovakia during the first 15 years after the Second World War was proof that the concept of the socialist health system for improving antenatal

15

Table 1. Comparison of perinatal and infant mortality in some countries (from WHO review, 1969)

Country	Antenatal mortality per mille	Early neonatal mortality per mille	Perinatal mortality per mille	Infant mortality per mille
Sweden	8	8	16	11
Finland	9	10	19	12
Denmark	9	10	19	14
Switzerland	9	10	19	14
New Zealand	10	9	19	16
Iceland	10	9	19	18
Bulgaria	10	9	19	25
Holland	12	8	20	12
Czechoslovakia	7	14	21	22
Norway	12	9	21	12
Canada	10	12	22	17
Australia	10	12	22	17
Salvador	10	12	22	47
Israel	11	12	23	23
Germ. Dem. Rep.	11	12	23	18
England	13	11	24	17
Poland	10	14	24	29
Rumania	13	11	24	42
Madagascar	18	6	24	102
France	15	10	25	17
Scotland	14	11	25	20
Belgium	12	13	25	20
Luxemburg	10	15	25	22
Kuwait	13	12	25	39
Ireland	14	12	26	23
Yugoslavia	10	16	26	32
U.S.A.	13	14	27	19
Malta	11	16	27	24
Germ. Fed. Rep.	12	15	27	23
Austria	10	17	27	26
Greece	14	14	28	27
Italy	18	16	34	28

and postnatal care was correct. In the first place, it included organizational measures (the establishment of a wide network of antenatal clinics, a progressive shift of all deliveries from home to hospital, with a several-fold increase in the number of available beds, close cooperation with the paediatrician immediately after birth). Secondly, it provided for the training of new medical and paramedical personnel. And last, but not least, it ensured a gradual transition from the predominantly mechanistic concept of obstetrics to a physiological concept and the formation of a new branch of paediatrics — neonatalogy. The subsequent rapid fall in perinatal mortality ranked Czechoslovakia among the first countries in the world in this respect. Since 1961, however, the decrease in perinatal mortality in Czechoslovakia has slowed down considerably and a number of other countries (in Europe the Scandinavian countries) have achieved still lower perinatal mortality, as seen from the abbreviated WHO survey for 1969 (Tab. 1).

Since it is well known that early neonatal deaths, in countries with a highly developed health system, account for about 50–75% of infant mortality, it can be stated with certainty that countries claiming a much lower early neonatal death rate do not include the early death of low birthweight foetuses in their figures for the WHO (Tab. 2).

Table 2. Comparison of proportion of early neonatal deaths in the infant mortality rate in various countries

Country	Early neonatal death rate (per mille)	Infant mortality rate (per mille)	Proportion of early neonatal deaths in infant mortality rate (per cent)
Sweden	8	11	73
Switzerland	10	14	71
Czechoslovakia	14	22	64
Bulgaria	9	25	36
Rumania	11	42	26
Salvador	12	47	25
Madagascar	6	102	0.6

The perinatal mortality figures given by these countries thus do not conform to WHO criteria and they therefore occupy an inappropriate place in the table. (For instance, Bulgaria ought rightly to show an early neonatal death rate of at least 15 per mille; this would correspond to 60 % of its infant mortality rate, so that its total figure for perinatal mortality would be about 25 per mille, which would bring it down to the 20th to 25th place. The same applies to Rumania, Salvador, Madagascar and others.).

The WHO analysis further shows that Czechoslovakia has the lowest antenatal death rate in the world, but that its early neonatal death rate ranks it the 16th among the 60 recorded countries. It would not be right to conclude from these figures that the standard of paediatric care on the first 7 days after birth is low there, however. The high early neonatal death rate is associated with the large number of infants with a birthweight of less than 500 g, which many countries do not include in their perinatal mortality statistics at all. It is clear from these examples that the existing definitions of the WHO for calculating perinatal mortality as a criterion of the quality of perinatal care when comparing it in different countries are no longer satisfactory.

17

POPULATION PROBLEMS

Perinatal medicine is also closely related to population problems. From the 1950's, the positive post-war population trend was succeeded by a decrease in the birth rate lasting up to 1967. Since then, there has again been a marked increase, which is related to parentage of the large postwar generation and mainly, since 1973, to the encouragement given by the Czechoslovak government. A few per mille decrease in perinatal mortality cannot significantly influence a population increment, but although good results in perinatal medicine cannot influence the population quantitatively, they have other, far greater possibilities for influencing it qualitatively.

In recent years, most of the advanced countries have come to realize that the prosperity of society is becoming increasingly dependent upon the proportion of mentally able individuals in the population. Extensive socio-economic studies in the U.S.S.R. demonstrated that raising a worker's education by one class helped him to master new techniques in half the time and increased his output by 2%. Different authors give different figures for the rough estimate of the proportion of individuals of low intelligence ($2 - 16$ %), according to their borderline criterion (different I. Q. levels, ability to complete different grades of schooling, etc). Today there are dozens of studies demonstrating that mental retardation is often caused by disturbances originating during the perinatal period, many of which could have been avoided. This makes perinatal medicine a very important branch of medicine, which could help to reduce this relatively high percentage of uneducable or only partly educable individuals and thus help to improve the quality of our population.

PERINATAL MORBIDITY

This is a new term covering different types and degrees of injury or disturbances of normal development originating in the perinatal period. The chief disorders are perinatal encephalopathies, mental retardation, sensory disturbances and epilepsy, but they also include certain congenital anomalies and minimal cerebral dysfunction. Their causal association with various pathological states of the mother during pregnancy or labour has already been demonstrated.

The recording of the individual disorders still leaves much to be desired and the data on their incidence in the population are thus incomplete. In the

U.S.A., for example, there are 2,624,000 severely mentally retarded individuals, 437,000 spastics and 428,000 epileptics (Wallace 1970). According to estimates, there are about 300,000 mentally deficient individuals in Czechoslovakia, 30,000 children attending schools for mentally deficient children and 50,000 attending schools for children requiring special care. Thousands of other children fail to complete primary school and finish in the 6th or 7th class (instead of the 9th). Still less is known of how many of these very grave conditions originated in the perinatal period. Isolated analyses (e.g. Bienkiewicz et al. 1970) indicate that the proportion must be at least 75 %. The economic, as well as the ethical, implications of these shocking figures are so grave that some of the more advanced countries have begun to take an active interest in them at the highest governmental level.

ECONOMIC CONSEQUENCES

A detailed study of the French Ministry of Health, worked out together, in 1970, by specialists in questions concerning perinatal medicine and economists, gives a model demonstration of the economic losses which perinatal mortality and morbidity mean for the state. Calculation of the losses was based on the following considerations:

(1) The large sums expended on the education or treatment of perinatally injured (handicapped) individuals.
(2) The very limited economic contribution of these individuals to the national income, owing to their low fitness for work.
(3) Perinatal deaths mean the loss of whole lives in the production process and hence of their contribution to the national income.

Calculated in this manner, the economic losses caused by perinatal mortality and morbidity in France, for example, amount to 10.5 milliard francs a year. In Czechoslovakia, a similar estimate, only for individuals with the severest perinatal injury, shows an annual loss of over 5 milliard crowns. Less severely afflicted individuals, of whom there are many times more, represent at least equals economic losses.

The French study submits two alternative solutions, with perspectives up to 1980, according to which every franc invested in perinatal medicine brings a profit of 5−10 francs to the national income. The health services can thus no longer be regarded as "unproductive", like they used to be − and unfortunately sometimes still are. In most of the more advanced countries, expenditure on perinatal medicine is today acknowledged to be not only the best investment for the future of the human race (Rauramo 1970), but also the best form of national investment.

FUTURE PROSPECTS

Perinatal care is a broad concept and any attempts to improve it must therefore be based on objective analyses, to ensure that investments made for its improvement are actually used where they are most urgently needed. There are dozens of such analyses, but they are practically entirely retrospective and cover only small series. As an example of a retrospective analysis on a national scale we have the analysis of all perinatal foetal and infant deaths in Czechoslovakia which is published annually by the Ministry of Health and which is unique of its kind. Such analyses are of great significance, since they reveal the most important causes of perinatal mortality or relevant deficiencies in perinatal care. The causes of perinatal morbidity can be studied only from prospective analyses, however. As examples, we have an English and an American analysis:

English analysis: In 1958, the British National Birth Trust Fund collected detailed information on 17,000 births over the whole of England in one week. The British National Child Development Study has followed up 14,000 of these children continuously since 1958 to the present day, precisely in association with complications which occurred in the mothers during pregnancy and labour.

American analysis: The National Collaborative Perinatal Project, initiated in 1964, continuously assembles data on the development of 60,000 children, like the English project, in relationship to pregnancy and labour risks, with special reference to perinatal morbidity and the mental development of these children.

In recent years the WHO has likewise held several conferences and working symposia on the analysis of the causes and the prevention of perinatal mortality and morbidity from the international aspect and has prepared, for this purpose, a number of separate international projects, which are at present being carried out in various parts of the world.

From the aspect of professional development in perinatology, the European Perinatological Society has become the European centre for the comparison of the latest diagnostic, therapeutic and preventive findings and of long-term results. Every two years it organizes European perinatology congresses

20

(the first in Berlin, 1968, the second in London, 1970, the third in Lausanne, 1972, and the fourth in Prague, 1974). These congresses were preceded by a similar one held in Prague in 1966, which was attended by delegates from 23 countries. Many European countries now have their own national perinatological societies, which regularly hold national congresses on the subject of perinatal medicine.

A French government-approved project plans an increase of 0.9 milliard francs in investments in perinatal medicine up to 1980. Of these, 10 million francs released in 1971 were spent as follows:

technical equipment of delivery theatres and neonatal intensive care units	. . . . .	2.8 million Fr.
training of specialists in perinatology	. . . . .	1.8
improvement of delivery theatre services	. . . . .	1.7
improvement of antenatal care services	. . . . .	1.5
vaccination against rubella	. . . . .	1.1
epidemiological studies and statistics	. . . . .	0.5

The relative distribution of these investments can be taken as a very good example, which, with various modifications, could likewise be suitable for other countries. In Czechoslovakia also, the technical equipment of some maternity hospitals needs to be supplemented by new, modern apparatuses. On the other hand, the problem of congenital developmental anomalies caused by rubella in the first 3 months (which in Czechoslovakia is resolved, in principle, by legal abortion) is of smaller significance and is replaced by the very important preventive campaign of inoculating all Rh negative women with anti-D globulin. In a lot of respects, perinatal care in Czechoslovakia is well ahead of many other countries (the wide network of antenatal and children's clinics, 99% of children born in hospital, close collaboration between obstetrician and paediatrician). This makes it all the more necessary to concentrate on the other sectors, the most important of which is modern, comprehensive care of high risk pregnancies in the obstetrical sphere and of high risk infants (specifically, early detection of psychomotor retardation) in the paediatric sphere.

SCREENING AND DIFFERENTIATION
OF THE HIGH RISK PREGNANCY

SCREENING OF THE HIGH RISK PREGNANCY

The history of this special obstetrical problem is closely associated with the development of obstetrics during World War II and in Czechoslovakia, as in other countries, with a high standard of medical care. "Foetal Traumatism", a clinical research campaign conducted in Czechoslovakia in the 1950's, which resulted in the characterization of the most serious and commonest causes of injury to the foetus or newborn infant, is one of the first analyses of this type ever to have been made anywhere. Since it was published only in Czech (1956), however, its international repercussions were minimal. It was not until 7 years later that Butler (1963), after extensive research over a large part of England, published an analysis of perinatal mortality from the aspect of the "high risk mother". He included under this term both labour complications and a large group of causes already present during pregnancy. Although most of the latter were already known previously and were mentioned in the above analysis, "Foetal Traumatism", in Butler's study they appear for the first time under the collective term "high risk pregnancy" – though still largely in connection with perinatal mortality. This makes the pioneer work of the Czech authors Znamenáček and Jirsová (1958), who, in association with the "Foetal Traumatism" campaign, carried out a three years' perspective follow-up and evaluation of the development of these "traumatized" children, even more outstanding. Today there are dozens of studies giving a prospective evaluation, from birth, of the development of children from high risk pregnancies, not only from the point of view of the paediatrician and the neurologist, but also of the psychologist and the pedagogue during the first years of school attendance.

In association with raised perinatal and infant mortality and perinatal morbidity, these "high risk mothers" can be defined as "any homogeneous subpopulation within which the probability of occurrence of perinatal mortality and morbidity is much higher than in the population at large". Reliable differentiation of these groups requires, in the first place, their exact characterization by identification of the various high risk factors.

A number of lists of these **high risk factors,** divided into several groups and varying in detail, but similar in principle, have been published on the basis of analyses of perinatal mortality (Butler 1963, Gold 1968, Wallace 1970). The Czech Society of Perinatal Medicine, on the basis of the experiences of three maternity institutions (the Institute for the Care of Mother and Child, Prague-Podolí, the Maternity Clinic, Prague, and the Maternity Clinic, Olomouc), likewise compiled a concise list of the most important high risk factors, which, since 1971, has been incorporated into the special identity card issued to pregnant women by the Ministry of Health. The potential seriousness and danger of some of these high risk factors (pathological states) for the foetus and the newborn infant is not so great as their danger for the maternal organism, however, and the two concepts must not, therefore, be confused. Although it is now common knowledge that a high risk pregnancy is a commoner cause of perinatal mortality, and even greater morbidity than any complications which may develop during labour, labour itself cannot be ignored as a risk, especially after a high risk pregnancy. A list of high risk pregnancy factors should thus be supplemented by high risk labour factors. The most important high risk pregnancy and labour factors are discussed successively in the following chapters.

Identification of the most important high risk factors and the registration of all women in whom one or more of these factors occurs is only the first requirement in the proper screening of a high risk pregnancy. Since these high risk factors do not all carry the same weight (i.e. do not form an equal danger for the foetus), we must know the reciprocal relationship of their "weight", i.e. we must quantify them. The elaboration of a reliable quantification of high risk factors ought to answer two basic requirements: a) perinatal mortality should not be the only criterion of seriousness, but it should also include different types and degrees of perinatal morbidity (perinatal encephalopathies, developmental psychomotor retardation), since it is fundamentally wrong to assume that the main causes of perinatal mortality and morbidity necessarily originate from the same groups of high risk factors (Butler 1969). b) In the evaluation of high risk factors determined in prospective studies, the "weight" of each factor should be estimated both singly and in correlation to others. In recent years, several points screening systems for high risk pregnancies have been published in the international literature (Tab. 3).

Table 3. Survey of scoring systems in perinatal medicine according to different criteria for quantification of risk factors

Criteria for quantification of risk factors	Scoring system of risk factors	
(1) Perinatal mortality	1965 Feldstein & Butler 1969 Butler & Alberman 1969 Effer 1973 Wilson & Sill	
(2) Infant mortality	–	
(3) Perinatal morbidity (early)	1967 Prechtl	(10 days)
(4) Combinations a) Perinatal mortality + early morbidity	1969 Nesbit 1969 Goodwin et al. 1970 Štembera	(Apgar score) (Apgar score) (Apgar score)
b) Perinatal + infant mortality + late morbidity	1972 Štembera & Zezuláková	(18 months)
(5) Maternal and infant mortality	1969 Perkin 1973 PAHO (Prindle & Gomez)	

The first studies of this type expressed the weight of a high risk factor only in relation to perinatal mortality or morbidity. In later studies, the authors tried to quantify the weight of the high risk factor simultaneously in relation to perinatal mortality and to the clinical state of the infant immediately after birth (evaluated by the Apgar score). A scoring system for the most serious high risk factors, representing the greatest danger for the life of the mother as well as of the foetus and infant, was elaborated with reference to family planning. The purpose of this system is screening for specific contraception precisely in these high risk groups and it is valuable chiefly in countries with a high birth rate and a high perinatal and maternal death rate.

Quantification of the weight of high risk factors together with perinatal mortality and morbidity (Štembera and Zezuláková 1976) and the classification of these factors into 4 main groups, i.e. history (including high risk factors in the general case history, the previous pregnancy and socio-economic factors), present pregnancy, labour and neonatal high risk factors, allowed the elaboration of a scoring system which can be used for the screening of high risk cases in any phase of development of the foetus and the newborn infant (Tab. 4).

The absolute and relative weight of the various high risk factors, determined from the perinatal and infant mortality rate and the perinatal morbidity rate in the given population and expressed by a points system, is associated with

Table 4. Applicability of scoring of "at risk" fetuses and newborns according to different groups of risk factors and to the time of their registration

Scoring according to groups of risk factors	Screening	
	when	for
H	First visit	Special antenatal care
H + P	a) Visits during pregnancy	(1) Special antenatal care (2) Hospitalisation
	b) At the end of pregnancy	(1) Intensive care during labour (2) Induction of labour (3) Selective Caesarian section
H + P + L	After delivery	(1) Observation of the newborn (2) Intensive care of the newborn
H + P + L + N	Before discharge from the hospital	(1) Neurolog.-psychic supervision (2) Rehabilitation

(H = history, P = pregnancy, L = labour, N = newborn)

a number of other factors, e.g. with the extent and quality of antenatal, natal and neonatal care, the state of health and the health consciousness of the population at large, nutritional factors, etc.

HIGH RISK PREGNANCY REGISTRATION AND DIFFERENTIATION

In Czechoslovakia, the excellent antenatal care system can be used as the organizational basis for the registration of high risk pregnancies.

The basic antenatal clinic

The antenatal clinic is the first (and only) place where high risk pregnancy screening commences. The ultimate result (the prevention of perinatal mortality and morbidity) depends primarily on how well it functions. The work of the obstetricians and midwives attached to these clinics can be improved and made easier by various organizational measures, but the final effect will always depend, in the first place, on their own qualifications and conscientious- ness. The Czech Commission for Perinatal Medicine has elaborated a new card for pregnant women, which will ensure, in the first stage, uniform determina- tion of the case history, with special reference to high risk pregnancy, at the very first visit (the most important relevant risk signs are simply marked off) (Tab. 5). These can be supplemented by further signs which may occur later

Table 5. High-risk-pregnancy screening in Czechoslovakia (taken from the card issued to pregnant women)

General history	Previous pregnancies
Primipara	Induced abortions } – 1, 2, more, complications
Age $\geq$ 30 years	Spotaneous abortions } – 1, 2, more, complications
Height $\leq$ 155 cm	Premature births – 1, 2, more, complications
Pre-pregnancy weight $\pm$ 10 kg from normal	child lived, died,
Essential hypertension I, II	traumatized
Chronic renal disease	Maintained } – by conservative methods,
Disturbances of menstrual cycle (treated)	pregnancies } by cerclage
Sterility $\geq$ 2 years	Infant > 4,000 g } died perinatally
Diabetes (diet, insulin)	Small-for-dates } traumatized
Heart disease (treated)	Rh (ABO) isoimmunization
Operations (uterine anomaly)	Toxaemia: oedema, proteinuria, hypertension
	Diabetes not util pregnancy (diet, insulin)
	Protracted pregnancy ($\geq$ 42 weeks)
	Surgical delivery (Caesarian, forceps, vacuum extractor)

Present pregnancy

Haemorrhage: single – slight repeated – severe before/after 28th week	Weight: excessive increment, over weight, under weight
Contractions: isolated – weak frequent – strong before/after 28th week	Toxaemia: oedema proteinuria hypertension
Cervix: contracted – relaxed, cerclage	Anaemia: Hb < 9 g
Rh (ABO) antibodies	Hydramnios
Infections – pyrexial, zoonoses (serum positive)	Twins
	Breech presentation
	Abnormal positions
Diabetes (diet, insulin)	Small-for-dates foetus (estimate)
Glycosuria	Protracted pregnancy ($\geq$ 42 weeks)

N. B. Underline appropriate risk factor(s), supplement at further regular check-ups during pregnancy, so that any health worker, in any pregnant woman, can make a first, rapid, rough evaluation of whether there is any danger to the foetus. In the next stage, when the individual risk signs are taken together with their weight, the evaluation of the high risk pregnancy becomes more exact. In the first, experimental study we found that, among the 25 – 33 % of all pregnant women in the population in whom a high risk pregnancy occurs, one third (i.e. 11 % of the total population) of these most serious cases, in which every second pregnancy terminated in perinatal mortality or morbidity, could be detected relatively very reliably by screening on a points system. Among the other 89 % (including the remaining 14 – 22 % high risk cases), which had a lower score, the infant was seldom traumatized. These 11 % pregnant women detected by means of the above screening method are precisely the ones who must be sent to special clinics for high risk pregnancies. At the same time, the screening results indicate the way in which labour and delivery should be conducted (Štembera et al. 1976).

The specialized clinic for high risk pregnancies

Whereas the main aim of the basic antenatal clinic is the screening of high risk pregnancies, the main function of specialized clinics is the further differentation of the 11 % pregnant women with a grave high risk pregnancy. The purpose of this differentation is to determine in which cases the foetus is in serious danger, so that intervention in good time can prevent its perinatal death or injury. This type of work not only makes greater demands on time for every case, but also requires the use of more complex methods (see chapter on methods). It thus entails close collaboration both with a laboratory and with a clinical department equipped with the necessary apparatus. The responsible obstetrician should likewise have a thorough knowledge of modern perinatal medicine. These specialized clinics are therefore, on principle, annexed to the matternity departments of large hospitals and institutes (in the first stage) and, in time, will be attached to large maternity hospitals. Another task which could be allotted to these clinics is the ante-conception care of infertile women.

The institute centralising high risk pregnancies

The immediate necessity, in the first stage, is to supplement existing institutions (maternity and gynaecology departments), so that the most serious high risk pregnancies (diabetes, Rh isoimmunization and cardiopathies) can be consistently centralized in every region. Centralization ought to cater for an area with about 10,000 – 15,000 births a year, so that each region would have 1 – 3 such institutes, according to its size. Other high risk pregnancies (in particular toxaemia and premature labour) from the immediate vicinity would naturally also be concentrated in these institutes. The chief demands which ought to be made on these institutes are as follows:

a) The closest possible contact (both personal and geographic) with the paediatric intensive care unit.

b) A 24-hour paediatric emergency service in the delivery theatre.

c) A delivery theatre equipped like an obstetrical intensive care unit (modern foetal monitors, Astrup equipment to hand, an ultrasound B-scan).

d) Closely coordinated collaboration with other, contiguous branches and departments (laboratory, X-ray and isotope departments, internal medicine, surgery, anaesthesiology).

e) The allocation of 20 – 30 beds for a high risk pregnancy ward (at least 1 bed per 100 births per year).

f) A medical and paramedical staff with a thorough knowledge of modern perinatal medicine.

In the second stage, the number of these institutes should be extended so as to allow the centralization of other high risk pregnancies, in particular EPH gestoses (toxaemia) and premature labour. These institutes should be governed by the same principles as those enumerated above, with a few slight modifications, e.g. the high risk pregnancy ward ought to have about 15 beds (at least 1 bed per 150 births per year). This type of centralization of high risk pregnancies ought not to be carried out in institutions with less than 1,200 births a year (uneconomical). At the same time, attention should be paid to its geographical situation in the region.

Both types of institutes for the centralization of high risk pregnacies should moreover carry out supplementary screening of these pregnancies for any further risk factors originating during labour and thus add to the accuracy of the infant's "obstetrical" prognosis. This is a great aid to the paediatrician in the screening of high risk infants for further neurological study, since repeated neurological examination of all infants will not be possible for a long time to come, because of the lack of paediatricians with neurological qualifications. We can pick out only 14 % of live born infants most seriously at risk by screening, however, and in this way, as we have had opportunity of convincing ourselves, we shall be able to detect 10 out of 11 infants in danger of future perinatal injury in time.

FURTHER AUXILIARY MEASURES

Postgraduate study

As a result of the hundreds of publications on advances in perinatal medicine which appear every year in Czechoslovak and other journals, and of the dozens of new methods and therapeutic techniques connected with the unprecedented development of medical electronics and biochemistry in recent years, most field workers have lost their bearings and are unable to distinguish essential from less important information. It is therefore necessary for the members of leading institutions, where the most important new findings can be tried out, to participate in postgraduate courses organized primarily for the workers in institutes intended for the centralization of high risk pregnancies and in paediatric intensive care units. In the next stage, these trained workers ought themselves to become organizers and teachers (aided, if need be, by the members of leading institutions) in similar regional postgraduate courses for field workers. Since team work in the delivery theatre means very close cooperation between obstetrician and paediatrician, it was found best for each to be kept well informed of innovations and progress in the other's sphere of work. As a result, joint postgraduate perinatology courses for obstetricians and paediatricians were instituted in Bohemia and Moravia in 1971. The first results indicate that this was a step in the right direction. The present monograph is intended to serve the same purpose.

The above remarks apply equally to the further training of paramedical staff, the midwives in the labour ward and the children's nurses in the intensive care unit. The work in both these places is becoming increasingly specialized, so that even the youngest students in the nurses' colleges can hardly acquire any detailed knowledge. Unless the paramedical staff is properly qualified, it is virtually impossible for these highly specialized departments to operate satisfactorily. The corresponding courses held in Bohemia and Moravia since 1972 have proved to be invaluable in this respect.

Documentation

New forms of work require new forms of recordkeeping. The first step is the card for pregnant women already mentioned. A suitable records system for specialized clinics, labour wards and delivery theatres is another categorical necessity. The basic conditions for these changes are:

a) Clear arrangement of the many recorded data (risk factors, results of laboratory and clinical examinations, data on the course of labour and delivery), to allow complex evaluation of the patient's immediate condition at any time.

b) The possibility of easy automatic processing of all these data in large series to obtain new information, e.g. on the use of new diagnostic and therapeutic techniques.

Educational work

The rapid progress made in perinatology ought not to be kept secret from the pregnant woman, since a well-informed patient is a more cooperative patient. It is hard to imagine the stress which many of the more modern examination methods utilizing the latest findings in medical electronics, or even just the term "high risk pregnancy" — so familiar to ourselves — means for some pregnant women. On the other hand, the woman ought to be kept better informed on how many of the risk factors which she herself can either prevent completely, or at least prevent from becoming worse by early treatment, could have dire consequences for her baby's life. In this respect, repeated radio and TV talks and discussions and popularly written articles in women's magazines have proved highly successful in Czechoslovakia.

GENERAL CASE HISTORY

This group of risk factors included chiefly those which, although not pathological states in the strict meaning of the term, have nevertheless been shown to have a close bearing on raised perinatal morbidity and mortality. Most of them typically exemplify the difficulties sometimes experienced in evaluating them separately and, conversely, how some of their combinations increase pregnancy risks. They are likewise examples of an adverse influence having effect (not primarily) but secondarily, and most often evidenced by a markedly high incidence of premature births.

AGE AND PARITY

Numerous studies of large series have demonstrated conclusively that perinatal mortality is higher among women under the age of 15 and over 35. Perinatal mortality rises even from the age of 30, however, compared with younger women (Tab. 6 and 7).

Table 6. Perinatal mortality, incidence of premature births and age distribution in population of 16,285 women giving birth in England in 1958 (no twin births)

Age	Percentage of prem. births	Perinatal mortality (per mille)	Distribution in population (%)
< 20	8.0	33.1	5.0
20 – 24	6.3	27.5	28.8
25 – 29	6.1	27.2	32.6
30 – 34	7.1	34.8	20.4
≧ 35	7.3	48.7	13.1

Table 7. Perinatal mortality and distribution in population in correlation to age — analysis of 137,427 births in Czech Socialist Republic in 1969

Age	Perinatal mortality		Distribution in population (%)
	absolute	per mille	
<15	4	133	0.02
15–19	269	17.3	13.8
20–24	1,188	20.2	50.6
25–29	621	23.2	23.4
30–34	274	29	8.2
35–39	152	38.9	3.3
≧40	66	64.5	0.8

This state is again largely associated with the familiar higher incidence of premature births in both very young and older women. Another, though less frequent cause in older women is the greater probability of an incidence of further risk factors, which increases with advancing age (essential hypertension, diabetes, renal diseases, sterility in women with a late first pregnancy, etc.). With older women, the probability of developmental defects in the offspring is also greater (see chapters on congenital anomalies). When evaluating the results of these studies, it is always important to compare them with the distribution of the given groups in the population, since this shows the number of women in the population in whom we can anticipate an incidence of certain risk factors; for instance, an age of 35 and over occurs significantly less often in the Czechoslovak population (4.1 %) than in the English population (13.1 %), while for the incidence of women under the age of 20 the reverse applies. Since an age of less than 20 years is not a risk factor in the Czech Socialist Republic (as seen from Tab. 5, except for very young girls), the pregnancy shift to the youngest age group in that country compared with England (though bearing in mind the time difference, i.e. 1958 and 1969) is actually a favourable phenomenon from the high risk pregnancy aspect.

Far fewer studies exist on the association between the women's age and perinatal morbidity, although here again there is a convincing direct connection (Štembera et al. 1972).

The influence of parity on perinatal mortality has been demonstrated in numerous analyses, which show that it is again the extreme groups, i.e. the primipara on the one hand and the multipara on the other, which are the most at risk. The same applies to these as to the extreme age groups as regards a raised incidence of prematurity (Tab. 8).

Table 8. Correlation of incidence of premature births to parity

a) England, 1958		b) U.S.A., 1958 (whites)	
Parity	% of premature births	Parity	% of premature births
I	7.6	I	7.2
II	5.4	II	6.5
III−IV	6.8	V	7.4
V	7.4		

Combination of these two risk factors (age and parity) is a typical example of how the risk in such cases is not merely additive (Tab. 9).

Table 9. Correlation of incidence of premature births to both parity and age (U.S.A., 1958 − whites)

Parity	Age	% of premature births	Parity and age	% of premature births
I	15−19	8.5	V-para	7.4
			15−19 years	8.5
I	25−29	6.9	V-para, 15−19 years	18.3
I	≧40	13.7		

PRE-PREGNANCY HEIGHT AND WEIGHT

The higher perinatal mortality demonstrated in several analyses among small women is again closely associated, as in the above two cases, with a raised incidence of premature births (Tab. 10). In many countries, this factor is closely related to the woman's socio-economic position (the lower the socio-economic group, the smaller the woman's average size). Close association of this factor

Table 10. Perinatal mortality and incidence of premature births in correlation to woman's height

a) England, 1958				b) U.S.A., 1958 (only I-paras in the same soc.-econ. group)		
Height inches	cm	% of prem. births	Perinatal mortality per mille	Height inches	cm	% of prem. births
≧65	159	4.7	25.3	≧64	156	5.6
62–64	151–156	6.1	29.4	61–63	154–149	7.8
<62	151	9.3	36.6	<61	149	11.7

with a higher incidence of premature births was, however, demonstrated in all socio-economic groups (Tab. 11).

Table 11. Perinatal mortality in correlation to woman's height and socio-economic position (England, 1958)

Height		Perinatal mortality per mille	
inches	cm	husband professional worker	unskilled labourer
≧65	159	19.4	31.5
62–64	151–156	23.5	38.5
<62	151	27.8	48.9

As for height, it is impossible to set an absolute high risk limit for the woman's pre-pregnancy weight (only a relative one, in correlation to height and age). The relationship of pre-pregnancy weight to perinatal mortality has therefore been studied in extreme cases only. Raised perinatal mortality was demonstrated among both markedly obese women (15–20 % overweight) and severely underweight women (10–15%), while a causal association of

Table 12. Incidence of premature births in correlation to woman's pre-pregnancy weight

a) Series of 87,858 births (Nyirjesy 1970)		b) U.S.A., 1958	
pre-pregnancy weight	% of premature births	pre-pregnancy weight	% of premature births
<45 kg	16.7	15% underweight	13.2
≧90 kg	3.8	normal or overweight	2.3

weight with a high incidence of premature births was demonstrated in underweight women only (Tab. 12). In obese women, we must therefore reckon with yet another causal factor in raised perinatal mortality (latent diabetes, some other endocrine disorder, etc.).

STERILITY

Reliably demonstrated and treated primary or secondary sterility of at least two year's duration (if treatment was followed by conception) is an acknowledged important high risk pregnancy factor. If these women do not have a spontaneous abortion (which is twice as frequent in these cases as in the normal population), the risk is manifested in raised perinatal mortality. This is demonstrated by an analysis of labour in 160 women treated for sterility (Havránek et al. 1967), in whom perinatal mortality (81 per mille) was fourtimes the value in the control group (the figure includes both antenatal and postnatal mortality). The increase was not due either to a raised incidence of premature births (6.9%), or to greater participation of premature neonates in perinatal mortality (69%). In these cases, we must therefore presume the existence of another causal factor, which at present is not altogether clear, but which is very serious (placental dysfunction due to altered placentation?).

CHRONIC DISEASES

The most important of these diseases, which may progress or become decompensated during pregnancy, so that they endanger the mother's life as well as the foetus's (diabetes, cardiopathies), or may give rise to superimposed toxaemia (renal diseases), are discussed separately in the chapter entitled "Present pregnancy".

DEVELOPMENTAL UTERINE ANOMALIES

This situation, which is a risk factor mainly because it involves raised predisposition to abortion or premature labour, is discussed in the chapter on repeated spontaneous abortion.

PREVIOUS PREGNANCIES

This second group of risk factors includes:

(1) Disturbances during a previous pregnancy and labour, of a type which could represent an increased risk for the development of the foetus and could be expected to recur. These are:

    a) certain pathological conditions of pregnancy (latent diabetes, EPH gestosis),

    b) disturbances of the duration of pregnancy, i.e. shortening (artificial or spontaneous abortion, premature labour) or protraction,

    c) a pathological course of labour, with surgical termination.

(2) Disturbances of development of the foetus in a previous pregnancy:

    a) nutritional (a small-for-gestational-age or over-weight foetus),

    b) damaged foetus (serious perinatal morbidity and congenital anomalies),

    c) perinatal death of the foetus.

Although factors from both these groups can often be combined, the second group, as a whole, carries a greater risk for the development of the present foetus than the first group.

Most of the above risk factors are discussed in the chapter "Present pregnancy". The present chapter deals only with artificial abortion, repeated spontaneous abortion and congenital anomalies.

ARTIFICIAL TERMINATION OF PREGNANCY

In this chapter, artificial termination of pregnancy is evaluated only as a risk factor, endangering the maternal organism in a subsequent pregnancy in association with a greater probability of perinatal mortality and morbidity.

We have omitted all the other possible complications resulting in an immediate disturbance (e.g. perforation of the uterus) or a delayed disturbance (e.g. inflammation or the formation of adhesions, leading to secondary sterility or a raised probability of spontaneous abortion).

The most frequent and most important complication after artificial termination of pregnancy is injury of the uterine cervix and its subsequent incompetence. The injury is usually latent and is not manifested until the next pregnancy, when it causes premature labour. Prior to 1958, the year in which the legal abortion bill was passed in Czechoslovakia, cervical incompetence was seldom a cause of premature labour. Today, after experiences with over 1 million legal abortions, cervical incompetence following legal abortion has become one of the main causes of premature labour.

Another, less common, complications is isoimmunization of a Rh negative woman during artificial termination of pregnancy. It has been demonstrated that only 0.25 ml foetomaternal transfusion during the actual operation can cause the woman to be sensitized. The literature puts the proportion of these cases at $4-18$ %.

Likewise we cannot exclude the possibility of injury of the deep layers of the endometrium and myometrium during the operation, which can cause anomalous placentation at these sites in the next pregnancy. This could lead to placental dysfunction in the last weeks of pregnancy and subsequently to a small-for-dates or hypoxic foetus. The raised incidence of stillbirths in women who have had an artificial abortion could be the outcome of this disturbance.

As a result of these possible complications, there is an increase in the international literature in the number of studies drawing attention to the close association between the artificial termination of pregnancy and the raised percentage of premature births and higher perinatal mortality in the next pregnancy. Indirect evidence is provided by the striking association between the legal abortion frequency and the frequency of premature births and high perinatal death rate in various parts of Czechoslovakia (Tab. 13). The raised perinatal death rate is due to the raised early neonatal death rate, which, in turn, is the outcome of a rising percentage of premature births. In any such detailed analysis, however, we must always take into account a number of different factors which may participate in the final result (whether this is the percentage of premature births or the perinatal death rate), e.g.

a) whether it was the first pregnancy which was terminated, or whether the woman had already given birth (the former is the more serious),

b) the week of pregnancy in which abortion was performed (the later the date, the greater the degree of dilatation of the cervix required and hence the greater the danger of the cervix being injured,

Table 13. Legal abortion frequency in certain regions of Bohemia in 1967 and frequency of premature births and the perinatal death rate and early neonatal death rate in these regions after a 4-year interval

	Number of legal abortions per 100 births (1967)	Frequency of prem. births (%) (1971)	Perinatal death rate (per mille)	Early neonatal death rate (per mille) (1971)
South Bohemia	56	5.5	18.5	12.4
West Bohemia	66	6.8	20.9	14.3
North Bohemia	76	6.9	22	15.1
Prague	101	7.2	23.5	16.3

c) the length of the interval between artificial abortion and the present pregnancy (the shorter the interval, the greater the risk),

d) the method used for abortion, i.e. abortion forceps and a curet, or suction (which requires smaller dilatation of the cervix and thereby reduces the risk),

e) the number of previous abortions (the greater the number, the greater the risk).

It was found that one abortion was followed by a complication-free pregnancy in 41% of the cases (i.e. by the birth of a term foetus without any preceding signs of threatened abortion or premature labour), while pregnancy after 2−4 abortions was free from complications in only 33% (Krátká 1967). After one abortion the percentage of premature births rose by 40% and after more than one by 70% (Dráč 1970). In Hungary, the percentage of premature

Table 14. Perinatal death in Czechoslovakia in 1970 according to birthweight in relation to number of preceding legal abortions

Number of preceding legal abortions	Absolute	Number of perinatal deaths percentage according to birthweight		
		< 1,500 g	1,500 − 2,499 g	≧ 2,500 g
0	2,244	31	33	36
1	667	50	25	25
2	217	55	28	17
3	97	60	24	16

38

births among women who have had one abortion is 14.4% and among those who have had 3 and more abortions it is 20.5% (Horský 1971). A nation-wide analysis of perinatal mortality in Czechoslovakia demonstrated that the greater the number of preceding abortions, the higher the percentage of perinatal deaths among infants with a birthweight of less than 1,500 g born to these women (Tab. 14).

If one or other of the above disturbances has already occurred, owing to previous artificial termination of pregnancy, successful prevention of premature labour requires early detection of cervical incompetence (see chapter Diagnostics — cervical index), followed by cerclage. The prevention of Rh isoimmunization after legal abortion is assured in Czechoslovakia by the administration of anti-D globulin to all Rh negative women immediately after the operation.

REPEATED SPONTANEOUS ABORTIONS

Many analyses have been published in the international literature, demonstrating that the probability of repeated abortion (or premature labour) increases in correlation with the number of previous abortions. We therefore consider ourselves justified in including previous spontaneous abortions among high risk pregnancy factors and in evaluating their importance in proportion to the number of previous abortions. The significance of this high risk factor is demonstrated by an analysis of the course of pregnancy, labour and the clinical state of the newborn infants of 178 habitually aborting women in the years 1966 to 1970. Twenty-two (12.4%) of these infertile women, to whom, after a detailed preconception examination and specific therapy, we recommended a further pregnancy, aborted again. The remaining 156 gave birth to an infant (Tab. 15).

The higher percentual incidence of premature births, higher perinatal mortality and more frequent marked postnatal depression of the newborn infant — evaluated from the Apgar score — confirm that pregnancy and labour risks are raised in infertile women (Zwinger et al. 1972).

The incidence of spontaneous abortions represents about one tenth of all births and fivefold perinatal infant losses in Czechoslovakia. According to the latest statistics, spontaneous abortion occurs in 25,000 – 30,000 pregnancies. The situation in other countries is similar.

It is generally almost impossible to form a correct conclusion about the cause of each individual abortion. With some couples, however, spontaneous

Table 15. Survey of perinatal mortality rate and postnatal depression of the newborn in 156 habitually aborting women with specific therapy

Weight of foetus (g)	Incidence (%)	Apgar score (%)			Perinatal mortality (per mille)
		10 − 9	8 − 7	6 − 1	
<2,500	8.6	64.3	21.5	14.2	428.5
>2,500	91.4	88	7	5	−
Total	100	85.9	8.3	4.5	38.4
Other births at ICMC*		93.7	3	1.9	24.8
Of these, <2,500	6.3				273

* Institute for the Care of Mother and Child

abortions are a regular occurrence and in these cases we are bound to assume that the premature termination of pregnancy is due not to random causes, but to relatively constant factors, i.e. that it is determined biologically. We know that an increase in the number of repeated abortions is accompanied, in one couple, by an increase in the percentual probability that the causes of the abortions are stable. Among all spontaneous abortions, habitually aborting women account for about 2%. In Czechoslovakia, this means that at least 500 infertile women miscarry every year. Generally speaking, the causal factors which lead to habitual abortion are the same as for random abortions (Fig. 1).

A combination of two or more possible causal factors is no exception. It is therefore essential, when assessing the importance of the individual factors in habitual aborters, to evaluate the clinical picture of previous unsuccessful pregnancies correctly.

In both random and repeated abortions, the factors causing premature termination of pregnancy can be either of ovular origin, or determined by the internal environment (the maternal organism) and the external environment, which acts on the development of the foetus. When attempting to detect them in habitual aborters, we concentrate primarily on the period before the next conception. The opportunities for studying them during pregnancy are greatly reduced and because of the maximally conservative methods used to treat an imminent or already started abortion, a pathomorphological search for primarily ovular causes in aborted products of conception is almost impossible, owing to degenerative changes in the ovum. The study of possible causes of pathological development of the foetoplacental unit is likewise virtually out of the question in this phase.

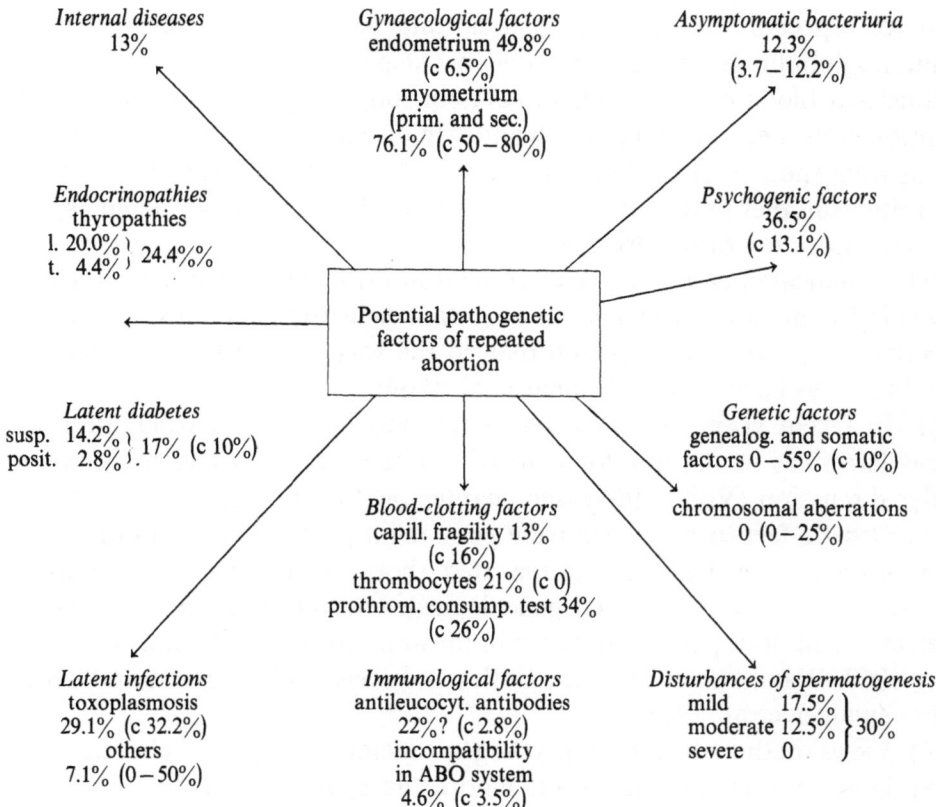

Fig. 1. Scheme of possible pathognetic factors determining repeated habitual abortion. Results of 5-year study. Percentual incidences cited in literature given in brackets. c = percentual incidence in control group (Zwinger).

Examination of habitually aborting women

The preconception investigation of external and internal maternal factors should include the following:

(1) A specific and detailed study of the **anamnestic data.** These furnish information on any negative factors in the aborting women's environment and regime, on the possible toxic effect of the most diverse substances and, of course, on all past systemic diseases whose sequelae might be damaging to physiological development of the foetus.

(2) A general **medical** examination allowing the infertile woman's actual state of health to be evaluated. Among laboratory tests we place emphasis on special **haematological** tests (raised capillary fragility and a deficiency of certain blood-clotting factors can endanger the development of the

embryo, especially in the early phases) and **haemato-immunological** tests (immunoglobulin levels, the possible participation of antibodies against corpuscular blood particles in habitual abortion). We have intentionally not mentioned the need for tests for Rh and ABO isoimmunization, in which the aetiopathogenesis is clear. Other tests, e.g. of the urine for **bacteriuria,** help to exclude another potential aetiopathogenetic abortion factor, i.e. an asymptomatic infection of the urinary tract.

(3) In indicated cases, the general medical examination can be individually supplemented by investigation of certain **endocrine** functions. From our experience, we are of the opinion that, at the very least, a thyroid disorder should always be excluded (Soumar et al. 1969).

(4) In recent years, the question of the possible broad participation of **latent infections** in the development of habitual abortion has again come under discussion (Vojta 1969) (see chapter on Infections).

(5) **Genetic factors** are a relatively permanent parental encumbrance and when investigating the causes of repeated abortion we must therefore look for any genetically determined genealogical, chromosomal and metabolic aberrations in both parents and also in the aborted ovum (Benirschke 1963, Carr 1967, Waxmann et al. 1967, Butler and Reiss 1970, Larson and Titus 1970, Zwinger et al. 1976).

(6) Views on the influence of **psychogenic factors** on repeated abortion are at variance. We cannot, however, ignore the raised activity of the myometrium of the non-pregnant uterus, which we found after psychogenic stress.

(7) A normal **general gynaecological examination** helps to detect certain other factors. Their direct pathogenetic role in abortion is sometimes unquestionable, but in other cases it has so far not been reliably demonstrated (vaginal and cervical biocenosis, chronic inflammations etc.). Special attention should be paid to detailed examination of the endometrium and myometrium.

(8) Only a functionally fit **endometrium** ensures an adequate medium for proper development of the fertilized ovum. If we find retardation of the secretory transformation of the endometrium, we should not only record the details exactly, but should also evaluate, in the endometrial glands and secretion, the presence and metabolism of carbohydrates, which we regard as the prime source of nutrition for the earliest stage of development of the fertilized ovum (Hughes et al. 1967, Luh and Brandau 1967, Zwinger et al. 1969 a, Douglas et al. 1970). A study of hormone levels, vaginal cytology and the phenomenon of arborization of the cervical mucus helps to determine whether delayed secretory transformation of the endometrium is due to deficient hormone production or to a non-receptive endometrium (Horský and Zwinger 1969).

(9) The **myometrium** is evaluated with reference to the anatomical structure of the uterus, which may display either primary or secondary anomalies, and to its functional quality, as manifested in the character of spontaneous and reactive motility.

Primary anatomical abnormalities of the uterus develop either during the embryonic phase (congenital developmental defects) or during sexual maturation, while **secondary abnormalities** are usually the outcome of previous gestations or intrauterine measures (**cervical incompetence**: basic studies by Palmer and Lacomme 1948, McDonald 1957; **intrauterine synechia**: Asherman 1950, Sweeney 1966). These pathological states are two of the commonest obstacles to a normal reproductive process in habitual aborters (Palmer et al. 1965, Zwinger et al. 1969 c), in whom hysterography is consequently an essential diagnostic operation (Zwinger et al. 1974).

The preconception determination of **myometrial functional insufficiency** by means of uterine tensiometry or electromyography (Sureau et al. 1965, Zwinger et al. 1969 b, d; 1970; 1972 a) may signal inadequate adaptability of the myometrium to the raised demands of pregnancy, which results, in given circumstances, to the development of habitual abortion.

(10) Failing to **examine the partner** of an aborting woman would be a grave error. In addition to haemato-immunological tests, to which he is subjected together with his partner, he should be examined for disturbances of spermatogenesis (Raboch 1965) manifested in aberrations of sperm morphology and biochemistry. The negative effect on the foetus of a delayed immunological reaction by the maternal organism to the sperms has not, so far, been reliably demonstrated.

The above enumeration of the diagnostic possibilities for determining the aetiopathogenesis of repeated abortions is doubtless not complete, but it shows the present means we have at our disposal for resolving this serious problem. Today, in a comprehensive evaluation of an infertile couple by means of the available methods, we are successful in over 80 % of the cases and in the same number of habitually aborting women we can ensure that the next pregnancy will have a successful course (Zwinger et al. 1972 a).

Treatment of women with repeated abortions

After a habitually aborting woman has been examined a large proportion of the therapeutic methods directed at the cause must be applied before the next pregnancy is commenced.

If therapy of a character other than gynaecological is required, we consult a specialist in the relevant field and follow his instructions. In other cases, the treatment is undertaken by the gynaecologist.

In demonstrated retardation of the secretory transformation of the endo-metrium, we administer **hormonal preparations** (steroids) for a few months (usually 3 cycles), inducing pseudopregnancy. As well as producing positive changes in the endometrium (Zander 1967, Schmidt-Matthiesen 1968, Horský and Zwinger 1969), this improves uterine motility and the recordings approach the findings in fertile women (Zwinger 1969, Zwinger et al. 1970).

Our studies show that the effect of hormonal therapy lasts about 3 months after discontinuing treatment. The optimal time for further conception is the second cycle after termination of therapy. In cases of marked retardation of secretory transformation of the endometrium, we continue hormonal therapy with gestagens – which are known not to have masculinizing effects on the foetus – during the first half of pregnancy. The administration of gesta-gens during pregnancy without repeated retardation of secretory transforma-tion of the endometrium having been determined prior to conception is, although often done, open to dispute (Zuspan 1969).

We assume likewise that hormonal therapy prior to conception (and in a fresh pregnancy) has a direct effect on the myometrium in certain serious primary uterine anomalies (marked hypoplasia). In bipartite types of uteri we have had good experience with **surgical repair of the uterus** (metroplasty) (Zwinger and Horský 1969). We also treat secondary lesions surgically. For intrauterine synechiae we use our own method, in which, after **breaking down the synechiae** by the vaginal route, we introduce an IUD into the in-trauterine cavity (Zwinger et al. 1969 c).

Cervical incompetence determined prior to conception should be corrected by the 13th week of pregnancy by **cerclage,** without waiting for clinical signs of incompetence. Only the most serious cases of cervical incompetence are operated on prior to conception. In some cases, tracheloplasty after Rubowits (1953) is supplemented by preconception cerclage of the cervix at the site of the internal os (Zwinger et al. 1973).

Where irregular function of the myometrium, manifested as hyperexcit-ability, is determined prior to conception, the normal depressant therapy is indicated, together with the timely **administration** of myovascular relaxants during pregnancy sometimes as early as at the beginning of the second tri-mester.

A **pregnancy** recommended, after preconception examination and treat-ment, to a woman with a history of habitual abortion, must, as a **high risk** pregnancy, receive exceptional care for its full duration. We check it dynam-ically once a week, not only by a **detailed clinical examination** (growth of the uterus, the state of the cervix), but also by means of **vaginal cytology** and the **arborization phenomenon** (both, in the first two trimesters, react very reliably to impaired balance of the hormonal regulation of pregnancy – Zwinger et al. 1968), by determining certain **hormone** (e.g. HCG, pregnanediol, serum progesterone, total oestrogen, oestradiol) and **enzyme levels** (e.g. thermostable alkaline phosphatase) and by studying the **vitality** and growth of the foetus by means of ultrasound, the foetal ECG, etc.

CONGENITAL ANOMALIES

The genesis of human offspring is affected by heavy losses right from conception. About 25% of zygotes die within 16 weeks and at least 5% of the survivors are abnormal. Congenital anomalies (CA) are responsible for a large proportion of early abortions and for abnormal development of the surviving foetuses. Their causes (Tab. 16) — teratogens, mutagens and can-

Table 16. Main complexes in the aetiology of congenital anomalies

Character of the aetiological factor and its proportion in the aetiological complex as a whole		Typical forms of congenital anomalies
Faulty (hereditary) information at **gene** level	20%	Achondroplasia Cleft palate
Faulty (hereditary) information at **chromosome** level	10%	Down's syndrome Klinefelter's syndrome
Viruses (and possibly some microorganisms)	10 – 20%	Certain heart anomalies Atresia, stenosis of ducts
Other and unknown factors chemicals, radiation	50 – 60%	Multiple malformations

cerogens — form a complex known as the **multifactorial (polygenic)** system which can impair the embryo's development after conception or affect the maternal or paternal germ cell before conception. The overall frequency of the individual types of defects cannot be expressed by an exact, constant figure. For instance, the risk of some CA depends upon ethnic group (anencephaly), consanguinity (CA determined by a double dose of recessive genes), advanced age of the mother (chromosomal anomalies) or the father (achondroplasia, trisomia 8, haemophilia), maternal diabetes (gross skeletal defects) and probably upon a number of other factors which have not yet been identified.

At present we cannot distinguish the main and less important factors or determine the mechanism of their action. The accepted model of the multifactorial (polygenic) origin of CA implies that many of them are the outcome of interaction of genetic and non-genetic factors which may, by themselves, be harmless. These factors induce genetic or somatic mutation and possibly, on occasion cause CA by acting at a level of cell differentiation other than through DNA or RNA.

Their permanent incidence in the newborn population suggests that **there is no effective way of preventing CA,** the main reason being a lack of knowledge of the intricate laws of teratogenesis and mutagenesis. Genetic counselling was consequently, for a long time, entirely dependent on the **indirect** method when computing the risk of the development of CA, i.e. on the application of the rules of statistical probability to a particular family. This was later augmented by the determination of a single dose of recessive genes – a method of detecting carriers which is being further elaborated. Chromosomal examination is another contribution to counselling. The last progressive method is **prenatal diagnosis,** which makes full use of all the known techniques of classic genetic counselling (and other, specific methods) for direct diagnosis of the state of the **embryo (foetus) in utero.** Prenatal diagnosis has developed remarkably (Tab. 17), especially in the past five years, in which it has been technically improved and has come into large scale use in an increasing number of laboratories.

Amniocentesis brought the first real progress in prenatal diagnostic. Experience with this technique since its first application in 1958 (Parish et al.) allows the following "axioms" to be formulated. Its use is recommended be-

Table 17. Methods and techniques of prenatal diagnosis

Method	Technique	Can be used from
Direct	X-ray of foetal skeleton	12th week
	X-ray of surface of foetus after pretreatment with contrast substance (foetography)	10th – 12th week
	Sonography, i.e. ACG and EEG	8th – 10th week
	Ultrasound and stereo-ultrasound	14th week
	Foetoscopy	16th week
	Aspiration of amniotic fluid and elements contained in fluid	10th – 12th week
	Biopsy of membranes, placenta and foetus	10th week
Indirect	Examination of mother's blood (urine)	any time

tween the 12th and 14th week of gestation. Before that, the amount of amniotic fluid is small (we require at least 2 ml, optimum 5 – 10 ml, sometimes up to 20 ml) and afterwards the proportion of living cells in the sample dwindles rapidly. Location of the placenta by ultrasound and exclusion of the presence of twins is desirable. Since (according to the type of test) we need 3 (sex chromatin) to 21 – 25 days (cultivation) before obtaining a result, therapeutic abortion can be carried out at about 16 – 17 weeks. This is acceptable to the woman, the doctor and the law. The samples should be evaluated in expert laboratories – preferably **in two** different places. Only skilled workers can avoid errors in the examination of enzymes, chromosomes and other types of biological material (Tab. 18).

Table 18. Examination of material obtained by amniocentesis

Material	Facilities for examination of	
Foetal cells	ABO groups Rh factor	Directly or after cultivation, which also allows cytogenetic examination and/or auto-radiography
Amnion elements	Sex chromatin Metachromasia	
Placental cells	Biochemistry Histochemistry	
Maternal cells (lymphocytes, reticulocytes)	Ultrastructure	
Amniotic fluid	Enzymes, steroids, proteins, amino acids	

If the customary rules are all observed, the proportion of unsuccessful samplings can be reduced to less than 5% and falsely positive (falsely negative) results to less than 1% (Nadler 1968).

Amniocentesis may provoke abortion; we should not forget that we are working in a period with a high frequency of spontaneous abortions (Fig. 2) and, moreover, with material with a high probability of congenital abnormalities (in fact, a suspected foetal anomaly is actually the reason for amniocentesis). A knowledge of these associations, i.e. that the foetus might well have been lost even without amniocentesis, will pacify the doctor's conscience if, as so often happens, he is blamed for inducing abortion.

Amniocentesis is indicated by a geneticist, a paediatrician and an obstetrician and the material is evaluated by a laboratory, with which agreement must be reached on the time of taking the sample, on its size and on the adjustments necessary for its analysis.

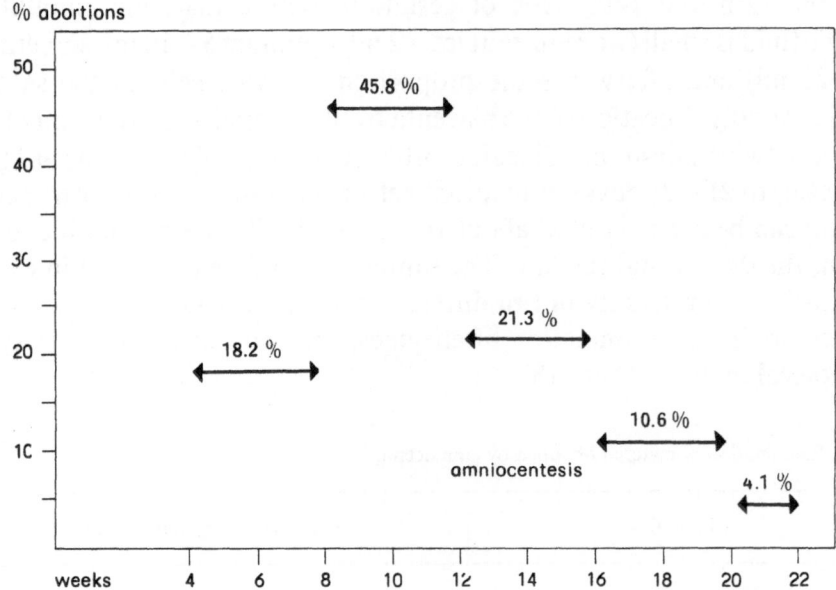

Fig. 2. Frequency of incidence of spontaneous abortions in individual weeks of pregnancy, showing best time for amniocentesis (Kučera).

Table 19 gives a list of groups of CA and of some individual types of metabolic CA which can be diagnosed prenatally. About 60 metabolic CA alone can be diagnosed, while the total number of all types of anomalies is in the region of 100 (Littlefield et al. 1974, WHO 1972).

Diagnosable CA's represent about 0.6 − 0.8 % of all births, but in fact the figure will be much lower. It is both technically and organizationally impossible to do a complete prenatal diagnosis in every pregnant woman, especially primiparas, who account for about 50% of all pregnancies. We shall thus be dealing mainly with women:

a) who have already been delivered of a child with a CA diagnosable in utero and carrying a recurrence risk of 1 : 10 and over,

b) who belong to families genetically at risk and have not previously given birth (or have had a healthy child),

c) whose husband is a close relative (e.g. first cousin),

d) who are known to be translocation carriers or carriers of recessive pathological genes and whose husband is the same type of carrier,

e) women over the age of 39 (or possibly 35),

f) infertile women (i.e. who have repeatedly miscarried or who have tried unsuccessfully for over a year to conceive).

The indication for prenatal diagnosis will be extended as new findings are made in biochemistry and other branches of science. This will mean an in-

Table 19. Some prenatally diagnosable congenital anomalies (Milunski et al. 1970, WHO 1972)

Chromosomal aberrations
    Autosomal
        trisomia
        deletion
        translocation
        breaks, e.g.
            Fanconi syndrome
            Bloom syndrome
            Louis-Bare syndrome

Amino acid metabolism
    : Maple syrup urine disease
    Methylmalonic aciduria
    : Cystinosis
    : Homocystinuria
    and 5 others

Carbohydrate metabolism
    Glycogenosis type II, III and IV
    : Galactosaemia
    : G-6-PD deficiency
    and 3 others
Lipid metabolism
    Gaucher's disease
    Generalized gangliosidosis
    Tay-Sachs disease (hexosaminidase A deficiency)
    Sandhoff's disease (hexosaminidase A + B deficiency)
    Niemann-Pick's disease
    Refsum's disease
    and 7 others

Mucopolysaccharides
    Hunter's disease
    Pfaundler-Hurler syndrome

Other congenital diseases
    : Cystic fibrosis of pancreas
    : Adrenogenital syndrome
    Lesch-Nyhan syndrome
    Lysosomal acid phosphate
    Xeroderma pigmentosum
    Acatalasaemia
    Chediak-Higashi syndrome
    Erythropoietic porphyria
    I-cell disease
    Orotic aciduria
    Sickle cell disease

The sign : in front of a diagnosis means that the examination must be exceptionally painstaking because of genetic heterogeneity of the disease.

crease in the annual number of operations and in the efficacy of diagnosis, which today is put at about 10%. The degree of efficacy depends upon the choice of the sample. In **routine examinations,** e. g. all women over the age of

45, we can detect up to 10 % foetuses with a chromosomal anomaly, whereas screening yields a substantially lower proportion of positive findings and a study focussed on women belonging to families with a positive history of a well defined entity reveals more than 20% among the cases under analysis.

Prenatal diagnosis cannot prevent all CA's and reduces only a small proportion of them, but it belongs integrally to the other, "classic", methods and however exclusive its exacting and responsible character may make it, it must be included among the routine methods.

PRESENT PREGNANCY

The negative effect of different pathological states during pregnancy often takes the form of chronic foetal distress lasting weeks or even months, which is of greater significance today than acute dangers. This group of high risk signs is consequently one of the most important. The signs discussed in detail in the first part of the chapter are the most serious.

DIABETES AND PREGNANCY

Pregnancy complicated by diabetes mellitus is a classic example of high risk pregnancy for several reasons:

(1) It is accompanied by high perinatal mortality, (2) complications of the neonatal period are so frequent that every such infant ought, on principle, to be treated in an intensive care unit, (3) various later psychosomatic anomalies directly connected with intrauterine development are also very common and (4) the sequelae of abnormal embryogenesis, in the form of different malformations, are about four times more frequent than in other pregnancies.

Incidence of diabetes

In 1966, 0.7% of the total Czechoslovak population was registered in diabetic clinics, but it is estimated that at least a further 1.3 % of the diabetic population is not registered, because the condition has not yet been diagnosed. These figures roughly concur with those for other countries. It is an alarming fact that the number of registered diabetics is increasing everywhere and we must therefore reckon with more diabetic pregnant women.

The proportion of pregnancies with diabetes in Czechoslovakia can be estimated at 1 to 1,000 births. To this we must add a given number of cases of latent diabetes. Diabetes mellitus is thus not the largest group of obstetrical pathological states, but it is a very important group because of the number of complications. According to a study carried out in 1965, about 170 – 180 diabetic women give birth annually in Czechoslovakia, i.e. 12 – 13 per million of the total population. In relation to the number of births, the frequency is 0.7 to 1,000, i.e. roughly 1 to 1,400 (not counting cases of latent diabetes).

Perinatal mortality

Today, perinatal mortality for diabetic pregnancies varies from 15 to 20 %, even in the largest centres:

Pedersen and Pedersen (1965):	17.8% (306 infants)
Worm and Jutzi (1966):	15.4% (622 infants)
Herre, Horký and Jutzi (1966):	18.9% (304 infants)
Constam, Rust and Willi (1971):	18.1% (127 infants)
Delaney and Makowski (1971):	18% (334 infants)

These authors agree, however, that perinatal mortality can be significantly reduced, if the pregnant diabetic woman is properly supervised. This is illustrated by the lists in which some authors divided their material into two groups according to the degree of control of diabetes during pregnancy (Tab. 20).

Table 20. Perinatal mortality for diabetic pregnancies with good and poor antenatal control

Author		Poor control		Good control	
		Number of infants	Perinatal mortality	Number of infants	Perinatal mortality
Pedersen and Pedersen	1965	–	–	176	7.9%
Delaney and Makowski	1971	92	33.6%	150	10.6%
Constam, Rust and Willi	1971	59	28.0%	68	9.0%

On the other hand a perinatal mortality of 2,1 % in a series of 92 newborns has been reported by Roversi (1972).

Table 21. Perinatal mortality for diabetic pregnancies in the Institute for the Care of Mother and Child

	Number of births	Number of infants	Losses				Total	
			before birth		after birth			
1952 – 1963	136	137	12	8.8%	14	10.1%	26	18.90%
1964 – 1966	110	111	6	5.4%	8	7.2%	14	12.61%
1967 – 1969	91	92	6	6.5%	6	6.5%	12	13.04%
1970 – 1972	205	209	11	5.3%	4	1.9%	15	7.20%
1973 – 1975	349	354	3	0.9%	11	3.1%	14	3.96%

The statistics in Tables 20 and 21 show that, with good control, an optimum limit of about 8 – 10 % can be reached, i.e. that in diabetes some losses are inevitable. The next paragraph gives causes, which, according to the results of a patho-anatomical and clinical analysis, can be regarded as unavoidable and shows which losses must be regarded as unnecessary.

Unpreventable antenatal losses:

Losses caused by severe complicating diseases such as glomerulonephritis or pyelonephritis, intercapillary glomerulosclerosis (Kimmelstiel-Wilson syndrome), with or without superimposed gestosis. The foetus usually dies before the induction of premature labour can even be considered.

Unpreventable neonatal losses:
a) losses caused by congenital developmental defects incompatible with life,
b) losses after spontaneous premature births, if the infant is too immature and dies at birth of CNS trauma or as a result of a pneumopathy.

Preventable antenatal losses:
a) losses caused by serious decompensation of diabetes during pregnancy,
b) losses due to "diabetic post-maturity".

Preventable neonatal losses:
a) losses after induced premature labour, if the infant is immature and dies as a result of immaturity of the lungs or of brain trauma,
b) losses caused by intranatal asphyxia.

Table 22. Analysis of perinatal mortality in diabetic pregnancies in the Institute for the Care of Mother and Child, from the aspect of avertibility

			Losses							
			unpreventable				preventable			
			before birth	after birth	total		before birth	after birth	total	
1952–1963	26	18.9%	3	7	10	7.2%	9	7	16	11.7%
1964–1966	14	12.6%	4	4	8	7.2%	2	4	6	5.4%
1967–1969	12	13.0%	3	4	7	7.6%	3	2	5	5.4%
1970–1972	15	7.2%	5	3	8	3.8%	6	1	7	3.4%
1973–1975	14	4.0%	1	10	11	3.1%	2	1	3	0.9%
Total	81				44				37	

Tab. 22 implies that 34 of the 67 infants who died around the time of birth could, theoretically, have been saved. At the present time, perinatal mortality can be improved only in the preventable losses group. It will probably not be possible to reduce perinatal mortality below 7% in adequately large, representative series (see total unpreventable losses: 7.2%, 7.2%, 7.6%).

Gigantism of foetus in diabetic mother

The infant of a diabetic mother differs at birth from a normal infant chiefly in respect of its birthweight, which is significantly higher than the weight of infants born to healthy mothers. The excessive birth weight is due to obesity (deposition of fat and glycogen).

The cause and pathogenesis of gigantism have not, so far, been definitively elucidated, but the theory that the changes in the foetus are due to maternal hyperglycaemia, leading first to foetal hyperglycaemia and then to foetal hyperinsulinism, with all the further metabolic consequences, is finding an increasing acceptance.

To prevent foetal gigantism, we keep the mother's blood sugar level, day and night, at values as near as possible to normal. A single blood sugar test first thing in the morning is definitely not an adequate guide. Tests of the diurnal blood sugar "profile" are indispensable.

Prevention of perinatal morbidity and mortality among the infants of diabetic mothers

The prevention of mortality and morbidity consists primarily in full compensation and the prevention of the keto acidosis. This requires very frequent diabetological check-ups, either in the out-patients' department or directly in a hospital. The danger of decompensation is particularly great in the vomiting period, i.e. during the first months of pregnancy, and in intercurrent pyrexial infections, e.g. influenza. It is very useful if the pregnant woman can cooperate by learning to test her urine regularly herself by means of Lestradet's reagent. She takes a knife point of reagent, places it on something white and drips 2 – 4 drops of urine onto the white powder. Violet coloration signifies the presence of acetone. The deeper the shade of violet the higher the acetone concentration in the urine. If the result is doubtful, the urine of a healthy individual can be used as the control. The prevention of a diabetic foetopathy consists not only in good compensation, but particularly in maintaining the mother's blood sugar level at values as close as possible to normal. The obstetrician and the diabetologist may sometimes be at variance on this point, since the latter may be content with a value of 180 – 200 mg% or even more, if the woman feels well, has no large losses and is free from acetone. It has been demonstrated, however, that a blood sugar level of over 150 mg% is injurious to the foetus. It should also be borne in mind that insulin resistance rises, especially in the second half of pregnancy, so that the previous dosage is no longer sufficient and must be raised.

Prevention of intranatal trauma

Because of the danger of mechanical trauma if surgical termination of the second stage of labour is found necessary, because of dreaded dystocia of the shoulders and because of raised capillary fragility, the maximum care should be taken during labour. If we consider that the infant might be injured if delivered by the natural route, we do not hesitate to terminate labour by Caesarian section. We regard the following as indications for Caesarian section in a diabetic woman: (1) a bad previous obstetrical history (dead foetuses, injured infants), (2) Caesarian section at the preceding delivery, (3) breech presentation, (4) severe toxaemia based on a chronic renal disease, (5) ophthalmological complications of diabetes (danger of amotio retinae, a diabetic retinopathy).

Lastly, in diabetic women we take all the other, normal obstetrical indications for Caesarian section with greater benevolence. We perform it in about one third of all cases — in half primarily and in the first or second stage of labour in the rest.

In surgical termination during the second stage, on principle, we give precedence to forceps over the vacuum extractor.

Latent (asymptomatic) diabetes

Latent (asymptomatic, chemical, subclinical) diabetes is defined as a genuine metabolic anomaly whose only difference from manifest, clinical diabetes is that the clinical signs and some laboratory signs, such as polyuria, polydipsia, glycosuria and fasting hyperglycaemia, are not yet manifest. The consequence of latent diabetes for the foetus are just as serious as those of manifest diabetes and perinatal mortality is actually higher, precisely because the diabetes is not diagnosed and treated. The newly introduced term ,,potential diabetic" is of practical significance for the screening of latent diabetes.

Potential diabetes

The obstetrician must always consider the possibility of latent diabetes if
(1) there is a history of diabetes in the woman's family,
(2) the woman has already had one or more stillbirths,
(3) the woman has already had one or more very large infants (over 4,000 g, but mainly over 4,500 g),
(4) the woman is obese,
(5) examination shows that the foetus is disproportionately large for the given week of pregnancy, or polyhydramnios is present,
(6) sugar is repeatedly found in the urine,
(7) the above signs are combined.
In all these cases further laboratory tests should be done to confirm or refute the diagnosis of latent (asymptomatic) diabetes.

Prediabetes

This term has been used as a synonym for latent diabetes, or as being virtually identical with "potential diabetes". Since it is a source of misunderstanding, the WHO has recommended that it should be reserved only for retrospective studies, e.g. if we are supplementarily interested in fertility in the period prior to the clinical manifestation of diabetes, without being able to determine whether a metabolic disorder was actually present at the time or not.

Laboratory diagnosis of latent diabetes

We pronounce a diagnosis of latent diabetes if the fasting blood sugar level is normal, but the blood sugar curve does not return below a given limit after a glucose load. The method used for determining glucose must be taken into account in the evaluation (with Hagedorn and Jensen's method the limit is $10-20$ mg % higher than for Nelson's method or enzymatic methods).

In agreement with the international literature, we should like to recommend the following simple test:

The first sample is taken first thing in the morning, before breakfast. Immediately afterwards the patient drinks 0.25 l cold water containing 100 g glucose and a pinch of sodium citrate to make it more palatable.

The second sample is taken 60 min later.

A third sample is taken 120 min later.

At the same time the patient collects her urine. The first urine, passed before taking the first blood sample, is not collected. Urine is then collected 60 min later in one vessel and after a further 60 min in another vessel and sugar and acetone are determined in both.

Evaluation of blood sugar curve

With Nelson's method, we regard
the first blood sugar value as normal if it does not exceed 100 mg%.

The second blood sugar value (60 min later) is the least important for the evaluation. Values of over 180 mg% are regarded as abnormal.

The third value (after 120 min) is considered to be abnormally high if it exceeds 120 mg%. Values of $120-140$ mg% are evaluated as mildly raised, while values of over 140 mg% are clearly indicative of latent diabetes if the fasting value is below 100 mg%.

Treatment of latent and manifest diabetes

Latent diabetes requires treatment just as much as manifest diabetes, the chief element being a diabetic diet. The difference is only quantitative. We must decide whether or not to use antidiabetics during the further course of pregnancy. Our aim is to reduce blood sugar values over the whole day, so that the mother does not overfeed the foetus in the uterus with carbohydrates from her blood and does not induce in it excess deposition of fat and glycogen with all the consequences of this process. Tests of the diurnal blood sugar profile decide whether a diet will be sufficient, or whether oral antidiabetics or insulin are necessary. There is no point in testing the fasting blood sugar level first thing in the morning, or the percentual 24-hour urinary sugar level, since they are altogether inadequate. In latent diabetes we expect the morning fasting blood sugar level to be normal anyway. It is therefore essential to test these values after meals during the whole day. We sometimes content ourselves with the morning, midday and evening profile, but it is far better to test the complete diurnal blood sugar profile, which informs us of the situation about 2 hours after each meal and of the morning fasting blood sugar levels.

Diurnal blood sugar profile

We determine the blood sugar profile by testing the blood sugar level at the following times: 7.00 – 10.00 – 12.00 – 15.00 – 18.00 – 21.00 – 23.00 – 7.00 hours. If none of the values exceeds 130 – 150 mg%, there is no need for a change in diet or medical treatment and it can be assumed that the foetus will not suffer from any pronounced diabetic foetopathy.

The type of insulin and the administration route and dosage which will give a satisfactory blood sugar profile are entirely individual. In general, however, it is best to divide insulin into 2 to 3 daily doses.

EPH GESTOSIS

Up to now, various terms have been used in the international literature to describe this condition (e.g. toxaemia, toxicosis, eclampsism, pre-eclampsia). Lately, the term EPH gestosis, suggested by the international organization Gestosis, which possibly gives the best characterization, has started to gain ground. It describes the gestation-associated condition manifested in the signs E (/o/edema), P (proteinuria) and H (hypertension). The term EPH gestosis also covers cases which may appear earlier than late in pregnancy and, conversely, excludes various other diseases of pregnancy not characterized by the signs E, P and H.

The diagnosis of EPH gestosis is based simply on the finding of the signs. It is sometimes difficult to decide whether or not the EPH signs are the signs of a disease from which the woman suffered prior to becoming pregnant. The diagnosis is thus established by exclusion.

Oedema of all types is found in about 30% of all pregnant women. It occurs mostly round the ankles or on the instep, appears in the afternoon and evening, especially in hot weather, and disappears during rest in bed. It is thus orthostatic in character. It is claimed that these types of oedema have nothing to do with EPH gestosis.

Only forms which do not disappear during the night, and particularly those which spread to the legs, the abdominal wall and the face are regarded as gestotic oedema. In extreme cases the oedema may be generalized.

It may be difficult to decide whether oedema is orthostatic or gestotic, because some oedemas of the legs, for example, disappear at night, at a rate in inverse proportion to their size. Oedemas which we pronounce to be gestotic, because they involve the legs, abdomen and face, may also disappear during rest in bed, without any treatment, thereby demonstrating their orthostatic origin. The decision of whether we should declare an oedema to be orthostatic or gestotic is thus a matter for arbitration and agreement.

The organization Gestosis suggests that at least pretibial oedema still demonstrated after a night's rest should be regarded as gestotic.

Relationship between the pregnancy weight increment and EPH gestosis

It is a general rule that pregnant women with signs of gestosis have a higher mean weight increment than pregnant women free from such signs.

It is also a general rule that greater weight increases are accompanied by a greater probability of signs of EPH gestosis appearing (Fig. 3).

The value of this claim in actual individual cases is very limited, however. We must bear in mind that the total weight increment at the end of pregnancy can have any value from 1 to 23 kg in women with no signs of EPH gestosis and any value from 1 to 28 kg in women with signs of gestosis (Fig. 4). Any total weight increase is thus compatible with a physiological course of pregnancy and, conversely, EPH gestosis can appear in the presence of any total weight increase. This means that the total weight gain, in an individual case, is of very little practical significance, since it merely draws attention to greater probability of signs of gestosis appearing.

Characteristics of physiological weight increase

A statistical analysis of a large number of patients showed that the curve illustrating the weight increase is mildly sigmoid and that it is linear between the 13th and the 37th week (Vedra 1969). The rate slows down somewhat towards the end of pregnancy. This curve represents growth of the ovum and the uterus, growth of the breasts, the increase in the size of the mother's fluid spaces and growth of the mother's energy reserves.

Knowledge of the growth curve in an individual case is of significance only if we know it beforehand. With some reservation, this is actually possible.

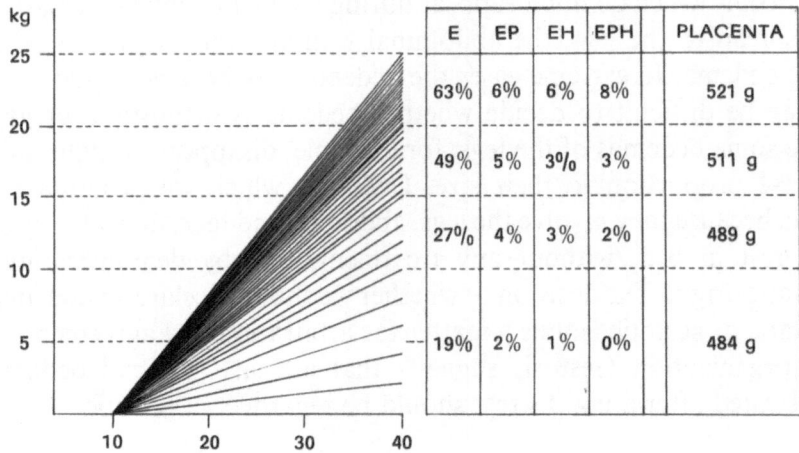

	E	EP	EH	EPH	PLACENTA
	63%	6%	6%	8%	521 g
	49%	5%	3%	3%	511 g
	27%	4%	3%	2%	489 g
	19%	2%	1%	0%	484 g

Fig. 3. The figure shows that the greater the weight of the placenta, the higher the weight increase and hence the more frequent the signs of toxaemia.

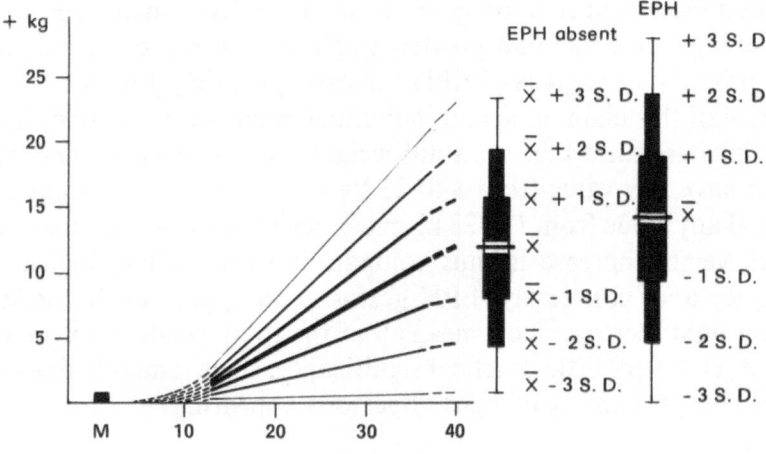

Fig. 4. The total weight increase in EPH gestosis at the end of pregnancy is higher than in healthy women, but the variances of the individual values largely overlap.

Mean $\pm$ 1 S. D. includes about 66% of all cases.
Mean $\pm$ 2 S. D. includes about 95% of all cases.
Mean $\pm$ 3 S. D. includes about 99% of all cases.

Fig. 5. Estimation of weight increase for the third trimester based on data between the 13th and 25th week.

Black circles – actual values measured between the 13th and 25th week.

Broken line – estimation by graphic extrapolation.

White circles – actual values measured in the third trimester. Matematical estimate:

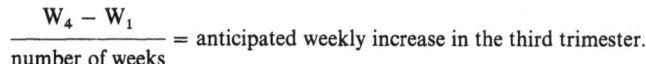

$$\frac{W_4 - W_1}{\text{number of weeks}} = \text{anticipated weekly increase in the third trimester.}$$

Fig. 6. Physiological and pathological weight increase.

Top curve: pregnancy with physiological course.

Bottom curve: shading represents pathological increase in the rate of weight gain or pathological fluid retention.

E – edema; P – proteinuria;
H – hypertension.

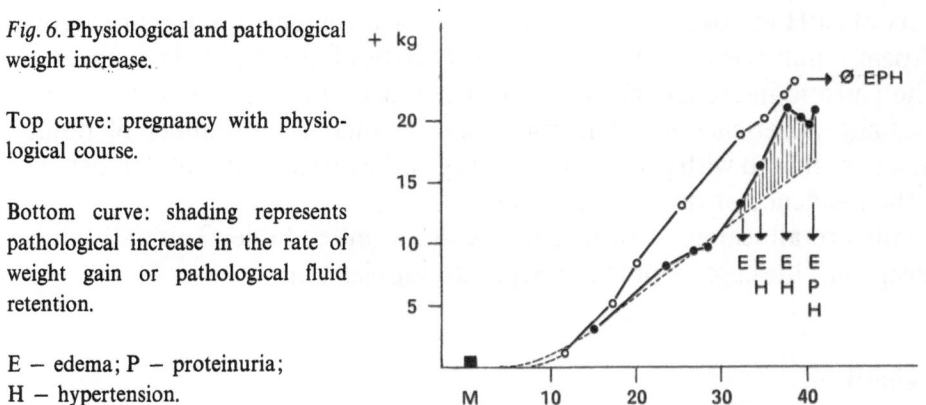

If we know at least 4 reliably measured values between the 13th and the 25th week, i.e. at a time when EPH signs occur only exceptionally, we can extrapolate the further course of the growth curve (weight increase) in a graph, or calculate the anticipated weight increase in subsequent weeks for the rest of pregnancy (Fig. 5). The only condition is that we must maintain standard conditions for measuring body weight, especially regarding clothing, the time of day, food, etc.

The weight increase can be regarded as physiological if it remains linear between the 13th and the 37th week.

Any appreciable deviation (plus or minus) means that growth of the foetal and maternal tissues is not following an absolutely physiological course.

Abnormal or pathological fluid retention is manifested in an increase in the rate of weight gain, usually as a precursor of generalized oedema (Fig. 6).

Conversely, cessation of the weight increase is often a sign of retarded growth of the maternal tissues and also of the foetal tissues, so that the foetus is small for the gestational age.

The above findings likewise imply that the determination of any upper limit for a "normal" weight gain rate, or attempts to restrict the weight gain, e.g. by a reducing diet or by saluretics, in fact constitute gross interference with the physiology of reproduction.

We must remember that the same weight increase, in different women, can in one case be absolutely physiological, if it remains linear from the 13th week of pregnancy, and in another denotes some pathological condition, if it deviates substantially from the linear in the second trimester.

Gestotic index

The purpose of the gestotic index is to allow quantitative evaluation of the gravity of EPH gestosis so as to permit reciprocal comparison. It is analogous to Apgar's numerical expression of the gravity of the asphyxia syndrome.

The gestotic index has been tested in practice in a number of European clinics and experience has confirmed that an increasing number of points correlate well both with perinatal mortality and with small size of the foetuses and the incidence of premature births.

Points are allocated according to a gestotic index table (Tab. 23) which we keep with the case records as a separate supplement.

Proteinuria

Since urine tested by the usual screening methods is always devoid of protein, any trace of protein in the urine must be regarded as a sign of a pathological condition.

Hypertension

The division between the physiological and the pathological, i.e. between a normal and a raised blood pressure, lies between 135 and 140 mmHg systolic pressure and between 85 and 90 mmHg diastolic pressure. A value of 140/90 is thus already pathological.

Table 23. Gestotic index

	0	1	2	3	Datum points	Datum points	Datum points
OEDEMA (after night's rest)	none	tibial	general	–			
PROTEINURIA (paper, sulphosal.)	none	±	+	+ +			
Esbach	≦0.4 per mille	0.5 – 2 per mille	2.1 – 5 per mille	> 5 per mille			
Biuret (% or 24 hours)	none	≦100 mg	101 – 250 mg	> 250 mg			
Systolic BP	< 140	140 – 159	160 – 179	≧ 180			
Diastolic BP	< 90	90 – 99	100 – 109	≧ 110			
				Total			

Explanation of points evaluation:

Oedema: no points given for oedema found only on the instep or ankles

Proteinuria: only one of the given methods is evaluated by points.

Points evaluation is carried out repeatedly during pregnancy, at regular intervals.

Classification of EPH gestosis

Since the clinical gravity of gestosis varies with the signs, different classification systems have been evolved. We give only the one suggested by the organization Gestosis (1970).

I. Essential EPH gestosis:
   (1) monosymptomatic
   (2) polysymptomatic (with two or three signs)
   (3) eclampsia imminens
   (4) eclampsia

II. Superimposed EPH gestosis based on:
   (1) chronic renal disease
   (2) chronic vascular disease

III. Chronic diseases with the signs E, P or H, as long as they do not deteriorate during pregnancy (i.e. not EPH gestosis).

Incidence of EPH gestosis

Since mild, monosymptomatic borderline forms (especially oedemas) are often evaluated very subjectively and are sometimes recorded as a gestosis, sometimes as the extreme limit of the physiological and sometimes (in the case of oedema) as non-gestotic oedema, it is hard to compare the incidence of EPH gestosis as a whole. The data on the incidence of eclampsia can be compared very well, however. The incidence of eclampsia is also a good criterion of the level of antenatal care and of prevention of the severest forms of EPH gestosis.

At the international symposium held in Basel in 1969, various European clinics gave widely differing figures for the frequency of eclampsia: 1 : 54 (Linz, Austria), 1 : 333 (Münsterling, Switzerland), 1 : 188 (Würzburg, German Federal Republic), 1 : 477 (Basel, Switzerland), 1 : 625 (Berlin), 1 : 1250 (Tübingen, FRG), 1 : 1899 (Mannheim, FRG), 1 : 2000 (Bamberg, FRG), 1 : 2200 (Second Clinic, Prague), 1 : 5081 (Postgraduate Medical Institute, Prague) (1966 – 1970), 1 : 5168 (Institute for the Care of Mother and Child, Prague, 1966 – 1970).

Incidence of eclampsia in the Czech Socialist Republic (Bohemia and Moravia):

```
1960   153 eclampsias out of 125,015 births, i.e. 0.12% ..........  1 :  833
1965   104 eclampsias out of 145,423 births, i.e. 0.07% ..........  1 : 1428
1970    99 eclampsias out of 145,535 births, i.e. 0.07% ..........  1 : 1428
1974    67 eclampsias out of 191,963 births, i.e. 0.03% ..........  1 : 3333
```

EPH gestosis as a high risk pregnancy factor

The danger of EPH gestosis for the foetus is proportional to the severity of gestosis, i.e. the greater its severity and the longer its duration, the greater the danger for the foetus. The risks are: a) high perinatal mortality, b) a small--for-dates foetus, c) the danger of premature labour and consequent immaturity of the foetus, d) neonatal morbidity.

a) *Perinatal mortality*

In 1967, EPH gestosis accounted for 8.6% of perinatal mortality, in 1968 for 8% and in 1969 again for 8%, more than two thirds of which came under antenatal mortality (5.2%, 4.9% and 5.1% respectively).

After the group "unknown causes", EPH takes second place among the causes of antenatal foetal losses.

Eclampsia and cases of gestosis superimposed on a chronic renal disease carry the highest perinatal mortality (chiefly antenatal).

b) *Small-for-dates foetus*

The birthweight of the small-for-dates foetus is significantly lower than the mean birthweight for the corresponding week of gestation. Five to ten percentiles are generally acknowledged to be the limits of normal weight and are given as such in the chapter on the small-for-dates infant.

c) *Prematurity and immaturity*

The proportion of premature births accounted for by EPH gestosis is not, *per se*, very high. Kotásek claims that signs of gestosis are present in about 12% of mothers who give birth prematurely. Butler (1963) estimated that mild gestosis accounted for 5.4% of premature births, moderately severe gestosis for 5.8% and severe forms for 18%.

EPH gestosis accounts for a relatively high proportion of premature stillbirths. Death of the foetus is the primary cause of premature labour, however, and expulsion before term is secondary.

d) *Neonatal morbidity*

The number of studies on the relationship between infantile neonatal morbidity and EPH gestosis of the mother (not counting small-for-dateness as an outcome of gestosis) is far too small. Infantile morbidity seems to be higher chiefly where the mother has superimposed gestosis.

In severe forms of gestosis the placenta may be abrupted, so that the foetus suffers from severe hypoxia. If the infant survives protracted hypoxia, it may be seriously damaged.

Prevention of foetal morbidity and mortality in EPH gestosis

The prevention of morbidity and mortality is associated with the prevention and treatment of gestosis. In this connection we refer the reader to the abundant international literature. Here we shall briefly survey the main principles of prevention only. They are:

(1) **Active detection** of pregnant women potentially endangered by EPH gestosis. They include women with a primarily large and rapid weight incre-

ment, women with a multiple pregnancy and with polyhydramnios and women with chronic renal or vascular disease (glomerulonephritis, pyelonephritis, diabetic nephropathy, essential hypertension).

(2) **Registration** and care of women with a rapidly mounting weight increase and with oedema. These women are examined at weekly intervals.

(3) **Hospitalization** if the blood pressure reaches 140/90 or when the first traces of albumin appear in the urine (we confirm that it in fact is albumin). Experience shows that the signs of EPH gestosis are to some extent reversible. If the blood pressure remains fixed at a high level, however, and if albumin is present in the urine in more than trace amounts, there is usually no hope of improvement. Hospital treatment, however, can prevent the signs from becoming worse.

For pregnant women with chronic renal disease we recommend a long preventive stay in hospital, even if there are not, as yet, any signs of superimposed EPH gestosis.

(4) **Induction of labour.** In severe gestoses with chronic proteinuria and fixed hypertension, the danger of antenatal death of the foetus or a small-for-dates foetus is high. When deciding whether to terminate pregnancy or let it continue, we have various tests and examination methods at our disposal:

a) the 24-hour urinary oestriol level, every day or every second day, or the oestriol level in 2-hour urine fractions after an i.v. injection of dehydro-epiandrosterone;

b) serial cytological tests of vaginal smears;

c) estimation of the maturity of the foetus from the creatinine concentration or from the amniotic fluid cytology (although the indication for amniocentesis for this purpose is still a matter of controversy);

d) amnioscopy;

e) the NPN or urea concentration in the maternal blood;

f) functional tests of the foetal sounds (step test, oxytocin test).

We induce labour before term if the objective findings lead us to conclude that the foetus is in danger of dying or of becoming relatively even smaller if left in the uterus. We do so mainly in the following situations:

a) fixed hypertension with diastole of over 110 mmHg in primary gestosis;

b) persistent and (mainly) increasing proteinuria;

c) an increase in the plasma urea or NPN level;

d) a progressive drop in the oestriol level;

e) poor results of functional tests.

We always induce labour if signs of EPH gestosis are present after the 40th week of pregnancy.

Rh IMMUNOLOGICAL CONFLICT BETWEEN MOTHER AND FOETUS

The immunological conflict between a rh negative mother and a Rh positive foetus can give rise, in the infant, to haemolytic disease, which, if not treated, is accompanied by high perinatal mortality and extremely dangerous morbidity in the form of nuclear jaundice (kernicterus). Rh haemolytic disease can be caused by isoimmunization not only with antigen D, but also with other, subsidiary antigens of the Rh system (see below).

Incidence in the population

About 13% of marriages in the Czechoslovak population are Rh incompatible (mother rh negative, father Rh positive), but the proportion of endangered children is far smaller, because a) not every child of a Rh positive father inherits the Rh positive factor, b) not every rh negative mother who gives birth to a Rh positive infant forms antibodies to the Rh factor, because compatibility in the ABO system provides some protection against Rh immunization, c) foetomaternal transfusion is not always large enough to cause a primary immune reaction.

Although 13% of marriages are Rh incompatible, therefore, only 8% of pregnancies are potentially endangered (mother rh negative, father Rh positive, partners compatible in ABO system). At birth, we find that some of the infants are rh negative. Only 5.6% are potentially endangered, but among these, Rh isoimmunization actually occurs in only one tenth. If we bear in mind that multiparas account for about 50% of the total number of births, it can be estimated that about 0.3% of all the infants born today in Bohemia and Moravia are in danger of Rh isoimmunization (given 180,000 births, proportion accounted for by multiparas 50%, 5.6% potentially endangered, 10% actually sensitized, we arrive at a final figure of 504 infants). In countries with a higher multiparity rate, the proportion of immunized infants will be larger (in West Germany, for instance, it is put at 0.8% of all births).

Haemolytic disease of the newborn takes different forms, whose severity varies according to the degree of haemolysis. The mildest form is anaemia (about 10% of all cases), icterus gravis haemolyticus (85%) is a severer form and the severest is hydrops foetalis universalis (5%). It is not known how often nuclear jaundice develops.

Active detection of high risk pregnancies

According to the directions of the Ministry of Health, the physician of any antenatal clinic in Czechoslovakia is obliged to seek out pregnancies with a danger of Rh isoimmunization. He must examine

(1) the woman's blood group and Rh factor at the first visit,

(2) the father's blood group and Rh factor if the woman is rh negative, and

(3) if the partners are Rh incompatible, he must test one blood sample for anti-Rh (anti-D) antibodies in each trimester.

Evaluation of serological results

The reading of the serological results can be hampered by the use of different symbols.

Antigens

When the Rh factor was discovered, blood containing this factor was said to be Rh positive and all other types Rh negative. Later, however, it was found that the Rhesus factor was not a single antigen, but a series of antigens forming a Rh system. This meant altering the symbols. The first antigens to be discovered were C, c, D, d, E and e, and then came others, such as F-f, V-v, C^W, C^X, E^W, D^U, C^U, E^U and further Rh antigens. The immunizing capacity of the various subsidiary antigens varies. The strongest is antigen D, followed, in descending order, by C, E, c, e.

Rh haemolytic disease can be caused by other subsidiary antigens, as well as by antigen D.

To give a concrete example; the infant of an A rh negative mother and an A rh negative father dies of Rh haemolytic disease caused by antigen C, because the mother's genotype was cde/cde and the father's CdE/Cde. The father was thus a rh negative CC homozygote.

Genotype

Determination of the father's genotype is sometimes of practical significance. If the father is a D (Rho) homozygote, all his children will be D (Rho) positive. If he is a D (Rho) heterozygote, half of his children are likely to be D (Rho) positive and half d (and hence rh) negative and not endangered by haemolytic disease.

Each chromosome carries three genes: C or c, D or d and E or e (or other, rare combinations of further subsidiary antigens). If both of a pair of chromosomes carry the same gene, the individual is a homozygote, e.g. D D or C C. If each carries a different gene, the individual is a heterozygote, e.g. Dd or Cc, etc.

Genotype can be determined only by a specialized laboratory equipped with the necessary testing sera. Since it is impossible to distinguish serologically whether a given case is type DD or D d (also written R R or R r), the laboratory result is modified in conformity with this limitation, i.e. the second letter is either omitted or is replaced by a dot. To put it more precisely, the laboratory is incapable of deciding whether the individual is a homozygote or a heterozygote. We know from genetic studies, however, that some subsidiary antigen combinations are far commoner than others and we can therefore estimate, with a given, sufficiently large margin of statistical probability, whether the combination in question is homozygous rather than heterozygous, and vice versa.

The following are the most frequent subsidiary antigen combinations, in descending order:

$CDe/c.e$ = $CcD.ee$ = $CcDee$ = probable R_1r heterozygote (about 33%)
$CDe/C.e$ = $CCD.ee$ = $CCDee$ = probable R_1R_1 homozygote (about 17%)
$cDE/c.e$ = $ccD.Ee$ = $ccDEe$ = probable R_2r heterozygote (about 13%)
$CDe/c.E$ = $CcD.eE$ = $CcDEe$ = probable R_1R_2 homozygote (about 11%)

Antibodies

There are two types of antibodies – spontaneous and immune. Spontaneous antibodies (isoagglutinins) occur in subjects whose history shows no cause of sensitization. The frequency of immune antibodies is as follows (in descending order): anti-D, anti-CD, anti-DE, anti-E, anti-c, anti-C, anti-e.

Anti-d, anti-F and anti-9 antibodies have not, so far, been found.

Antibodies are determined the most frequently by the following methods:

(1) The salt test. This is not very sensitive and detects complete antibodies, most of which do not cross the placental barrier and are thus mostly incapable of causing haemolytic disease.

(2) The albumin test detects incomplete antibodies, which have no difficulty in crossing the placenta.

(3) The globulin (anti-human globulin), or Coombs test, which has two forms (direct and indirect).

In the newborn infant the direct Coombs test is used to demonstrate erythroblastosis.

The indirect Coombs test is one of the most sensitive tests for the presence of antibodies.

(4) Ferment tests, which detect incomplete antibodies.

69

The antibody titre is expressed either semi-quantitatively, by 1 – 3 crosses, or quantitatively, as the actual titre (1 : 2, 1 : 4, 1 : 8, etc).

In practice, it is very important to realize that the same serum may give a negative result in one test and a positive result in another [e.g. in pregnancy, the papain test positive (titre 1 : 1), the indirect Coombs test negative. In the newborn infant the direct Coombs test positive. Mild haemolytic disease in the infant treated by replacement transfusion].

Evaluation of antibody titre

Views on the significance of the antibody titre for infantile morbidity vary. In general, it can be claimed that the antibody titre in the mother's serum is of only limited significance for determining the gravity of the condition of the foetus or the newborn infant, although it is true that a high titre represents a greater danger for the foetus. If the titre in the indirect Coombs test does not exceed 1 : 16, the infant is probably not in serious danger. A great deal, however, depends on the sensitivity of the titration sera which the laboratory has at its disposal.

An increase in the antibody titre during pregnancy is not of practical significance, since it can occur even when the foetus is rh negative (nonspecific reaction).

Spectrophotometry of the amniotic fluid

The presence of antibodies in the pregnant woman's serum constitutes a danger for the foetus and makes certain preventive or therapeutic measures necessary, but the first thing is to estimate the degree of the risk. The method of choice is spectrophotometric determination of the bilirubinoid pigment concentration in the amniotic fluid, which is directly proportional to the degree of danger (see chapter on diagnostic methods).

Treatment and prevention of haemolytic disease of foetus during pregnancy

The presence of antibodies in the pregnant woman's serum signifies that the foetus is jeopardized. The presence of bilirubinoid pigments in the amniotic fluid (demonstrated by spectrophotometry of the fluid) demonstrates haemolysis of the foetal RBC. The extent of haemolysis, and hence the degree of danger, is read from a Liley nomogram or from the table used by Freda. We must then decide on our subsequent action.

If the foetus is in grave danger and is sufficiently mature for a real hope of survival, we induce premature labour. Today we can base our decision on ultrasound estimation of the size of the foetus.

If the foetus is immature and spectrophotometry indicates grave danger, the only possibility is to give the foetus a transabdominal intrauterine transfusion. The purpose of this is to help the foetus overcome the danger of haemolytic anaemia and consequent hypoxia until there is a chance of its being sufficiently mature to survive the neonatal period.

Transabdominal intrauterine transfusion of the foetus is an exceptionally exacting operation, which only a team of highly qualified specialists can perform. Details will be found in the specialist literature.

The purpose of inducing premature labour is to prevent further maternal antibodies from reaching the foetus, i.e. to prevent haemolytic disease from progressing. It is thus prophylactic, and not therapeutic, in character.

Transabdominal intrauterine transfusion is basically symptomatic, and not causal, treatment, because it gives no protection against futher haemolysis. Its purpose is to prevent anaemia-induced hypoxia.

No causal therapy exists, because we still cannot remove antibodies effectively from the mother's serum. All experiments to date attempting this proved inefficacious.

Icterus neonatorum can be caused by subsidiary antigens other than antigen D (Rh_0), with equally devastating results.

Prevention of Rh isoimmunization

In the Czech Socialist Republic the prevention of Rh isoimmunization has been compulsory since January 1, 1972, its aim being to prevent primary sensitization. This is possible if anti-D antibody prepared from high titre serum from immunized pregnant women is administered within 72 hours after the infant's birth. An anti-D immunoglobulin G preparation (IgG Anti-D) is obtained from this serum by fractionation. An i.m. injection of $200-300$ µg of the active substance, administered within 72 hours after delivery, adequately prevents primary sensitization by eliminating Rh positive foetal RBC from the mother's blood stream.

Indications for prevention of Rh isoimmunization

According to instructions issued by the Czechoslovak Ministry of Health, since January 1, 1972, all primiparas fulfilling the following conditions are compulsorily protected against Rh isoimmunization: (1) mother rh negative,

(2) infant Rh positive, (3) infant and mother compatible in ABO system, (4) direct Coombs test in infant negative.

After the birth of an infant to a rh negative mother, therefore, the obstetrician must see that the relevant tests are carried out. If the conditions are met, 1 ampoule of an IgG Anti-D preparation is injected intramuscularly within not more than 72 hours.

PREMATURITY

According to WHO standards, on which statistical analyses in Czechoslovakia are also based, the criterion of prematurity is a birthweight of under 2,500 g. This has the advantage that it can be measured objectively, and the disadvantage that it also covers mature, but small-for-date infants, the proportion of whom is by no means negligible (see chapter on the small-for--date foetus). When evaluating statistical analyses, this fact must be borne in mind. It is true that the difficulty is abolished by the criterion evaluating prematurity by the length of the gestation period (limit 37 weeks, i.e. less than 259 days), but this cannot always be determined objectively with sufficient reliability.

A nation-wide analysis started is 1965, when Czechoslovakia adopted WHO criteria of perinatal mortality, shows that the **incidence** of premature births has not changed and is still about 6%. Perinatal deaths among premature foetuses and infants account for more than 67% of **total perinatal mortality,** however (Tab. 24), and in large towns and industrial areas for up to 80%. If perinatal mortality is to be significantly reduced, therefore, the first thing to do is to lower the incidence of premature births.

As well as being the chief cause of perinatal mortality, prematurity is also a decisive factor in **perinatal morbidity.** Numerous modern studies have demonstrated that a close association exists between prematurity and neurological disorders and different degrees of mental retardation (including minimum brain damage) during subsequent development.

Among children treated for perinatal encephalopathy during the past few years in the Železnice Rehabilitation Centre, Czechoslovakia, the number with a birthweight of under 1,500 g was 6.3 times greater, and with a birthweight of 1,500 – 2,000 g 2.2 times greater, than the incidence of these weight groups in the general population (Tišer et al. 1974). In Prague, where the proportion of premature births is 8%, the proportion of these children in normal elementary schools is only 5.3%, while in schools for mentally defective

Table 24. Incidence of premature births and their proportion in perinatal mortality in Czechoslovakia (1965 – 1972)

Year	Total births	Premature births		Perinatal mortality	
		Total	%	Prem. births (%)	Total per mille
1965	227,222	13,111	5.8	67.7	22.9
1966	218,705	13,283	6.1	67.7	22.7
1967	213,081	12,494	5.9	67.0	21.6
1968	212,995	12,308	5.8	67.3	20.9
1969	219,269	12,887	5.9	65.3	20.7
1970	223,958	13,364	5.85	65.8	20.4
1971	233,663	14,290	6.1	65.9	20.6
1972	247,819	14,940	6.0	67.4	20.4

children it is 10% and in children's mental institutions 20% (Gutvirth et al. 1972). A detailed analysis of a group of 10-year-olds whose birthweight was under 1,000 g showed that not only did more of them have a low IQ than full-term children, but that the concentrating capacity of their kidneys was also lower (Syrovátka et al. 1972). It is true that the many other factors by which the child is influenced long after birth must also be taken into account in such analyses, but prematurity undoubtedly plays the decisive role, as seen from an analysis carried out during the first year of life (Tab. 25).

Table 25. Correlation of retarded development and neurological disorders to birthweight and gestation age, determined in infants under the age of one year (Bishop et al. 1964)

Weight (g)	Gestation age (weeks)	Percentage of cases with disorders		
		Mental score 75	Motor score 27	Neurological disorders (%)
≦2,500	<37	39.0	33.3	4.2
≦2,500	≧37	17.4	14.8	2.8
>2,500	<37	12.7	10.1	1.8
>2,500	≧37	7.7	6.2	1.2

Many retrospective analyses have been carried out in an endeavour to determine the **causes of premature birth.** Pre-pregnancy states and complications of pregnancy were found to be the commonest. Since these are also high risk pregnancy factors, they are analysed in detail in the relevant chapters. They include:

Personal history factors:

(1) Age
(2) Parity
(3) Height
(4) Pre-pregnancy weight
(5) Legal or spontaneous abortions, premature births
(6) 1 – 2-year interval between births
(7) Uterine malformations and tumours

Current pregnancy factors:

(1) Number of examinations during pregnancy
(2) Nutrition
(3) Anaemia
(4) Infections
(5) Toxaemia (EPH-gestosis)
(6) Cardiopathies
(7) Multiple pregnancy
(8) Placenta praevia
(9) Smoking
(10) Employment and sociological factors

These factors do not all act separately, but are often combined, so that it is difficult to assess the importance of their role in the case of premature labour. The number and/or importance of these factors also changes with the passage of time. For instance, good antenatal care and prompt registration has led to a decrease in severe forms of toxaemia. On the other hand, in women in danger of habitual abortion, exact determination of the causes and specific therapy enables some of these pregnancies to be carried through to a later gestation period, when they terminate in premature labour, however.

The first step in the **prevention** of premature labour, therefore, must be to detect women with the above risk factors at the earliest possible stage of pregnancy and register them at once. Such screening, through evaluation of the importance of the various factors concerned, allows individual determination of the premature birth risk coefficient, which forms the basis of subsequent treatment. Papiernik-Berghauer et al. (1970) successfully prolonged pregnancy in this manner and obtained a mean foetal weight increment of 800 g. In cases of previous premature births or abortions, pre-conception examination is necessary, followed by the appropriate treatment (see chapter on infertility).

Since the causes of premature labour are very varied, its successful and **early diagnosis** requires more than one examination technique. With registered women, the first requirement is regular palpation control of the cervix. An attempt to classify these findings objectively, in index form, is given below (Tab.26).

Table 26. Danger of premature labour (cervical palpation findings: 0 – 10 points)

Points	0	1	2
Length	normal	shortened	< 1.5 cm
Passage	external os closed	open for part of finger	open for whole finger
Position	in posterior vaginal vault	in middle of vault	anteriorly
Consistency	tough	semi-tough	soft
Presenting part	vaginal vaults empty	engaging	lower segment dilating

Women with a shortened, open cervix (a high index) should not only be sent to hospital for a detailed diagnosis, followed by treatment, but in very severe cases there should be no hesitation in performing cerclage, even at a late stage (unless it was already done in the first trimester). An analysis of the causes of premature labour showed that, in many cases, contractions occurred when no changes could be found in the cervix (Hodr 1970). All registered cases should thus be subjected to a further, special examination with the aim of differentiating the most serious ones.

The finding that the incidence of premature births and small-for-date foetuses among pregnant women with a cardiac output of less than 380 ml/m² was double the normal rate prompted Räihä et al. (1956, 1967) to carry out an early diagnostic study of the danger of premature labour in a relatively large population series.

Although their findings were both confirmed (Boensen et al. 1958, Backman et al. 1963, Bishop 1964) and refuted (Knapp et al. 1969), they stimulated the study of changes in the uterine circulation in association with different pathological states of pregnancy, including premature labour. Tracer studies demonstrated a decrease in the uterine blood flow after physical exercise in cases of severe toxaemia (Morris et al. 1956, Weis et al. 1958). Since in earlier retrospective analyses, this was given as one of the commonest causes of premature labour, interest soon centred round changes in the uterine circulation in cases with a danger of premature labour, with reference to their possible diagnostic uses (Bruns et al. 1957, Lysgaard et al. 1965). The finding that abortion or premature birth also occurred in 2/3 of cases of experimental uterine ischaemia (Hodari 1967) provided yet another stimulus.

In an attempt to imitate a normal day's work load by means of the step test, it was found, in cases in danger of premature labour, that the foetus reacted to a temporary decrease in the uterine blood flow, with a raised blood flow in the skeletal muscles, by a change in the frequency of the foetal heart sounds as well as of foetal movements (Hodr et al. 1967). The heart sounds diminished most markedly in cases in which treatment was unsuccessful.

Vaginal cytology is another valuable and simple method (see chapter on diagnostic methods). The more the vaginal smear loses its uniform character typical for pregnancy and approximates to cytotype II or III before the 40th week, the greater the danger of premature labour (Židovský 1967, 1970).

As knowledge of the pathogenesis of premature labour progresses, symptomatic therapy retires from the scene, to be replaced by **causal and preventive methods** aimed at:

a) anticipating in the mother environmental factors and pathological states known to be possible causes of premature labour;

b) ensuring that stimuli originating from uterine activity do not affect the uterine muscles.

Metroplasty for developmental uterine abnormalities and operations for cervical incompetence prior to pregnancy abolish only a small proportion of the causes of premature labour.

Hormonal (progesterone) therapy, stimulated by the progesterone block theory (Csapo 1954, 1955), did not come up to expectations in clinical practice.

Phenothiazine and diazepam derivatives (Valium, Librium) abolish the perception of contractions in some cases, either through an analgetic effect or by inhibiting the limbic system, thereby creating the impresion that the contractions have stopped. Objective recordings demonstrated that the amplitude and frequency of the contractions were unaltered, however (Jung et al. 1966, Wolff 1968).

The synthesis of isoxsuprin (Vasodilan, Duvadilan), which has an inhibitory effect on the uterine and vascular smooth muscles and acts via beta-receptors, was an effective stimulus for utilization of the relaxant action of this substance in the prevention or treatment of incipient premature labour. A decrease in uterine activity was demonstrated objectively in cases both of toxaemia and of threatened premature labour by intrauterine pressure changes of up to 25% (Hendricks et al. 1961) and an increase in the uterine blood flow (measured by the thermistor method). Isoxsuprin has certain side effects, however, i.e. a drop in blood pressure and tachycardia, which produce disagreeable symptoms in most pregnant women (palpitations, headache, sweating). In some cases the symptoms are so intense that the effective dose has to be reduced or even discontinued.

Further beta-mimetics, with much milder side effects, were prepared by combining isoxsuprin with specific antidotes. These produce a much better therapeutic effect, with arrest of uterine contractions. They include Alupent (Brugger 1966, Eskes 1970), Dilydrin (Eggimann 1969), Dilatol (Neumann et al. 1971), Orciprenalin (Poseiro et al. 1969, Baillie et al. 1970, Cobo et al. 1970), Ritodrine (Baumgarten 1970, Wesselius et al. 1971), Th 1165 a = Berotec (Gamissans et al. 1968, Baumgarten 1969, Mosler 1969, Boden 1970, Štembera 1972 b) and Partusisten.

Beta-mimetic therapy always starts in the form of an infusion, which should be continued until the contractions stop altogether, but in any case for not less than 12−24 hours. Peroral administration should be started before completing the infusion; some authors recommend intramuscular before peroral administration. When used preventively (e.g. for reinforcement before and after cerclage for cervical incompetence at the end of the second or the beginning of the third trimester), beta-mimetics are administered only per os.

The dosage must be decided individually for each separate case. It is regulated by the tocolytic effect and by the undesirable side effects produced by different doses of the given beta-mimetics (Tab. 27).

Table 27. Comparison of intravenous inhibitory doses of different beta-sympathomimetics and of their side effects on the maternal organism (Hüter et al. 1972)

Beta-mimetic	Intraveneous inhibitory dose (μg/min)	Percentual decrease in maternal B. P.		Percentual increase in maternal heart rate
		systol.	diastol.	
Th 1165 a	1.5− 3	17	22	24
Ritodrine	250−400	10	10	35
Dilatol	150−250	21	27	37

The sooner **beta-mimetic therapy** is instituted (i.e. while the uterine contractions are not too long or too intensive and as long as there are no produced changes in the cervix), the more effective the dose (beware of underdosing!) and the longer the treatment is continued after the symptoms have subsided (several weeks' peroral therapy), the greater its success. When evaluating this form of treatment, one should not forget the psychological effect of the actual administration of the drug. Only comparison with the effect of a placebo can give reliable evaluation. For instance, success with Ritodrine was reported in 80% of cases in which the amniotic fluid had not escaped, compared with 40% given a placebo (Wesselius et al. 1971); Alupent was able to prolong pregnancy by 28. 7 days in cases in which the amniotic fluid had not escaped (19.6 days after a placebo), while in cases in which the fluid had escaped pregnancy was prolonged by 8 (as against 0.8) days (Eskes 1970). Beta-mimetic therapy is unsuitable if the cervix is dilated to 4 cm or more and we likewise do not employ it after the 37th week. The question of the maintenance of pregnancy after the amniotic fluid has escaped is discussed in the chapter on premature escape of the amniotic fluid.

Beta-mimetic therapy is absolutely contraindicated in cases of diabetes (manifest and latent), cardiovascular disease and intraovular infection. We neither found any side effects on the foetus ourselves, nor found any description of them in the literature.

The therapeutic use of ethyl alcohol (Fuchs 1967) is based on its presumed inhibition of oxytocin secretion by the neurohypophysis. A 9.5% infusion arrested uterine activity in 60 % of cases of premature labour and prolonged pregnancy up to at least the 37th week (Fuchs et al. 1967). Good success was also reported with the attainment and prolonged maintenace of a 0.1 per mille alcohol concentration in the blood. It should be borne in mind, however, that the foetus possesses no enzyme systems capable of breaking down any alcohol which may cross the placenta. This treatment is also often accompanied by side effects (nausea to pernicious vomiting, hypotension).

In countries in which abortion was made legal for a relatively wide range of indications, an increase in the number of women with cervical incompetence (as a cause of premature labour) was found after a few years. In these cases, cerclage of the cervix, in various modifications, is the causal treatment. Incompetence determined prior to conception is corrected by cerclage in the 13th week, without waiting for the clinical signs. If the patient was not examined before conceiving and the signs of incompetence do not appear until the second trimester, cerclage, reinforced by the administration of beta-mimetics, can still be carried out at even this advanced stage of pregnancy and, if the patient's history warrants it, at the beginning of the third trimester. If the indications for this treatment are properly regarded, the proportion of failures is very small. Its percentual use depends primarily on the frequency of cervical incompetence in the population. In Czechoslovakia, cerclage is performed during pregnancy in $1 - 3\%$ of all pregnant women, but we still have no reliable comparison of the frequency of premature births among women with cervical incompetence treated by cerclage and other methods.

The modern approach to the reduction of prematurity is characterized by a shift of the obstetrician's attention from maximum technical care during premature labour (on which emphasis was formerly placed) to effective comprehensive prevention. The new approach can be successful only where there is the closest cooperation between the obstetrician in the antenatal clinic and the hospital (maternity home) obstetrician. This method of preventing prematurity has already borne the first objectively demonstrable successes in some parts of Czechoslovakia, not only by halving the percentage of premature births (Kolář et al. 1972, Štembera 1972 b), but also in a shift from low birthweight premature foetuses to groups with a higher birthweight (Štembera 1974).

SOME INFECTIONS DURING PREGNANCY

Anthropozoonoses are among the infections most frequently discussed during the past decade in association with perinatal mortality or damage. During that time, the once overrated significance of zoonoses — specifically **toxoplasmosis** (TX) — has been succeeded by equally erroneous underestimation of the importance of this infection. This is the outcome of many still unresolved questions. Today, it is generally acknowledged that acute TX in the mother can lead to acute TX in the infant. It is not yet clear, however, whether chronic (latent) TX in the mother, which appears to have been demonstrated, can also affect the foetus (Kouba 1970). Since the incidence of TX (which rises with age and is relatively high in central Europe — about 40 %) is about 20 % in young, fertile women, only a small proportion of whom contract the infection during or shortly prior to pregnancy, and since transmission to the foetus is estimated to occur in only 5 per mille of these cases (Kräubig et al. 1965), it seems correct to put the incidence of congenital TX in infants at about 1 − 3 per mille. Various authors have confirmed that TX is associated with abortion and premature labour, but again, their data on incidence vary considerably. The source of the infection is not only domestic animals (cats), but can come also from eating raw meat ("tartar" beef sandwiches, rare beefsteaks). The diagnosis and treatment of zoonoses have undergone similar changes in opinion during the same period. Today it is generally held that a mere positive skin test (IDT, erythema of more than 15 mm) should no longer be an indication for treatment, as it is merely an expression of contact with the disease. In a woman with a suspicious history (previous miscarriages, premature births or perinatal injury of the foetus), only raised titres (CFR 1 : 80 and over — Bozděch et al. 1961) and the three signs: cephalgia, fatigue and afternoon subfebrile temparatures ought to be accepted as evidence of latent TX and as an indication for preconception treatment. In treatment with Daraprim, sulphonamides and antibiotics, toxoplasmin vaccination is also recommended (Vojta 1969). Daraprim should not be used during pregnancy, however, or at least not in the period of organogenesis. Similar principles apply in the case of **Listeria** and **Brucella** infections (Duniewicz et al. 1964).

Infectious hepatitis is a rare disease during pregnancy, but it is characterized by high perinatal mortality and morbidity, as demonstrated by an analysis of 69 cases concentrated in the Bulovka Hospital, Prague, in 1961 – 1965 (Bernard et al. 1967). From the aspect of treatment, it is important, though sometimes difficult, to differentiate the aetiology of jaundice in pregnancy. More than half of these cases are accounted for by infectious hepatitis, while the other half comprise cholestatic hepatosis and jaundice of pregnancy associated with severe toxaemia. In all these types of liver diseases, perinatal mortality can be as much as 10%, mainly owing to the raised incidence of premature births (up to 25% of all cases).

Rubella is the prototype of our knowledge of the direct effect of an infection on the foetus:

a) in respect of its teratogenic action in correlation to the time of infection. For infection in the first month of pregnancy the proportion of developmental defects (mainly of the heart) is given as 50% (Siegel et al. 1960). In the second and third month it drops to 20% and later to a mere 1%.

b) in respect of retarded growth. In a series of 68 cases in an epidemic in the U.S.A. in 1964, 60% of the foetuses were small-for-dates, with a mean weight of 2,200 g at 40 weeks (Cooper et al. 1965).

If infection of the mother in the first trimester is demonstrated, therefore, we recommend termination of the pregnancy for health reasons.

Views on the influence of **influenza** on perinatal mortality and morbidity are very varied. Some large statistical analyses performed with reference to influenza epidemics demonstrate a 2- to 3-fold increase in the incidence of premature births, with raised neonatal morbidity, in cases in which the mother had influenza during the first trimester (Hardy 1965).

NUTRITION AND PREGNANCY

Nutritional disturbances during pregnancy, as a high risk pregnancy factor, can be divided into two groups:

Disturbances of the mother's nutrition

Marked deviation (plus and minus) of the woman's weight from normal at the outset of pregnancy was discussed as a high risk factor in the chapter "General case history". Here we analyse the negative effect of incorrect nutrition, or an insufficient increase in weight during pregnancy (an excessive increase was discussed in the section on toxaemia).

Under physiological conditions, the pregnancy-related increase in tissue weight averages 9 – 10 kg (foetus 3,500 g, placenta 650 g, amniotic fluid 800 g, uterus 900 g, breasts 400 g, blood 1,800 g, interstitial fluid 1,200 g – Hunscher et al. 1970). The different mean weight increment curves for the individual months of pregnancy were based on these data. Bearing in mind the wide scatter, which towards the end of pregnancy amounts to ± 6 kg for a mean increment of 13 kg, an increase of less than 7 kg during the whole of pregnancy, with a normal initial weight, must be evaluated as a risk factor. In such cases we found that the incidence of small-for-dates foetuses doubled.

The calorie consumption of the pregnant woman must ensure:
a) increased growth of the given tissues,
b) the basal metabolism of the given organism,
c) energy requirements (according to employment, age, etc.).

If the calorie supply is inadequate, it is reflected

a) partly in low foetal weight; a typical example of this is the mean 7% drop in the birthweight of infants born in Rotterdam in 1944, when food supplies were very short and the mean maternal weight increment during pregnancy was only 2 kg.

b) markedly in a raised incidence of premature births; typical examples of this are the 49% incidence of premature births during the siege of Leningrad in 1942 and the increase in the number of premature births in occupied Bohemia during the Second World War.

Although we no longer encounter this type of undernutrition in Czechoslovakia, we find other causes, e.g. pernicious vomiting, *prolonged emesis* and the desire to stay slim, which are sometimes responsible for an inadequate increase in weight during pregnancy. A wrong choice of diet is even more important than too few calories. A drop in the daily protein intake below 50 g is closely associated with a 3-fold increase in premature births. Another well known factor in Czechoslovakia is that pregnant women take too few vitamins (especially vitamin C), particularly in winter. This is not only because their fruit and vegetable intake is inadequate, but is also due to wrong preparation of vitamin-rich foodstuffs, mainly in canteens, restaurants, etc.

Disturbances of foetal nutrition — the small-for-dates foetus

This section analyses the small-for-dates foetus only in association with pregnancy; the small-for-dates neonate is discussed separately, in the paediatrics section.

Foetal nutritional disturbances actually stem from pathological states which cause:
– a low concentration of essential nutrients in the mother's arterial blood,
– depression of uteroplacental circulation,
– a decrease in the effective surface area of the placental membrane,
– impairment of diffusion or active transport across the placental membrane.
The pathological states causing these disturbances include:
– malnutrition of the mother (specifically protein deficiency),
– toxaemia and essential hypertension,
– severe or recurring haemorrhage during pregnancy.
According to the time, intensity and duration of these disturbances, they can be classified as:
– acute distress, usually manifested in intranatal hypoxia; in these cases we must therefore decide to deliver much earlier by Caesarian section,
– subacute (a few days') deprivation of the foetus prior to birth, when the foetus is normal, but consumes its fat reserves, and is therefore "long and thin" at birth,
– chronic malnutrition, lasting for weeks, which causes retardation of growth, so that the weight/length quotient is maintained, but the foetus is lighter and smaller than it should be for its gestational age, i.e. it is a genuinely "small-for-dates" foetus.
The primary outcome of intrauterine malnutrition is a several-fold increase in perinatal mortality, as seen from an English analysis of foetuses of over 38 weeks (Tab. 28):

Table 28. Perinatal mortality in mature small-for-dates foetuses and a control group

	Small-for-dates foetuses	Control group
Mortinatality	93.6 per mille	10.9 per mille
Postnatal mortality	54.4 per mille	6.4 per mille

Another outcome is raised morbidity, not only in the postnatal period, when the prognosis for these infants is actually better than for premature infants with the same birthweight, but also later, owing to impairment of psychomotor development (Schulte et al. 1967) and a low IQ, especially if retarded growth and immaturity are combined (Minkowski et al. 1968). Severe intrauterine malnutrition can cause a decrease of as much as 60% in the number of brain cells (Winick et al. 1969). As already mentioned, not every form of retarded foetal growth has such bad effects on perinatal mortality, however. For instance, the infants of small mothers and twins often come within the small-for-dates group because of their weight and gestational age but their perinatal mortality is far lower.

At present in the prevention of retardation of foetal growth, we concentrate on early diagnosis and treatment of the primary cause, or on more rest, to improve the uteroplacental circulation. The first reports on the possibility of intrauterine nutrition of the foetus by the transabdominal route, through the amniotic fluid (Renaud et al. 1972) and by the administration of repeated, slow glucose infusions to the mother several weeks before delivery (Šabata et al. 1973) are surprisingly promising.

CARDIOPATHIES

Cardiopathies are one of the most serious complications of pregnancy from the aspect of maternal mortality. Compared with 1956 – 1961, when cardiac defects accounted for 12.3% of maternal mortality in Czechoslovakia, in the next 5 years the figure rose to 15.3%. Today, cardiopathies rank second among the causes of maternal mortality and in obstetrical practice they are therefore counted among the most serious pathological conditions.

From the aspect of perinatal mortality and morbidity, the situation is different and the significance of this risk factor is smaller than in maternal mortality. This is borne out firstly by its relatively small percentual incidence (compared, for example, with premature labour or toxaemia), because the proportion of women who start pregnancy with heart disease today is $1 - 2\%$. Secondly, the not greatly raised perinatal mortality, which is given as $30 - 50$ per mille (Cannel et al. 1963, Ehrenfeld et al. 1964, Niswander et al. 1968), is due largely to a roughly double incidence of premature births (Barnes 1963, Schaefer et al. 1968). The incidence of neurological abnormalities during the first year of life in the children of these mothers is actually not different from the findings in a normal population sample (Niswander et al. 1967).

Discussion of the main principles of the treatment of cardiopathies during pregnancy, labour and the puerperium are outside the scope of the problems of high risk pregnancy as examined in this monograph. In this connection, the most important factors are a responsible decision by the physician at the outset of pregnancy whether to let it continue or to terminate it and early admission of the woman to hospital at the first signs of heart failure (cyanosis), which very often leads to premature labour and hypoxia of the foetus. The same applies to a timely decision to terminate pregnancy in the last trimester.

TWINS

The incidence of twins in central Europe is given as $1.08 - 1.2\%$, i.e. an average of one in 82 births. Raised perinatal mortality in twins is associated with various factors, the chief being a more frequent incidence of premature births. Twins (specifically the second one to be born) may also be exposed to a greater danger of acute intranatal hypoxia, as confirmed by the results of an English analysis of perinatal mortality and by statistical analyses in Czechoslovakia. Raised perinatal mortality among twins is also associated with relatively frequent poorer development of one of the twins owing to chronic distress caused by unequal transplacental nutrition, which is often reflected in survivors in a subnormal IQ (Babson et al. 1966, Willerman et al. 1969). A subnormal IQ, unrelated to prematurity, was also demonstrated in the other twin, however, on an average at the age of years 4. In an attempt to explain this finding, the possibility of raised, and not always fully met, protein requirements should be considered (Holley et al. 1969).

The main form of prevention of the perinatal risk entailed in a multiple birth ought thus to be good, specifically protein, nutrition of the mother during pregnancy and concentration on the raised danger of premature labour, with immediate admission to hospital on the appearance of the first signs.

ANAEMIA AND BLEEDING DURING PREGNANCY

When differentiating these two high risk pregnancy factors, which, in most cases, are directly associated with each other, "anaemia" applies only to cases of chronic anaemia, while "bleeding" also includes forms of acute anaemia.

The borderline for **chronic anaemia in pregnancy** — if we take this pathological state as a factor exercising a negative effect on development of the foetus

– is most frequently given as 8 – 10 g% Hb. Since 50% of women with 9 – 10 g% Hb do not actually have anaemia, but pregnancy hydraemia this limit can be moved to values below 9 g%, the incidence of which, in the Czechoslovak population, does not exceed 1 – 2 %. The negative effect of chronic anaemia is reflected mainly in a raised (about doubled) incidence of premature births.

Bleeding during pregnancy is one of the most serious signs of high risk pregnancy. Its danger for development of the foetus is determined by various factors, e.g. the time at which it occurs, its intensity and recurrence or persistence of bleeding, so that there can be no unequivocal criterion of its gravity. From the chronological or causal aspect, these cases can be divided into two groups:

a) Bleeding in the first trimester (heavy or repeated), which has a frequency of about 3% (see chapter on repeated abortions). If the woman does not miscarry, the incidence of premature births is more frequent in these cases (8% as against 5%). The incidence of severe intranatal hypoxia requiring delivery by Caesarian section is also more frequent (5% as against 2%) and perinatal mortality is consequently likewise higher (50 per mille as against 20 per mille).

b) Bleeding in the second and third trimester, the frequency of which is again given as 3%, and which can be divided into 3 subgroups, according to its cause, frequency and gravity:

Abruption of the placenta — 25 % of all haemorrhages — 50 % of perinatal mortality

Placenta praevia — 15 % of all haemorrhages — 13 % of perinatal mortality

Indeterminate causes — 60 % of all haemorrhages — 8 % of perinatal mortality

Although the absolute value of the above percentages may vary in different, similar series, these figures nevertheless give us a very clear idea of the extreme danger for the foetus and a reciprocal comparison of the gravity of these pathological states which cause bleeding in the second half of pregnancy and are thus a very dangerous high risk pregnancy factor.

ASYMPTOMATIC BACTERIURIA

The risk for the foetus associated with asymptomatic bacteriuria, which occurs in $5-7\%$ of all pregnant women, consists of

a) its potential danger for the maternal organism; asymptomatic bacteriuria is defined as a preclinical stage of pyelonephritis, which, if not treated in time, has a 50 % chance of developing into manifest disease during pregnancy;

b) a danger of *E. coli* endotoxin acting directly on the myometrium and hence the possibility of premature induction of uterine activity (Kass 1962, Henderson et al. 1962).

Most of the workers who tested Kass's conclusions failed to confirm a raised incidence of premature births in simple asymptomatic bacteriuria (Monzon et al. 1963, Prát 1967) but it is known that there is an association between the incidence of premature births and the presence of a manifest infection of the urinary tract during pregnancy.

Although the actual diagnosis of asymptomatic bacteriuria during pregnancy is methodologically not particularly exacting, if it were to be used as a screening method for all pregnant women it would nevertheless place a considerable strain on antenatal clinics and laboratories (reliable estimation of the middle urine flow, immediate storage on ice, the need for laboratory tests within not more than $1-2$ hours after collection). Specific examination for bacteriuria is a suitable screening method for selected women with a history of such infections, however, a prompt treatment of positive cases can help to prevent the development of pyelonephritis during pregnancy, when it is a high risk factor.

PROTRACTED PREGNANCY

Practically all our obstetricians are today agreed that mere prolongation of pregnancy beyond 294 days (about 4% of all pregnancies) does not necessarily endanger the foetus, but there are very few who deny in principle the significance of protracted pregnancy as a risk factor. The reasons for including protracted pregnancy among risk factors include the objective demonstration of a 3 times higher incidence of intranatal hypoxia characterized by a more frequent incidence of the classic signs, i.e. bradycardia and turbidity of the amniotic fluid, a more frequent need for surgical delivery based on foetal indications, more frequent postnatal depression of the infant (Nyklíček et al. 1969, Poradovský et al. 1969, Štembera et al. 1969), a low pH in the cord blood (Stříbrný et al. 1969), a raised incidence of signs of placental dysfunction (after Clifford) in the newborn infant (Soukup et al. 1969), or a marked increase in perinatal mortality (Tab. 29). Perinatal morbidity (both the severest forms and forms with minimum brain damage) is also increased in protracted pregnancies.

Table 29. Perinatal mortality in Czechoslovakia (total and divided according to the number of weeks from the 39th) (Nyklíček et al. 1969)

Weeks of pregnancy	Number of births	Perinatal mortality per mille
39 – 40	184,444	5.6
41	7,796	16.8
42	5,807	34.6
Czechoslovakia 1966, total	224,429	22.1

Many misunderstandings were abolished when the time aspect was dropped to second place and the functional aspect for both mother and foetus promoted to first:

a) the biological readiness of the maternal organism for labour,

b) the functional state of the placenta and foetus (the foetoplacental unit).

This approach led to the following differentiation, both in Czechoslovakia and in other countries:

(1) Physiological protraction of pregnancy (hypermaturity): the biological readiness of the maternal organism is delayed, but foetoplacental function is unimpaired; the foetus is healthy, its weight and length are usually over average and it is not endangered by hypoxia.

(2) Pathological protraction of pregnancy (postmaturity): foetoplacental function is impaired, further high risk pregnancy signs are generally present, foetal weight and size are often disproportionate, the foetus is endangered by varying degrees of hypoxia, but despite all this, triggering of the labour mechanism is delayed.

There are several methods by which these states can be distinguished:

a) Methods determining whether the maternal organism is ready for labour (palpation of the cervix, Smith's oxytocin test), which indicate whether there is any hope of success should labour be induced.

b) Methods determining placental dysfunction or danger to the foetus (amnioscopy, the step test, oestriol/24 hours, oestriol after DHEA-S).

c) Methods which, in some respects, provide an answer to both the preceding questions (gestational cytology, cardiotocography).

Today, many Czechoslovak laboratories combine these methods in varying ways for protracted pregnancies (Dlhoš et al. 1969, Horák et al. 1969, Hudcovič et al. 1969, Poradovský et al. 1969, Šikl et al. 1969, Štembera et al. 1969). Any decision to terminate pregnancy should be based on a clinical analysis of the case, and on at least two of the above methods for determining placental dysfunction. If the maternal organism were simultaneously found to be ready for labour, this would, of course be ideal, but even if it were not, this should never be allowed to bar the termination of pregnancy where the foetus is seriously endangered. The form of delivery is a different question (see chapter on the induction of labour). If the above criteria are observed, induced labour for prolonged pregnancy does not amount to more than 1% of all deliveries, i.e. about 20 − 25% of all pregnancies lasting more than 294 days (Horský et al. 1969) and in this way raised perinatal mortality in prolonged pregnancies can be virtually abolished (Štembera et al. 1969).

SMOKING AND PREGNANCY

It is stated in the literature that smoking during pregnancy reduces the foetus's birthweight. Frazier's analysis (Frazier 1961) clearly demonstrates a direct correlation between birthweight and smoking intensity: over 10 cigarettes a day lowers birthweight by an average of 200 g. Since a direct association has been demonstrated between smoking during pregnancy and a raised incidence of premature births (Tab. 30) and raised perinatal mortality (Tab. 31), smoking must also be included among the high risk pregnancy factors.

Table 30. Comparison of incidence of premature births among smokers and non-smokers

Author	Year	n	% of premature births: mother	
			smoker	non-smoker
Frazier (U.S.A.)	1961	2,042	18.4	11.2
Herriot (Scotland)	1962	2,745	12.6	6.3
NINDB project (U.S.A.) 10 hospitals	1966	7,018	11.3	7.7
Trča (Czechoslovakia)	1975	1,920	11.2	6.1

Table 31. Comparison of perinatal mortality among smokers and non-smokers

Author	Year		Perinatal mortality per mille		
			antenatal	postnatal	total
Butler	1958	smoker	27.6	17.2	44.8
		non-smoker	19.3	13.1	32.4
Frazier	1966	smoker	15.5	27.5	42.5
		non-smoker	6.4	23.3	29.7
Baršić	1975	smoker	19.1	9.2	28.1
		non-smoker	12.1	10.6	22.5

INTERVAL BETWEEN PRESENT AND PRECEDING PREGNANCY

Attention was already drawn 20 years ago to the more frequent incidence of premature births in pregnancies less than 2 years removed from the previous one. Since then, this finding has more than once been verified (Bishop 1964, Page 1970, Döring 1965) and has thus been confirmed as a high risk pregnancy factor. Recently, its significance was further emphasized by low IQ findings in 4-year-old children born less than 2 years after the preceding pregnancy.

ANTENATAL CARE

In western analyses, inadequate antenatal care is often given as a cause of high (up to 10-fold) perinatal mortality (Page 1970, Wallace 1970), mainly in association with high prematurity. Czechoslovak analyses also show that perinatal mortality among women without any antenatal care (who number just under 1 %) is 5 times higher. Although this is plainly an extremely important factor in perinatal medicine, as soon as attendance at the antenatal clinic has reached a given number of visits (in Czechoslovakia the mean number is 8), a mere further increase in the number of visits, without a basic change in the quality of the diagnosis and treatment, as ought to be provided by special clinics for high risk pregnancies, will not reduce perinatal mortality any further.

COMPLICATIONS DURING LABOUR

Labour itself is a physiological process and ought not, per se, to be a risk factor. Physiological labour in a woman with a high risk pregnancy is a different situation, however, since this physiological process, lasting several hours, may constitute the final acute stress which exhausts the last mechanisms compensating the many chronic stresses produced by her pregnancy. This is doubly the case in pathological labour. If the foetus dies during labour, or if we find trauma of the newborn infant immediately after delivery, we should not look for the cause **solely** in labour, until we have excluded or evaluated all risk factors in this and previous pregnancies and in the woman's history in general. This is the only way to determine the primary cause and to estimate the true proportional role of labour in perinatal mortality and morbidity.

BREECH DELIVERY

Although spontaneous breech delivery (Bd) belongs to the physiological delivery group, it is nevertheless included among risk factors, because it is more often accompanied by labour complications than vertex delivery.

Perinatal mortality: Although the mean frequency of incidence of Bd is about 5%, it accounts for fully 25% of intra- and postnatal deaths (Czech perinatal mortality figures, 1969). Total perinatal mortality in Bd (which is about 80 per mille for the whole country and is thus 4 times higher than for other presentations) is not an adequately reliable criterion for comparing the medical handling of Bd in different hospitals, for two main reasons:

a) the incidence of Bd rises sharply in inverse proportion to birthweight, so that immaturity may be the actual cause of death, and the frequency of premature births in different hospitals varies considerably,

b) antenatal mortality and the congenital malformations incompatible with life included in perinatal mortality distort the final figure still further.

Intra- and postnatal mortality among term foetuses without malformations would thus be a far more reliable criterion.

The same applies to the long-term study of **perinatal morbidity.** In studies of the frequency of the traumatization of infants born by Bd, the figures are much higher than for other births and range from 5% to 20% (Andreas 1959, Bolte et al. 1968, Russell 1969). Most of these cases are associated with surgical Bd by the vaginal route. The trauma is not always only of a motor type (e.g. spastic diplegia), but also includes mental disorders (Millar 1969, Wallace 1970) and epilepsy (Churchill 1959).

The warning figures for these last two indexes give food for thought on the **conduct of Bd.** We are not concerned here with discussing the advantages of spontaneous condutct of Bd after Covjanov or Bracht, but rather with considering how to reduce the high percentage of vaginal operations in Bd. In most of our hospitals, 14–20% of Bd are at present concluded by extraction (3–8% by complete extraction). One way is to ensure good uterine function in time by infusing oxytocin and the other to extend the indications for Caesarian section (see chapter on therapy). The utilization of these two solutions will reduce not only the percentage of extractions, but also perinatal mortality (Tab. 32).

Table 32. Effect of extending indications for Caesarian section in Bd on proportion of extractions and perinatal morbidity (Kittrich 1970)

Year	1954–1961	1966–1969
Number of cases	627	179
Spontaneous after Covjanov	71.9%	76.6%
Extraction	16.6%	6.1%
Caesarian section	11.5%	17.3%
Perinatal morbidity amoung foetuses and neonates >2,500 g	15.6 per mille	6.3 per mille

Primary Caesarian section should be undertaken in all cases of breech presentation with a high risk pregnancy (e.g. diabetes), during the first stage of labour, and, in good time, in high risk cases in which uterotonics fail to control uterine activity completely. A frequency of 8% Caesarian sections for breech presentations in the normal population and double that number in hospitals where high risk pregnancies are concentrated, is not an exaggerated demand if we are to combat perinatal mortality in Bd seriously.

PROTRACTED LABOUR

Only 10 years ago, this risk factor accounted for a high proportion of intranatal mortality in Czechoslovakia. Progressive shortening of the length of labour in a steadily mounting number of cases, from the increasing use of oxytocin infusions in most of our hospitals, has greatly reduced the participation of protracted labour in perinatal mortality (Tab. 33).

Table 33. Participation of protracted labour in intranatal mortality in Czechoslovakia

Lenght of first stage of labour in hours	Distribution of number of intranatal deaths (%) according to length of the first stage of labour			Total (absolute number)
	-8	$8-16$	$16+$	
Year 1962	31	37	32	304
1972	61	28	11	253

Protraction of the second stage of labour has an equally important — and for the foetus harmful — effect. Study of the pH in microsamples of foetal blood showed a marked increase in foetal acidosis precisely in this stage (Saling and Kubli — see Methods). The second stage ought therefore not to exceed 60 minutes, in any labour, and especially not after a high risk pregnancy. Among labours with intranatal death of the foetus, we nevertheless find 10% with a second stage of over 1 hour (Perinatal mortality in the Czech socialist Republic, 1972). The above improvement in the medical conduct of labour ought therefore to be applied to all other protracted labours.

PREMATURE RUPTURE OF THE MEMBRANES

If uterine activity does not commence within 24 hours after premature rupture of the membranes, the foetus is potentially exposed to greater danger from a possible intraovular infection. In such cases, the preventive administration of antibiotics to the mother (usually penicillin in a dose of 1.2×10^6 units/24 hours) is a generally recognized principle. Today, however, in view of the considerable changes in the microbial spectrum found in these infections, we are faced with the question of whether penicillin is a suitable anti-biotic and whether it ought not to be replaced by antibiotics with a wider spectrum, but not harmful to the foetus (e.g. Ampicillin).

With reference to the above risk, practically all hospitals are agreed that, in pregnancies of over 37 weeks, labour should be induced after 24 or 48 hours (see Induction of labour). The same problem in younger pregnancies is discussed in the chapter on premature labour. This state is even more serious in cases in which the amniotic fluid is turbid (meconium). This is a sign of intrauterine hypoxia and the possibility of the aspiration of such fluid increases the danger of early RDS for the foetus. There is also a danger of rapid development of infection, as demonstrated by *in vitro* experiments with amniotic fluid to which meconium was added. In such cases, therefore, the immediate induction of labour ought to be a categorical requirement.

FEVER DURING LABOUR

This state increases foetal risk in two ways:

a) through the transmission of a pathogen from mother to foetus, with subsequent adnatal infection of the newborn infant,

b) by interfering with the mother's metabolism and circulation, thereby negatively influencing the metabolism of the foetus; intrauterine hypoxia is consequently much commoner in these foetuses.

The danger to the foetus must therefore be provented by specific and intensive treatment of the infection in the mother and by shortening labour.

UMBILICAL CORD COMPLICATIONS

Umbilical prolapse is one of the most serious complications of labour, as it causes severe acute hypoxia in which only rapid termination of labour (practically always surgical) can save the foetus's life. Even so, there is always the danger that this severe acute hypoxia may result in perinatal injury to the infant.

Twisting of the umbilical cord round the foetus's neck cannot really be regarded as a risk factor, since it is virtually impossible to demonstrate it reliably prior to labour. We nevertheless consider it necessary to discuss this "complication" briefly, because its frequency in the population is high (23%) and its significance in perinatal mortality is sometimes overrated. This erroneous view, which prevailed in many studies, was reliably refuted in the past decade by statistical analyses. We likewise confirmed in metabolic and circulatory studies that the primary source of danger to the foetus in most cases with a twisted cord were other high risk pregnancy factors and that a twisted cord was only a secondary factor. We found that isolated twisting of the cord merely produced brief, mild acute hypoxia in the last phase of the second stage of labour and that this was manifested in only mild depression immediately after birth (Apgar score $8-7$ points/1 min), with normalization within 5 minutes (Štembera 1972). These conclusions concur with long-term studies of perinatal morbidity in cases with a twisted cord, in which no increase in the frequency of psychomotor injury was found.

SIGNS OF HYPOXIA DURING LABOUR

Clinical signs of hypoxia rightly belong to risk factors. Since their gravity is determined not only by their type, intensity, time of appearance and duration, but also by objective recording, so that they are likewise a diagnostic sign, they will be discussed in detail in the chapter on diagnostics.

SURGICAL DELIVERY

Labour is terminated surgically according to the foetal indications because the life of the foetus, or the future health of the infant, is endangered. It is thus (or ought to be) an operation which benefits the foetus and does not cause it further injury. From this aspect, therefore, surgical delivery ought not to be a risk factor, since the latter is actually the pathological condition endangering the foetus. These types of surgical delivery are consequently discussed in the chapter on therapy.

ANAESTHESIA AND ANALGESIA

Anaesthesia for Caesarian section

If actual surgical delivery ought not to constitute a danger to the foetus, then the same should also apply to anaesthesia, which is employed most often in Caesarian section. Again setting aside any risks entailed for the mother, we shall pay attention only to the risk of anaesthesia for the foetus. The conditions imposed by this risk in obstetrics are quite different from those in normal surgery. For one thing, it is essential to achieve adequately deep anaesthesia, but of only short duration, for the first 5 – 10 minutes (until the foetus is delivered), so that the foetus is affected as little as possible (or so that the effect of anaesthesia can be readily and quickly abolished immediately after its delivery). For another, we must bear in mind that there is a basic difference between the effect of an anaesthetic on a healthy foetus (or on one endangered only by a chronic risk) (e.g. Caesarian section indicated by the mother's condition – diabetes in the mother) and on a hypoxic foetus in which, owing to circulatory changes, more blood, and hence more anaesthetic, reaches the vitally important organs, i.e. the heart and the CNS (Kralert 1970). The CNS is more susceptible to the depressant action of barbiturates especially in acute hypoxia and this can lead during delivery to depression of vitally important centres or to further intensification of hypoxia-induced depression, with acidosis of the foetus. In such cases, therefore, methods are being sought for substituting other, non-barbiturate, substances for Thiopental, the previous standard, in the **induction of anaesthesia.** In this respect, good results have been obtained with Epontol, for example (Kralert et al. 1970). The question of **relaxants,** which are commonly used in modern anaesthesia, is no less important. The most satisfactory of these is succinylcholine, rapid depletion of which in the mother's blood largely limits its transport across the placenta to the foetus. The best **anaesthetic** to follow induction is another question, to which the same conditions apply as for induction (Sirotný et al. 1970), in a comprehensive series, discussed the wide and continuously supplemented range of anaesthetics at present in use or on trial, together with their advantages and disadvantages. Another danger is the possibility of acidosis of the foetus being aggravated from prolonged, regulated **hyperventilation with oxygen** when initiating anaesthesia (Saling 1967, Moya et al. 1965), if performed by someone insufficiently versed in obstetrical anaesthesia. These perils all show the need for having a permanent 24-hour anaesthesiology emergency service thoroughly acquainted with the special problems of obstetrical anaesthesiology.

95

Analgesia

Various, often widely differing techniques are used for analgesia during labour, but, as distinct from anaesthesia, the given substance acts on the foetus for a significantly longer time, although in lower concentrations. Many authors consequently regard analgesia as a much greater risk for the foetus than anaesthesia. In our opinion, such general condemnation is wrong, if only because of the wide variations between analgetic techniques, of which we give the following examples: **Neuroplegic mixtures** of different compositions and administered in different forms have steadily spread in Czechoslovakia during the past 5 years because of their minimal adverse effect on the foetus. Adequately intensive uterine activity — either spontaneous, or reinforced in good time by an oxytocin infusion when administering the mixture (Kotásek et al. 1968) is an important condition for their use.

A paracervical block, which is not much used in Czechoslovakia, but is commonly used in western countries, often reduces uteroplacental blood circulation, with consequent acidosis of the foetus (Teramo 1967, de Mot et al. 1971, etc.).

Inhalation anaesthetics used intermittently, always during a contraction, in lower than anaesthesiological concentrations, produce retrograde amnesia in the mother and are not supposed to be harmful to the foetus, even after several hours' administration. At present, we have little experience with the latest of these preparations (e.g. Pentran) in Czechoslovakia.

METHODS FOR DIAGNOSING
DANGER TO FOETUS
AND PLACENTAL DYSFUNCTION

The rapid development of biochemistry and medical electronics during the past few years has produced a spate of new methods, most of which require the use of modern apparatus or complicated laboratory techniques. This means that the majority of small institutions are unable to verify these methods themselves. This chapter therefore aims at giving the reader a survey of the most important of these methods and attempts to submit an objective evaluation of them. The size of the monograph does not allow every method to be described in detail, so each is accompanied by the most important references (original publications, special monographs).

RECORDING THE FOETAL HEART RATE (FHR)

Although the first, primitive attempts date back to 1892, foetal cardiography did not really begin to develop until the second half of the present century. These studies were all carried out with research prototype apparatus, however, and it is only during the past 10 years that their commercial production has been possible. The basic demands made on such a recording apparatus are:

The possibility of equally reliable recording of the FHR during both pregnancy and labour.

Evaluation of the frequency/min of the FHR simultaneously with its recording.

Evaluation of changes in FHR frequency in the shortest possible interval, preferably within the range of two cardiac cycles ("beat to beat").

Recording of uterine activity simultaneously with the FHR.

Adequate sensitivity of the apparatus and abolishment of background interference.

Miniaturization of the detector, to allow the woman freedom of movement in bed.

Simple operation, easy maintenance and a minimal break-down rate of the apparatus.

The equipment types so far produced are based on 3 different principles of obtaining information signals for recording the FHR:

a) the actual sound of the action of the foetal heart (phonocardiography). Substitution of recording of the time distance between two cardiac cycles for the sound signal has abolished some of the disadvantages of this FHR recording method (Hammacher 1962) and has resulted in a good serially produced foetal monitor;

b) the R wave in the whole foetal ECG complex (see the chapter on the foetal ECG);

c) ultrasound detection of foetal systole on the principle of the Doppler effect.

Method of evaluating the monitored FHR

Classic evaluation (bradycardia and tachycardia) has now been supplemented, in FHR monitoring, by a number of further findings. "Beat to beat" monitoring, as well as augmenting our knowledge of the physiology of the action of the foetal heart, has also added new diagnostic possibilities.

The mean FHR/min, which is evaluated over a period of 10 min and is termed the baseline, still remains the basic value. The results of cardiographic examinations have confirmed earlier experience that a mean FHR of 120 to 160 beats/min is the normal range for the foetal heart. An increase in baseline frequency to over 160 is defined as mild, and to over 180 as severe tachycardia, while a drop below 120 is defined as mild, and below 100 as severe bradycardia. Brief deviations from the baseline (from a few dozen seconds to several minutes) are defined as acceleration if the FHR rises and as deceleration if it falls, but the baseline remains the same. Obstetricians formerly defined these changes as alteration of the FHR. If the change in frequency lasts more than 10 min, however, it is defined as a rise (fall) in the baseline.

In addition to these changes in the FHR, in beat to beat recording we further distinguish very rapid fluctuation of the FHR (within a range of only a few seconds) from the baseline, both in amplitude and in frequency/min. These changes in the FHR are described as rapid fluctuation (Caldeyro-Barcia) or oscillation (Hammacher), or as baseline irregularity (Hon).

Both these forms of deviation of the FHR from the baseline are utilized today in the antenatal and intranatal diagnosis of an endangered foetus.

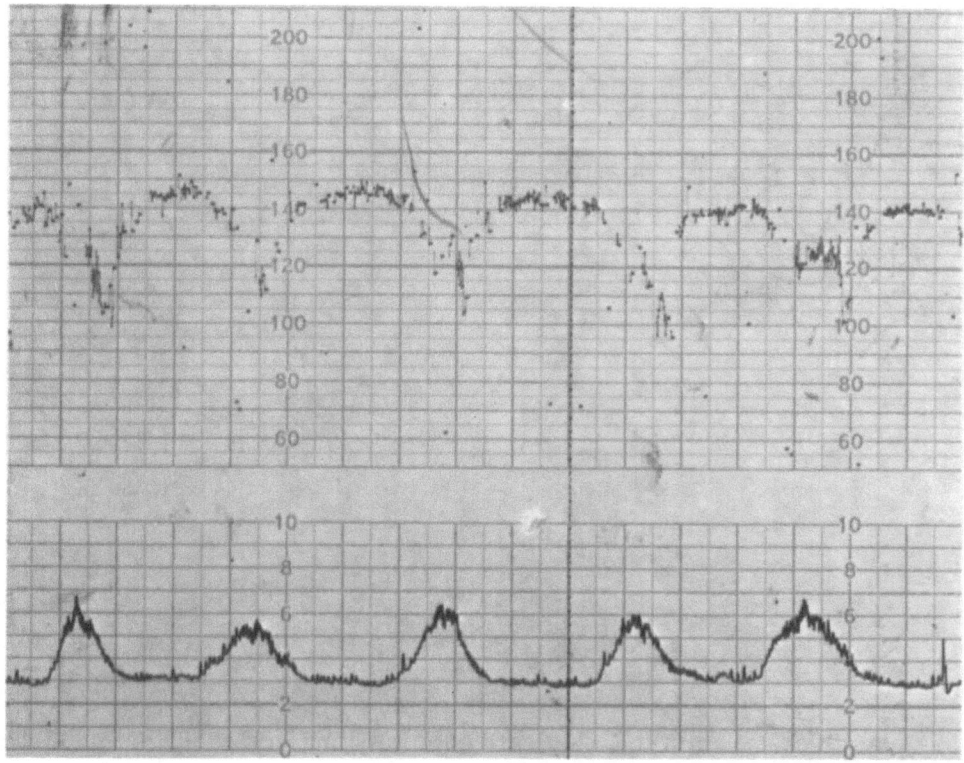

Fig. 7. Original cardiotocogram. Top curve: FHR — "Early deceleration, Dip I". Bottom curve: uterine contractions.

(1) The principle of the first form is the reciprocal relationship of slow changes in the FHR and uterine contraction and is therefore suitable mainly for diagnosis during labour. It distinguishes:

a) Early deceleration, HC = head compression (Hon et al. 1968), Dip I (Caldeyro-Barcia et al. 1964).

The FHR slows down at the beginning of a contraction and returns to normal by the end of the contraction; deceleration is caused chiefly by compression of the head owing to raised intrauterine pressure during contraction (Fig. 7).

b) Late deceleration, UPI = uteroplacental insufficiency (Hon et al. 1968), Dip II (Caldeyro-Barcia et al. 1964).

Deceleration occurs during a contraction, but persists for some time after it ends. It is caused by foetal hypoxia (lowering of Po_2) and is connected with acidosis of the foetal blood. It usually occurs in association with tachycardia between contractions, so that the FHR does not necessarily drop even to 120 beats/min (Fig. 8).

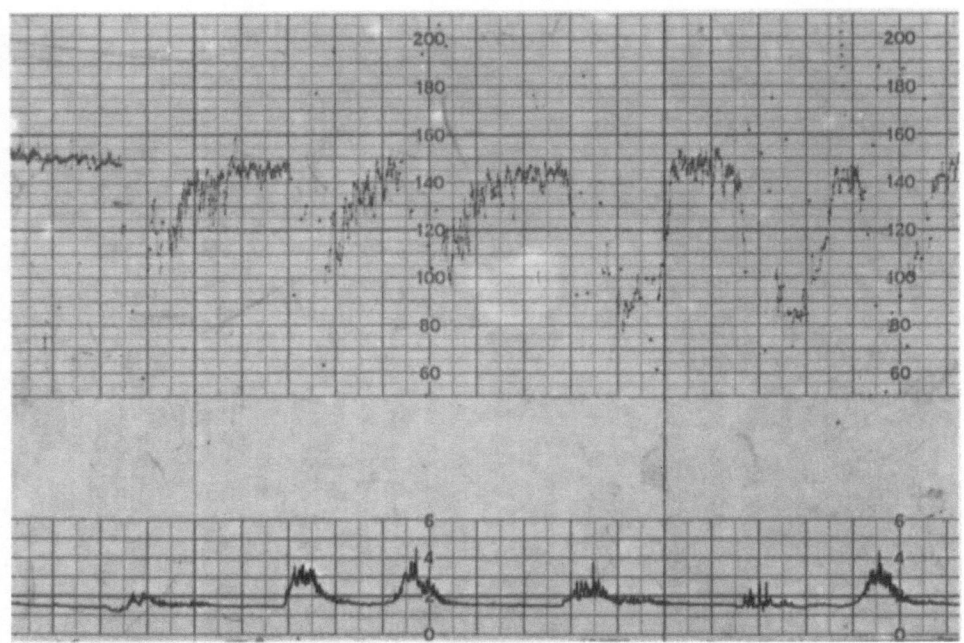

Fig. 8. Original cardiotocogram. FHR — "Late deceleration, Dip II".

c) Variable deceleration, CC = cord compression (Hon et al. 1968), Dip 0 (Caldeyro-Barcia et al. 1964).

Deceleration occurs in different phases of contraction and lasts 10 – 60 s. It changes with the mother's position. It is usually found in association with bradycardia and the FHR may fall as low as 60/min. A cord complication is the commonest cause (Fig. 9).

(2) The second form of evaluating the FHR utilizes the recording of rapid changes in the FHR, with reference to their amplitude and their rate, i.e. their number per minute. Since these changes take place independently of uterine contractions, they can also be used for antenatal diagnosis. As regards **amplitude** changes, Hammacher distinguishes 4 types of oscillations:

a) Type 0 — a "silent" FHR, i.e. fluctuation of the FHR within a range of 0 – 5 beats/min. If we exclude possible inhibition of the foetus by some drug (e.g. pethidine) and if this type lasts for at least 10 min, it is evidence of impaired adaptability of the foetal circulation to stress and of increasing metabolic acidosis of the foetus.

b) Type 1 — a "narrowly undulating" FHR, i.e. fluctuation of the FHR within a range of 5 – 10 beats/min. If we again exclude drug-induced inhibition of the foetus, this type denotes incipient depression of CNS regulatory mechanisms for adaptation of the foetal circulation, owing to incipient me-

100

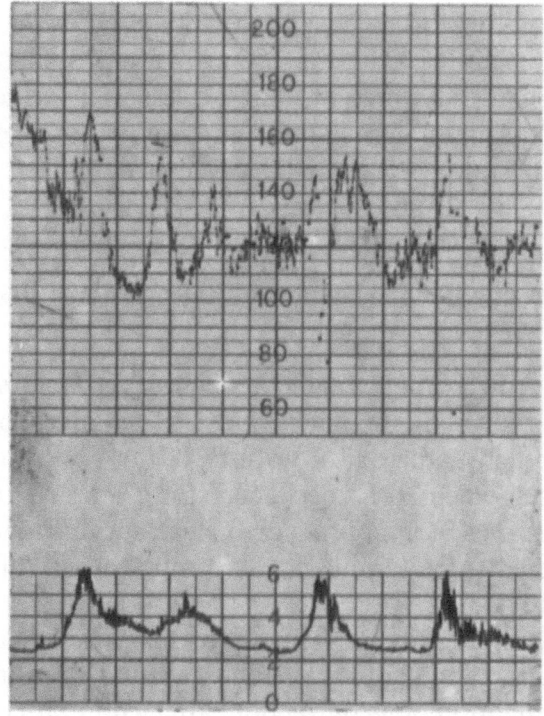

Fig. 9. Original cardiotocogram. FHR —
"Variable deceleration, Dip 0".

tabolic acidosis. From the aspect of the differential diagnosis it may also be "physiological sleep" of the foetus, in which case, after the foetus has been woken (by mechanical stimulation in the form of vaginal or external examination), type 1 changes to type 2.

c) Type 2 — an "undulating" FHR, i.e. fluctuation of the FHR within a range of 10−25 beats/min. This is evidence of a healthy foetus, especially if any movements of the foetus are accompanied by a transient rise in the baseline FHR, or by an increase in oscillation amplitude.

d) Type 3 — a "saltatory" FHR, e.i. fluctuation of the FHR, within a range of over 25 beats/min. This is indicative of a foetoplacental circulatory disorder and is a sign of danger to the foetus from hypoxia (often in association with a cord episode).

Hon divides short-term FHR fluctuation into 5 groups, according to their amplitude height; he relates amplitude height to baseline height and expresses it as a percentage of the absolute height of the FHR:

a) "No irregularity" means absence of any signs of fluctuation.

b) "Minimal irregularity" if the oscillations are less than 3% of the baseline frequency.

c) "Average irregularity" if fluctuation amounts to 4−9% of baseline frequency.

101

d) "Moderate irregularity" if it attains 10−15% of baseline frequency.

e) "Marked irregularity" if it exceeds the baseline by more than 15%.

Another criterion for evaluating oscillations is the **rate** at which they change. At present, this is a less well verified criterion, according to which a mean of 5 oscillations/min is a sign of a healthy foetus, while a decrease in this rate is a warning of intrauterine danger.

Reliability of evaluation of the monitored FHR

Today, the baseline frequency *per se* plays a smaller role in the diagnostics of foetal risk than it used to, and acquires significance only in association with other, pathological features of the FHR. Simple tachycardia is regarded as a compensatory mechanism for given stress of the foetus. Views on the significance of mild bradycardia are not unanimous, but it is usually not considered to be serious unless combined with other pathological features of the FHR.

Marked acceleration is of significance mostly as a demonstration of the adaptability of the foetal organism to various stress situations (e.g. after termination of a contraction, after Dip I, after examination by the obstetrician owing to pressure on the head, etc).

Deceleration of the Dip I type is primarily an expression of physiological changes in the foetal circulation during labour. These increase during labour; about 10% of all the contractions occur with up to 4 cm dilatation of the isthmus and minor engagement of the head in the superior pelvic canal, while up to 50% occur in the last phase of stage I (Althabe 1969). The importance of Dip O, which is one of the commonest forms of deceleration (Berg, 1972, found that it occurred in up to 90% of all labours) and is most frequently an expression of an acute decrease in the uteroplacental blood flow, should be evaluated in different ways − from its duration, a drop in its amplitude, a change in baseline frequency, its combination with a different oscillation type, etc. From this aspect, Kubli (1969) distinguished a mild form, which does not affect the foetal pH, a moderately severe form and a severe form, in which foetal acidosis of varying degrees of severity occurs.

Of all the forms of deceleration, Dip II is the most important indicator of placental dysfunction of the type of impaired O_2 and CO_2 exchange between mother and foetus, with resultant foetal acidosis (Tab. 34).

The gravity of Dip II can also be differentiated, according to the deceleration amplitude, as mild (decrease < 15 beats/min), moderately severe (15 to 45/min) and severe (> 45/min).

102

Table 34. Reciprocal association of foetal gas metabolism and FHR disturbance of Dip II type (Caldeyro-Barcia et al. 1968)

	O_2 saturation		P_{O_2} in mmHg		P_{CO_2} in mmHg		pH	
	<31%	>31%	<19.9	>19.9	<58.4	>58.4	<7.21	>7.21
Dip II pos.	7	0	5	0	9	5	20	8
Dip II neg.	2	28	2	29	8	32	4	89

The close association between Dip II and foetal acidosis is also confirmed by other authors (Hon 1967, Newmann et al. 1967, Wood et al. 1967, Lepage et al. 1970, Pendleton 1970). In a series of 1,500 cases in which the FHR was monitored, there was not a single case of foetal acidosis without Dip II (Lepage et al. 1970). On the other hand, an incidence of over 20 Dip II during labour was always accompanied by depression of the newborn infant (Caldeyro-Barcia et al. 1968). In addition to the depth of deceleration, a high incidence of Dip II also gave warning of increased danger to the foetus (Mendez-Bauer 1969).

An incidence of 30% Dip II in the presence of normal uterine activity can thus be regarded as the approximate diagnostic limit of foetal distress (Tab. 35).

Table 35. Reciprocal relationship between Dip II frequency during labour and postnatal depression of newborn infant

Dip II incidence	Apgar score
≦10% of contractions	10 – 7
11 – 31% of contractions	6 – 4
>31% of contractions	4

Diminution of oscillation amplitude is not only an expression of foetal hypoxia, but can also be caused by sleep and by CNS-inhibiting drugs administered to the mother, while augmentation of amplitude can be due to movement of the foetus or to external interference (e.g. examination, etc). Amplitude magnitude is also decided by the signal used by different types of foetal monitors. The amplitude range cited for Hammacher's types 0 – 3 applies to the phonocardiographic recording. The amplitude of the signal obtained from the electrocardiograph is lower and in evaluation after Hammacher corresponds to the nearest lower type. The oscillation amplitude obtained with an ultrasonic recorder varies according to whether the movement of the foetal heart, aorta or ductus arteriosus is detected. Diminishing oscillation amplitude or a decrease in the oscillation frequency per minute are, by themselves, only a warning signal in the diagnostic of foetal danger and do not indicate marked deterioration of the prognosis for the foetus unless they are combined. The most serious type of oscillation is thus type 0 ("silent"), with an oscillation frequency of < 2/min (Rüttgers et al. 1972, Kubli 1972, Fischer 1973).

Simultaneous evaluation of all these changes in the FHR, as they are combined in each individual case, makes foetal cardiotocography a valuable diagnostic method. Its monographic elaboration in the form of an atlas (Fischer 1973) is a great help for mastering this technique successfully.

Simplified FHR "monitoring" by means of auscultation

The successes of FHR monitoring led to the idea of utilizing the merits of this recording method for institutions not possessing the necessary equipment. Starting from the instant when a contraction ends, the examiner listens to the FHR with a stethoscope at 5-s intervals for 1 minute. In this way it is possible to imitate the evaluation of Dip II described above (Whitfield 1969, Štembera 1972), although it is obviously less precise and much more exacting for the personnel than monitoring.

FUNCTIONAL TESTS

The principle of these methods, which are also known as "loading" tests, is to expose the organism to stress imitating stress situations encountered in real life. Functional capacity reserves in the relevant systemic region are then evaluated from the subsequent reaction, the character of which is closely associated with the way in which the organism copes with the stress. The diagnosis of placental dysfunction is based on this principle. The uteroplacental circulation is exposed for short periods to different forms of stress, which, in the presence of placental dysfunction, causes temporary reduction of the foetal oxygen supply or the accumulation of metabolic degradation products in the foetus. The foetal circulatory system responds to this not only according to the intensity of the disturbance, but also according to its own adaptability to hypoxia.

104

Oxygen test

A 15 minutes' increase in the oxygen supply through a well-fitting mask markedly raises the P_{O_2} in the maternal blood and hence, in part, in the umbilical vein as well. Discontinuation of inhalation produces not only a several minutes' decrease in the foetal blood oxygen level (= stress) below the initial level (Štembera 1956), but also an increase in the lactate level (Marx et al. 1964), within 4—5 minutes. The FHR is monitored both during and for 15 minutes after discontinuing oxygen inhalation. If placental function and the adaptability of the foetus to hypoxia are good, the FHR does not change when oxygen inhalation stops. The greater the intensity and the duration of bradycardia after discontinuing inhalation, the greater the danger to the foetus (Štembera 1956). This method, which can be used both before labour and during the first stage of labour, has been verified and confirmed in many institutions in other countries (Tosetti 1958, Reygaerts et al. 1960, Rendina et al. 1967).

Effect of short-term administration of oxytocin on FHR

The typical changes in the FHR after uterine contraction (Dip II) in hypoxic foetuses were also utilized for the dignosis of foetal risk during pregnancy. A few contractions (= stress) are induced by administering oxytocin to the woman, either in 6 i.v. doses of 0.005 µg at 1-min intervals (Hammacher 1966) or in the form of a 30-min i.v. drip, until contractions of 30 mm Hg intensity are attained (Pose et al. 1970). The resultant changes in the FHR are evaluated in the way described in the chapter on FHR monitoring. Simultaneous recording of uterine sensitivity to exogenous oxytocin (see the oxytocin test) and the recording of changes in the monitored FHR in relation to induced contraction (see chapter on evaluation of the monitored FHR) is not only a loading test of placental function or adaptability of the foetus to stress, but is also a test of the likelihood of success of induced labour.

Step test

Three minutes' walking up and down low steps by the pregnant woman (= stress), with simultaneous F-ECG recording to diagnose placental dysfunction (Hon et al. 1961), demonstrated marked changes in women with EPH-gestosis (toxaemia), diabetes, essential hypertension and protracted pregnancy. Similarly, if the FHR was monitored instead, the same exercise,

105

in some cases of high risk pregnancy, demonstrated typical changes in the FHR indicative of danger to the foetus (Štembera et al. 1967). If the step test was replaced by pedalling on an ergometer bicycle specially modified for

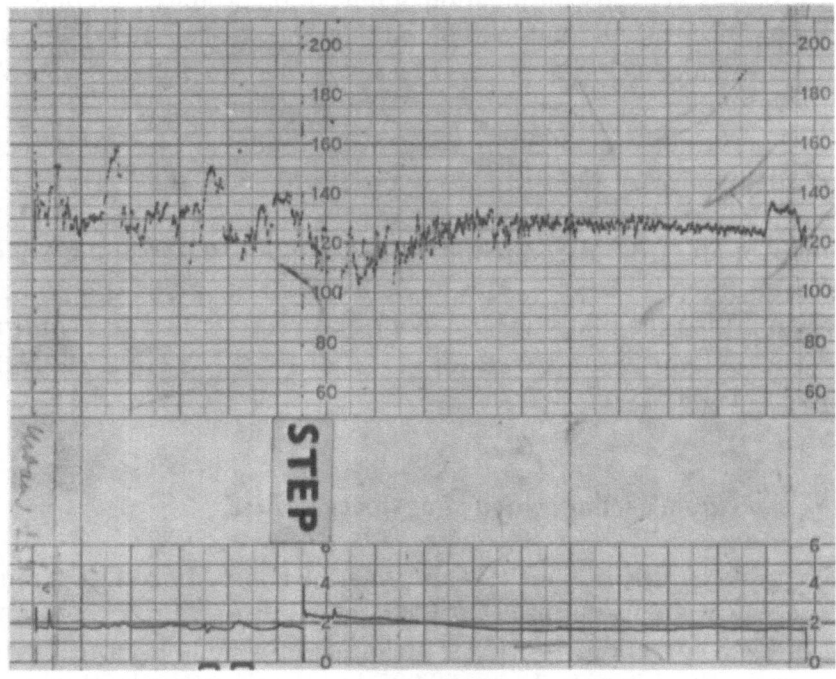

Fig. 10. Original cardiogram (absence of uterine contractions). FHR: in left half "type 3" (saltatory); in right half, after step-test, mild deceleration lasting 2 min, followed by "type 1" (narrowly undulating) lasting 5 min (Štembera, own material).

examining the pregnant woman in bed, with simultaneous recording of the FHR, it was found that the changes did not occur until towards the end of stress and that they persisted into the resting phase after stress (Štembera et al. 1967). The clinical diagnosis of foetal danger was therefore simplified by using FHR monitoring 10 min before and 10 min after a 3 minutes' step test of the pregnant woman on 2 steps, with a rhythm of 80 steps/min. Changes in baseline frequency, the type of oscillations or acceleration or deceleration are compared in the cardiographic recording (Fig. 10 and 11). Every one of these changes is evaluated by points, according to clinical experiences (perinatal mortality and a low Apgar score) acquired in several hundred cases (Štembera 1973). The sum of the points, corresponding to all the determined changes, represents the gravity of the danger to the foetus. The greater the number of points, the greater the probability that the foetus is endangered.

The reliability of the test is enhanced if it is repeated after an interval of 1–3 days. Persistence of a high points value of the test, or a progressive increase in the points value in repeated tests, means increased probability

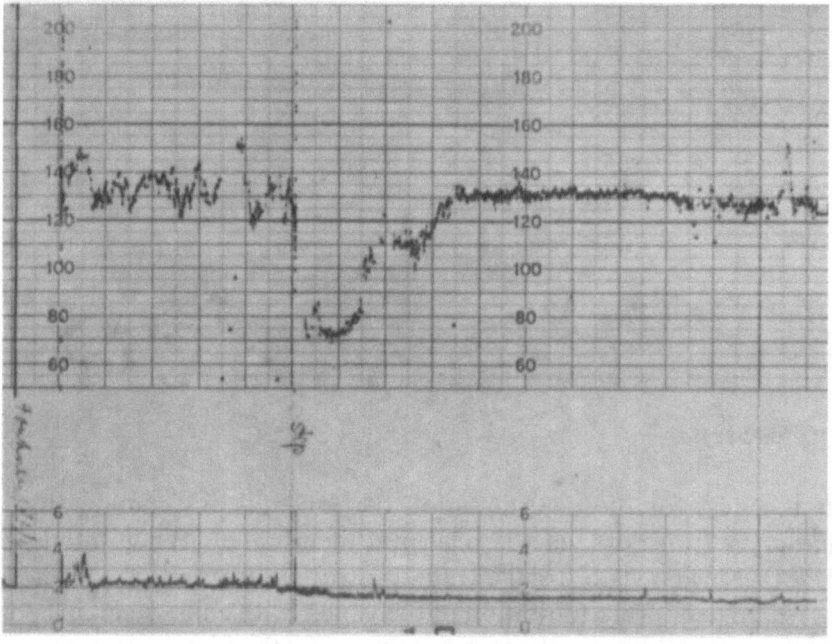

Fig. 11. Original cardiogram (absence of uterine contractions). FHR: in left half "type 3" (saltatory FHR); in right half, after step-test, pronounced deceleration lasting 2 min, followed by "type 0" (silence) lasting 5 min (Štembera, own material).

of danger to the foetus. Conversely, persistence of a low points value, or a decrease from a raised to a lower value and subsequent persistence at the low value, is evidence of normal development of the foetus, or of passing distress which does not endanger the foetus. The results of the step test correlate very well not only with the perinatal mortality rate or with postnatal depression of the newborn infant, but also with serious perinatal morbidity (Tab. 36).

The step test is indicated, from the 37th week, in high risk pregnancies in which placental dysfunction or impairment of the utero-foeto-placental circulation can be presumed.

Table 36. Relationship of different points values of step test in 208 foetuses on last days before birth to psychoneurological findings in the same children at 18 months (Štembera et al. 1973)

Step test points	Psychoneurological state of children at 18 months (number of children)			
	total	ICP	neurol. psychol. disorders	no signif. pathol. findings
≧ 14	6	2	4	0
10−13	12	0	3	9
4− 9	55	0	13	42
0− 3	135	0	3	132
Total	208	2	23	183

The atropine test

This is a test for the determination of placental dysfunction (impaired circulation or transport via the placental membrane). When administered to the mother in an i.v. dose of 0.01 mg/kg, atropine crosses the placenta to the foetus, where temporary inhibition of the vagus, with consequent preponderance of the sympathico-accelerator system, raises the foetal heart rate (FHR) by 10−35 beats/min (Soiva et al. 1959). The time needed for this reaction is given as 2−15 min. Its protraction or disappearance has been demonstrated in EPH gestosis (Hellmann et al. 1965) and other pathological states, as an expression of placental dysfunction. It can be employed during pregnancy. Reliable evaluation of the test requires basically objective recording of the FHR. With the elaboration of new diagnostic methods, the significance of the atropine test has diminished in recent years and it is gradually falling into disuse.

FOETAL ELECTROCARDIOGRAPHY

The first attempts at foetal electrocardiography (F-ECG) date back to 1906, but it was almost half a century before the findings could be utilized in practice.

F-ECG recording technique: Two types of recording techniques are used today: the external−indirect and the vaginal−direct technique, each of which is of value in somewhat different ways.

a) The external – indirect method is similar to the one for the adult ECG, except that four electrodes are placed on the mother's abdominal wall, the negative electrode on the lumbar region and the sixth (an earth) on the thigh (Bolte 1969). Bipolar conduction of all the electrodes against each other gives rise to 8 different leads. Since the amplitude of foetal heart potentials is very low, the use of an 8-channel, serially produced ECG apparatus with a sensitivity of 10 µv/1 cm recording width is recommended (Bolte 1969). Amplification of the potentials, on the other hand, is attended by disturbances caused by the muscle potentials of the mother's abdominal wall, the uterus and the foetal movements and by the mother's own ECG. The external method seldom detects P and T waves, but gives a good recording of the R wave. It can be employed during labour as well as during pregnancy.

b) The internal – vaginal method: The active electrode is placed on the foetus's head, the negative electrode on the mother's lumbar region and the earth on her thigh. The first vaginal electrode for attachment to the head of the foetus had the form of decompression suction discs, the size of which was gradually reduced until they could be introduced by means of an amnioscope. Hon's clip electrodes proved to be the most reliable, however, largely owing to the material from which they are made (silver – silver chloride; Hon 1967). The whole PQRST complex can be recorded by this method, but it cannot be used until the amniotic fluid has escaped and the cervix is sufficiently dilated.

Utilization and evaluation of the F-ECG: The uses of the F-ECG cover 3 diagnostic spheres:

a) Utilization of the R wave as a FHR monitor signal. Its advantage compared with phonocardiography is that the signal is not disturbed by background noises (see chapter on monitoring of the FHR).

b) The demonstration of a live foetus, its position and multiple pregnancy is more an auxiliary form of diagnostic utilization of the F-ECG. Breech presentation is determined from the direction of the main vector and its reliability, as in the diagnosis of twins, is small (about 80%). The diagnosis of a live foetus is highly reliable (98%) from the 37th week, but the examination must be carried out several times. At 33 – 36 weeks its diagnostic reliability is only 92%.

c) The third sphere is the diagnosis of foetal age, placental dysfunction and an endangered foetus.

Foetal age can be determined from the value of the R wave potential by the external method, since the height of the potential alters during pregnancy in accordance with given laws. The relationship is not linear, but displays two maxima. The first, at 25 – 26 weeks (25 µv), is followed by a drop, with the minimum at 29 – 30 weeks (11 µv), after which there is a gradual ascent up to the 37th week (20 µv), followed by an abrupt one up to the 40th week

(40 µv). The individual values vary within limits of $\pm$ 10%. The potential decrease at the beginning of the third trimester is due to the isolating effect of the vernix caseosa, which is formed during this period. A single examination is not very reliable, but 3 – 4 examinations over a period of 2 – 3 weeks detect potential changes and are thus more reliable. Even a single examination in the third trimester, showing a potential of over 20 µv, will exclude the possibility of an immature foetus, however (Bolte et al. 1966).

d) The fourth important sphere is the diagnosis of placental dysfunction in protracted pregnancy. Contamination of the amniotic fluid with meconium was found more frequently if the R wave potential was over 40 µv, while if it rose to 60 µv, signs of placental dysfunction also often appeared in the newborn infant (Bolte et al. 1966, Srp et al. 1970).

e) Danger to the foetus: The external method allows the electric axis of the foetus to be determined from the height of the amplitudes measured in the individual leads and danger to the foetus can be estimated from its deviation (Larks 1962). Excessive dextrodeviation is a sign that the right ventricle is overloaded owing to raised peripheral resistance in the foetoplacental bed (Srp et al. 1970).

f) Many studies have been carried out on changes in the foetal PQRST complex, because of the possibility of utilizing them to diagnose danger to the foetus. On correlation various changes in the monitored FHR or biochemical changes in the foetal blood with different F-ECG findings (Hon 1967, Pardi et al. 1971), it was found that:

if the FHR was normal, no changes were demonstrated in the F-ECG,

if bradycardia during contraction was present, but the biochemical findings in the foetal blood were normal, a biphasic P wave, or flattening of the P wave with shortening of the PQ interval, was demonstrated,

in foetal acidosis and myocardial hypoxia, the T wave was inverted or biphasic and the ST interval was shortened or prolonged.

A number of authors still – and quite rightly – warn against over-estimation of the importance of "pathological F-ECG complexes" when diagnosing danger to the foetus (Hradecký et al. 1964, Srp et al. 1970, Heinrich 1970). Another drewback is the impossibility of evaluating F-ECG complexes over a long period of time (in 1 hour we obtain 9,000) without having to resort to specifically programmed automatic computers (Hon 1967).

110

DETERMINATION OF FOETAL BLOOD pH FROM SKIN OF FOETUS'S HEAD

Since this method was first evolved (Saling 1961), it has spread rapidly all over the world, as seen from the dozens of studies commending it. It is based on the finding that, if the foetus is endangered, acidosis of the foetal blood usually increases, owing to the accumulation of acid metabolites in the foetal organism. It cannot be used until the amniotic fluid has escaped and the cervix is sufficiently dilated to admit a wide amnioscope. The foetal blood pH determined from skin on the foetus's head is intermediate to the pH in the blood in the umbilical vein and artery. Since the method itself is familiar from a host of publications, we think that it is more to the point to mention the most important sources of the errors which can occur on using this method (Kubli 1966, Brescher 1969).

Before making the microincision, hyperaemia of the skin of the head must be properly induced (differences of up to 0.07 pH).

The microincision must be made outside the area of the fontanelles, with a special lancet ensuring a maximum incision depth of 2 mm.

The blood must always be collected at the peak of a contraction (between contractions, or at the end of a contraction, the foetal blood pH is inconstant).

The blood should be collected into a glass capillary (in PVC capillaries the P_{CO_2} quickly falls, the P_{O_2} increases and the pH consequently rises).

The drop of blood should be aspirated within $2-3$ s (later, the P_{CO_2} falls and the P_{O_2} increases).

When examining the actual pH, the blood should be aspirated into the capillary without air bubbles.

Collection into 2 capillaries is preferable, as it reduces the possibility of error.

The blood should be examined within not more than 10 min after collection.

In work with an Astrup pH-meter, the potentiometer should be calibrated every 12 hours.

The actual tests (of the pH) can be done by the doctor on duty, but the error is greater than if they are done by a skilled laboratory assistant, and the apparatus is also more likely to be damaged (Bretscher 1969). If the above rules are observed, in clinical practice the error can be reduced to 0.05 pH.

In the foetal blood we can examine the **actual pH,** a decrease in which is evidence of acute acidosis (usually respiratory and metabolic combined), and the **equilibrated pH,** which corresponds to a constant P_{CO_2} of 40 mm Hg and is a reliable index of metabolic acidosis produced by an increase in the proportion of anaerobic metabolism. Other indexes of foetal acid-base balance (BE and StB) can also be calculated from this result.

Since the foetal blood pH falls during labour (especially in the second stage), all data on physiological or critical pH values must be expressed in relation to the given chronological phase of labour (Tab. 37).

Table 37. Mean physiological foetal blood pH values during labour (Fischer 1965, Saling 1966, Kubli 1966, Wulf 1967, Berg et al. 1970)

	Stage I (dilatation in cm)			Stage II	
	0 – 2 cm	3 – 5 cm	6 – 8 cm	beginning	end
pH max.	7.39	7.38	7.36	7.34	7.32
pH min.	7.29	7.27	7.26	7.25	7.21

The determination of borderline (critical) values is based on the percentual incidence of intranatal deaths and postnatal depression of the newborn infant (Tab. 38, Fig. 12).

Table 38. Correlation of foetal blood pH during first stage of labour to postnatal depression of infant and intranatal mortality (Wood 1968)

pH in stage I	Apgar score of 1 to 3
7.2	12% of cases
7.1 – 7.2	41% of cases
7.1	16 intranatal deaths per mille

The above analyses indicate that borderline foetal blood pH values determined in this way are too low, because the percentage of infants with postnatal depression is too high. Saling (1968) therefore raised the critical borderline values, although by so doing he also raised the percentage of wrongly positive results (see Fig. 12). He recommended:

at pH 7.25 taking further samples every 30 min,
at pH 7.2 terminating labour by Caesarian section, and
at pH 7 he regarded the foetus as lost.

While we admit that every evaluation of different methods by the above criteria has its errors, the given analyses indicate that the reliability of this method is good (about 82%).

The proportion of complications on using this method is less than 1%. One of the most serious is haemorrhage from the foetus's head after microin-

112

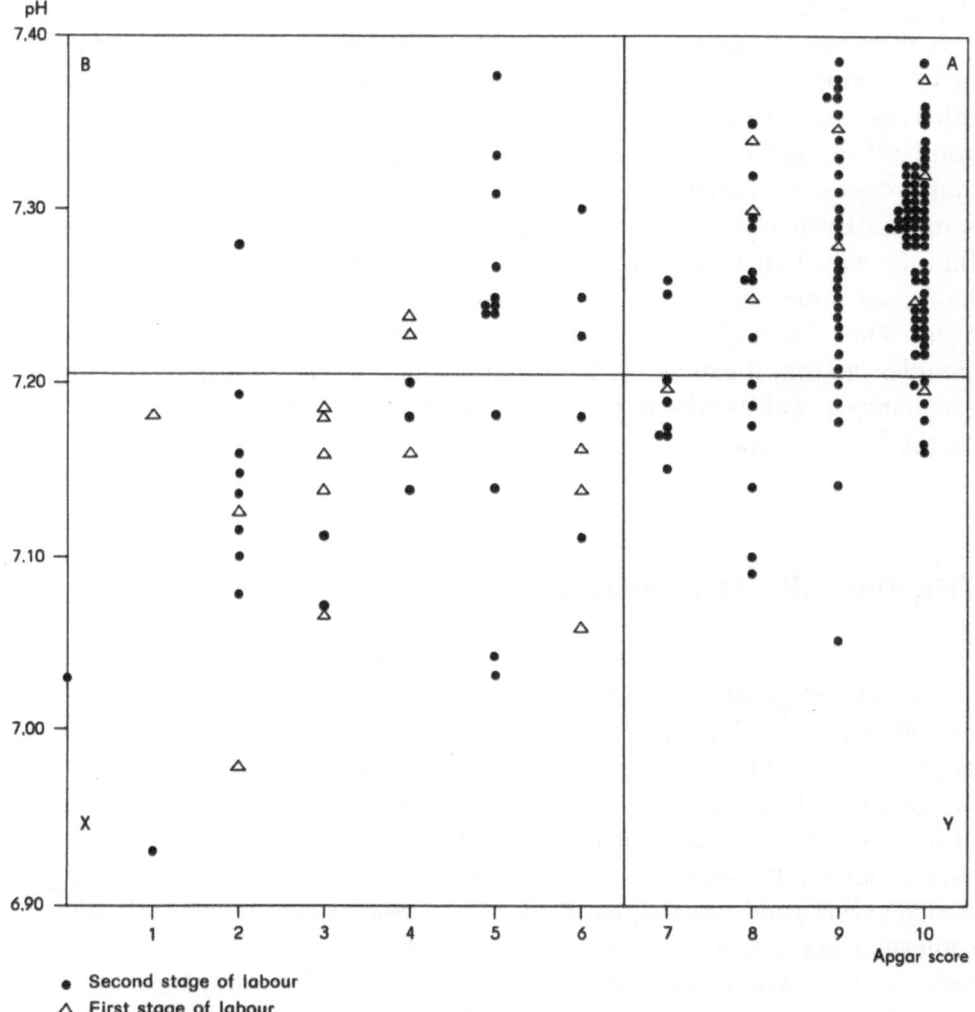

Fig. 12. Correlation of postpartal depression (<7 Apgar points) to foetal acidosis (pH ≤ 7.2 in foetal blood obtained by microsampling). Cases in square B wrongly negative, in square Y wrongly positive.

cision. Beard (1968) described two fatal cases and several others of severe haemorrhage in which the infant was saved by a transfusion immediately after birth. After collecting microsamples, therefore, any haemorrhage from the vagina, however slight, must be checked very carefully. One must also remain on the alert during the first hours after birth, since hypoxia-induced vasoconstriction, which occurs during labour, can afterwards be followed by haemorrhage from the microincision site.

An infection of the mother is a contraindication for the collection of micro-

113

samples. The vacuum extractor should not be used after microincision, since it increases the danger of haemorrhage and abscess formation.

It is wrong to set methods determining danger to the foetus by means of FHR monitoring and determination of the foetal blood pH against each other, as is sometimes the case. The two methods are complementary and not competitive, although the progressive development of foetal cardiography is narrowing the range of indications for the testing of foetal blood micro-samples. Even today, however, there are still some foetal cardiographic findings which are obscure and hard to interpret, and in these cases the foetal blood pH value can help to make the diagnosis of the state of the foetus more exact. The advantages of FHR monitoring over the testing of blood micro-samples are that it can be used before the amniotic fluid escapes, i.e. during pregnancy as well as labour, and that it provides a steady flow of information on the foetus's condition.

THE URINARY OESTRIOL LEVEL

The advantage of this method, whose possibilities were already pointed out 30 years ago (Koller 1941) is that it determines the intensity not only of placental function, as originally supposed by Diczfalusy et al. (1961), but of the whole foetoplacental unit, since foetal metabolism also participates in the production of the oestriol excreted in the mother's urine. Among the various known methods, the ones most commonly used in Europe today are Ittrich's (1960) and, less frequently, Brown's (1968). Both of these methods are somewhat exacting as regards apparatus, however, and are time consuming (working time in the laboratory, collection of 24-hour urine samples). Attempts have therefore been made to simplify them, either by examining only the morning urine, or by semi-quantitative determination − in both cases at the expense of accuracy, however. Since different authors use different methods and these are often further modified according to the conditions in each laboratory, it is very difficult indeed to fix a uniform ciritical limit indicative of danger to the foetus. The values given as normal towards the end of pregnancy cover a very wide range (12 − 50 mg/24 hours) and the lower limit of normal values also varies. Some authors put it at 15 − 20 mg/24 hours, while others put the critical limit at under 10 mg/24 hours or even at 5 mg/24 hours. Some claim that this limit represents only impairment of placental function and is not a sign that the foetus is in immediate danger; others, on the other hand, demonstrated oestriol levels above this limit in the presence of a dead foetus. All authors are agreed that the reliability of the method is increased by the repeated finding of low values or by the finding of an abrupt drop. Although we examine the oestriol concentration every day, this drop is sometimes hard to distinguish from pronounced diurnal fluctuation, which may attain, in the same woman, as much as 50% of the mean excretion value.

The cases most suitable for the diagnosis of foetal risk by means of oestriol are pathological states which impair the metabolism of the placenta or the placental circulation (toxaemia, a small-for-dates foetus, protracted pregnancy); cases in which the primary cause of the disturbances is not associated with placental dysfunction (Rh isoimmunization, diabetes) are less suitable. The authors sometimes used perinatal mortality or a low Apgar score as the criterion of the reliability of the method, sometimes only signs indicative of danger to the foetus. A few significant, but so far isolated, reports describe a close association between a low oestriol level during pregnancy and an incidence of mental retardation or neurological damage in later life (i.e. in the children) (Wallace et al. 1966), or even an association with a low IQ in these children at the age of 5 – 7 years (Coyle et al. 1970.)

Despite all the above difficulties and any discrepancies in the findings, there are still quite a number of authors who regard determination of the oestriol level in the woman's urine as a very good method for determining placental insufficiency, because the repeated finding of high values is evidence, in over 90% of the cases, of physiological development of the foetus, while low or falling values spell danger to the foetus in 50%.

The urinary oestriol level after DHEA-S

This method is based on the finding that the precursor of oestriol is dehydroepiandrosterone sulphate (DHEA-S), 20% of which comes from the mother and 80% from the foetus. Foetoplacental unit function was originally evaluated from the increase in the 24-hour oestriol level following the i.v. administration of DHEA-S to the mother (Lauritzen 1967), Dässler (1967) achieved the same effect by giving the mother ACTH; this stimulated DHEA-S production and thus raised oestriol synthesis. The determination of raised oestriol production after the administration of 30 mg DHEA-S was later supplemented by determination of the time needed for the foetoplacental unit to metabolize exogenous DHEA-S to oestriol (determined in four 2-hour samples after the administration of DHEA-S). The attainment of an excretion peak 2 or 4 hours after administration is evidence of very good function and at 6 – 8 hours of depressed function, while no increase is a sign of poor function of the foetoplacental unit (Kaiser 1970, V. der Craben 1969). In this way the proportion of wrongly positive results was reduced to 24% and of wrongly negative results to 3% of all the cases investigated. In a further elaboration of this method, we evaluate the mean initial value (from two 2-hour urine samples prior to administering DHEA-S), the time of peak elimination, the height of the peak in relation to the initial value and the total increase in the amount recovered in four 2-hour samples after the administration of DHEA-S in relation to the initial level, expressing all four data in the form of a points evaluation system (Tab. 39). A total of over 15 points means that the foetus is healthy; 7 points or less is a sign that the foetus is in grave danger. This modification greatly improves the accuracy of the method (Štembera 1973).

Table 39. Scoring system for each of the four parameters of the DHEA-S test

Parameters	Points												
	0	1	2	3	4	6	8	10	12	14	16	18	20
Initial oestriol value (mg) (+20%)	<0.5	0.5 −0.9	1 −1.4	1.5 −1.9	2 −2.4	2.5 −2.9	3 −3.4	3.5 −3.9	4 −4.4	4.5 −4.9	5 −5.4	5.5 −5.9	6 −6.4
Time of peak oestriol elimination (hours)	0	8	6	4	2								
Height of peak (mg)	0	0.1 −0.4	0.5 −0.9	1 −1.4	1.5 −1.9	2 −2.4	2.5 −2.9	3 −3.4	3.5 −3.9	4 −4.4	4.5 −4.9	5 −5.4	5.5 −5.9
Total oestriol recovery (mg)	0	0.1 −0.4	0.5 −0.9	1 −1.4	1.5 −1.9	2 −2.4	2.5 −2.9	3 −3.4	3.5 −3.9	4 −4.4	4.5 −4.9	5 −5.4	5.5 −5.9

In concluding this evaluation, it can be claimed that determination of the urinary oestriol level is a good method for screening foetoplacental unit function, in which the repeated finding of values of over 20 mg/24 hours confirms, with a high degree of probability, that the foetus is developing physiologically. If the value is lower, or if an abrupt drop occurs (even with high values), tests of the oestriol level after administering DHEA-S to the mother will yield more exact information.

For the determination of oestriol in the amniotic fluid, see the chapter on examination of the amniotic fluid.

The urinary pregnanediol level

Since only the placenta, and not the foetus, participates in pregnanediol production, its determination in the urine is a less reliable test of foetal risk than the determination of oestriol, so that today it has only a few supporters.

VAGINAL CYTOLOGY IN THE THIRD TRIMESTER

This diagnostic method covers two wide spheres:

(1) Determination of the **biological readiness** of the organism for labour. In this respect, vaginal cytology is today accepted as a reliable diagnostic method for determining term.

The first authors to mention the possibilities of vaginal cytology for determining term were Lemberg and Stamm (1954). Židovský (1955) demonstrated the dynamics of changes in the vaginal cytology picture towards the end of a normal pregnancy. He distinguished 4 diagnostic cytotypes, I – IV (Fig. 13a–d), and demonstrated their time limit in correlation to the onset of spontaneous labour.

(2) Determination of **placental dysfunction** or **foetal risk** in protracted pregnancy. Two concepts exist in this indication sphere:

a) A specific concept (Ezes 1954), in accordance with which diagnostic, pathognomonic conclusions are drawn on pathological protraction of pregnancy, with a risk to the foetus, from spceifie, "postpartum" findings in the cytogram, which is characterized by the presence of a large number of parabasal-postpartum cells.

b) A dynamic concept (Židovský 1957), in accordance with which diagnostic conclusions are drawn from a dynamic study of a series of vaginal smears and from their evaluation according to the four cytotypes mentioned above. Persistence of the "term" cytotypes III and IV for more than 6 and 3 days respectively is evidence of placental dysfunction or of danger to the foetus.

Today, most authors everywhere incline to the dynamic concept, although some are in favour of synthesis of the two concepts. Although originally a supporter of the specific concept, J. P. Pundel (1966), the well-known cytologist, wrote in his latest monograph:

"(1) A vaginal smear of the "pre-term" type (I and II) allows injury to the foetus caused by protraction of pregnancy to be excluded unreservedly, so that it is possible to wait until the smear is of the "term" type.

(2) A "term" type of smear (III and IV) means that labour should start within the next five days. If this interval is exceeded, experience shows that the pregnancy is genuinely protracted in over 90% of the cases, especially if the oestrogen test is positive. The danger of injury to the foetus increases with prolongation of this interval beyond the 5-day limit, even without a change to a regressive type (parabasal cells).

(3) If the smear (term) changes to a regressive type, it is a sign that the foetus is in danger, even though the clinical picture may still be normal.

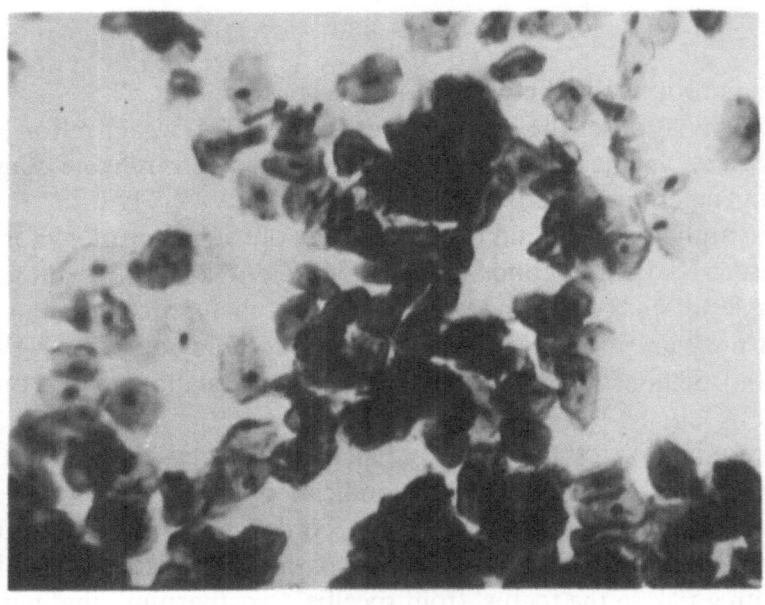

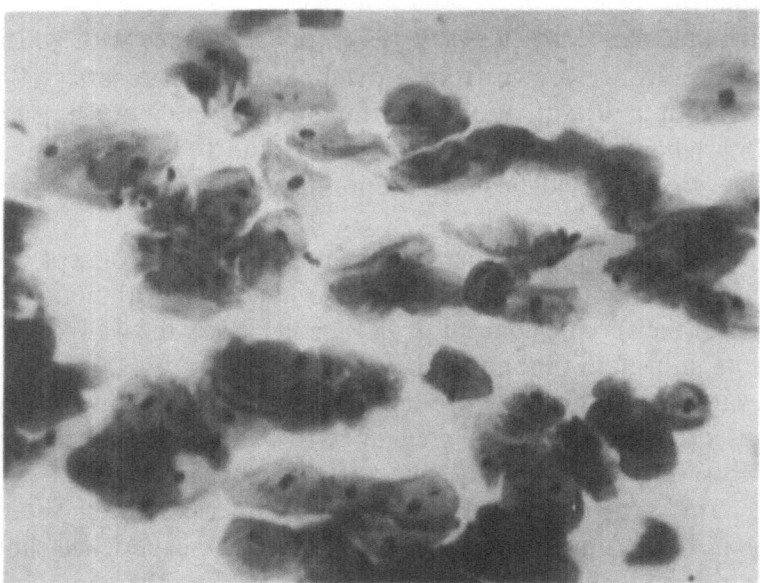

Fig. 13a. Cytotype I — "advanced pregnancy". Predominance of navicular cells in typical clusters. Ratio of navicular to intermediary cells 3 : 1. Practically no superficial cells. Leucocytes and mucus absent. All cells in smear intensely cyanophilic (Židovský).

Fig. 13b. Cytotype II — "shortly before term". Ratio of navicular to intermediary cells 1 : 1. Small number of leucocytes sometimes present, mucus absent. Slight intensely cyanophilic (Židovský).

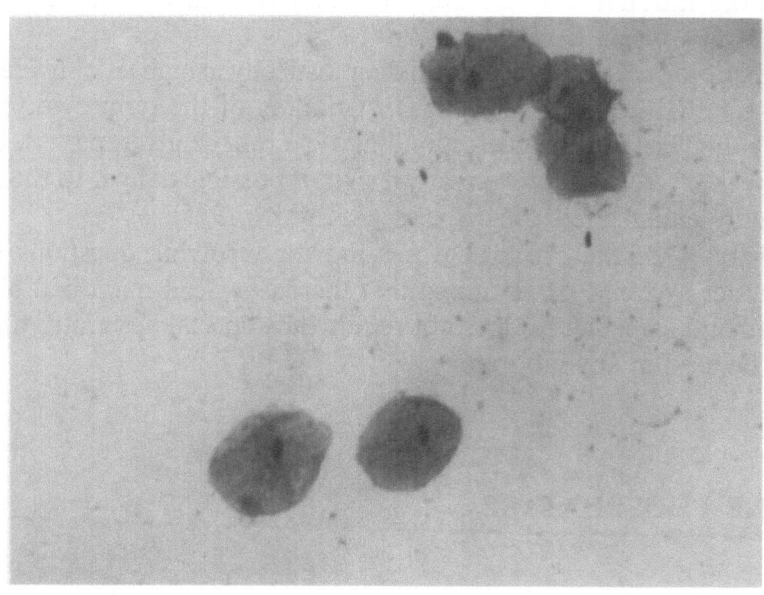

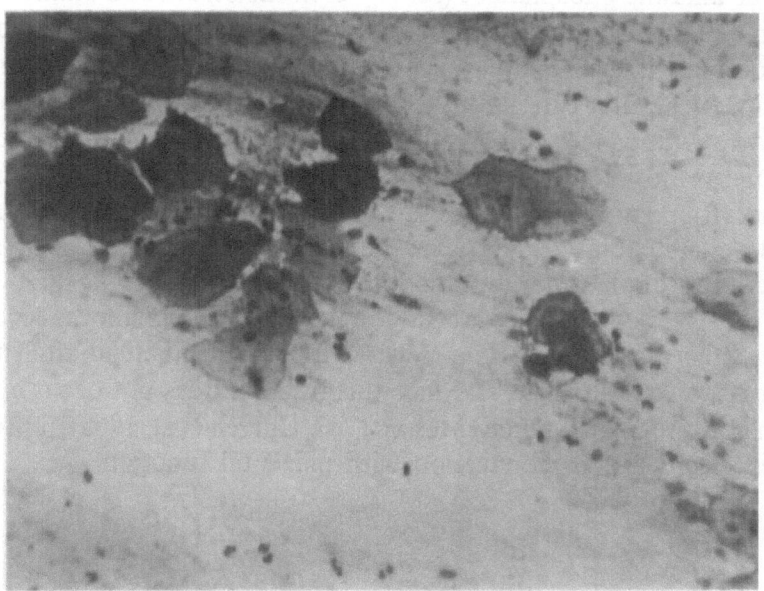

Fig. 13c. Cytotype III — "term". Predominance of intermediary cells (60 – 80 %) and increase in number of superficial cells. Navicular cells reduced to 5 – 10%; disappearance of typical clusters, cells separate, isolated. Some cells (about 10%) eosinophilic (Židovský).

Fig. 13d. Cytotype IV — "explicitly term". Navicular cells entirely absent, marked predominance of superficial cells (50 – 80%), often eosinophilic. Cytoplasm stained less intensively. Maximum separation of cells. Mucus and large quantities of leucocytes sometimes appear. Pyknotic nuclei predominate (Židovský).

119

It is therefore rational to terminate pregnancy if, clinically, it has reached term."

Vaginal cytology can also be utilized diagnostically in high risk pregnancies, especially in EPH gestoses (toxaemia). A finding of the term cytotypes III and IV, i.e. higher than the corresponding type for the given period, before the 36th week of pregnancy, is already a sign of possible danger to the foetus in potentially endangered pregnancies (Židovský 1975).

The reliability of the cytological method for resolving questions in the third trimester is over 80% assuming that there is a clean microbial picture. Its great advantage is that it does not require any special apparatus and can therefore be used in any laboratory.

ALKALINE PHOSPHATASE

Since the alkaline phosphatase (AP) level in the serum and amniotic fluid rises during pregnancy, the origin of the increase is ascribed to the placenta, so that a decrease in the AP level suggests a diagnosis of placental dysfunction. The physiological values given for the serum AP level towards the end of pregnancy have a wide range: $10-24$ King-Armstrong units or $4-12$ Bodansky units. Some authors confirmed that the AP level fell in placental dysfunction, while others found no such drop. Compared with determination of the urinary oestriol level, the total AP level in pregnancy serum is described as less reliable as a test of placental dysfunction.

About $60-70\%$ of the raised AP value at the end of pregnancy is accounted for by the "thermostable fraction", the value of which is read after heating 30 min in a water bath at 56°C. Since this fraction does not occur either in men or in non-pregnant women (Messer 1967, Curzen et al. 1968), it probably originates specifically in connection with placental function.

HUMAN PLACENTAL LACTOGEN (HPL)

Human placental lactogen (HPL), more recently designated as human chorionic somatomammotrophin (HCS), which was isolated from human placenta in 1962 (Josimovich and MacLaren), is formed entirely of syncytio-trophoblast. Its level in pregnancy serum rises from the 5th month of pregnancy and attains its maximum at 36 weeks. Its absolute value in µg/ml varies with the method (whether purely immunological or radioimmune assay) and also with the individual (from case to case). Low values (< 4 µg/ml from the 35th to 40th week) or rapidly falling values in the third trimester are evidence of placental dysfunction, but not of a disturbance affecting the whole foetoplacental unit, since the foetus does not participate in HPL (as distinct from oestriol) metabolism (Sciara 1963, Spellacy et al. 1966, Lindberg et al. 1972, etc). As with oestriol, the diagnostic value of the determination of only a single HPL value is far smaller than repeated determination of the HPL level (Chard 1973 – Tab. 40).

Table 40. Percentual risk of foetal distress and/or neonatal asphyxia in 225 clinically normal pregnancies in which HPL levels were estimated between the 35th and 45th week

	<4 µg/ml	$4-5$ µg/ml	>5 µg/ml
Number of patients in whom 1 or more HPL estimates fell into 1 group	30%	13%	8%
Number of patients with 2 or more corresponding serial HPL estimates	50%	13%	6%
Number of patients with 3 or more corresponding serial HPL estimates	71%	12%	4%

The two methods supplement each other very well, so that a simultaneous low oestriol and HPL level increase the probability of danger to the foetus, while high values mean greater probability of normal development. The advantage of HPL over oestriol assay is that there is no 24-hour urine collection and that the results can be obtained 90 minutes after taking the blood sample.

AMNIOSCOPY

The dozens of studies published every year in the international literature since this method was first discovered (Saling 1962) and the thousands of sets of results of amnioscopic examination are evidence of the great contribution this method has made to perinatological practice. The well known clinical significance of contamination of the amniotic fluid with meconium for perinatal mortality has in recent years likewise been demonstrated, in large series, for postnatal depression of the newborn infant (Tab. 41).

Table 41. Raised incidence of low Apgar score in association with contamination of amniotic fluid with meconium before onset of labour (Kubli 1969)

| Amniotic fluid | n | Number of cases (%) | | | Perinatal mortality | |
| | | Apgar score after 1 min | | | | |
		0 − 3	4 − 6	7 − 10	absol.	per mille
Clear	1,153	1.2	2.8	96.0	5	4
Turbid	163	6.1	6.8	87.1	10	61

The chief merit of this method is that contamination of the amniotic fluid with meconium can be determined before labour begins. Its incidence varies (from 6 to 20%), according to the proportion of high risk pregnancies in the given series. In addition to regular amnioscopic examination of high risk pregnancies on the last days before labour, it is therefore equally important to carry out introductory amnioscopy, i.e. at the outset of labour after admission to the labour ward, or if uterine activity is slow in commencing, when contamination of the amniotic fluid rises to 21.5% of all cases (Browne 1969). Another advantage of amnioscopy is the possibility of easy rupture of the amniotic sac when inducing labour in diabetic primiparas, which must often be done before term, when the cervix is still frequently long and narrow.

There is no need to describe how to perform amnioscopy, seeing that its use has now spread to most of the institutions concerned. The disadvantages of this method are minimal (artificial rupture of the sac in 1 − 3% of the cases, impossibility of using it after the 36th week of pregnancy because of an occluded cervix in 3%). Any increase in subfebrility in the postpartum period (Teramo 1969) can be prevented by strict asepsis. The reliability of a finding of meconium-contaminated amniotic fluid is high. The proportion of false positive findings is about 5% (Kubli 1966), while with a little experience false negative determination is virtually impossible. The remarks of those authors who do not agree with the inclusion of amnioscopy among preventive diagnostic methods are undoubtedly justified, because the presence of meconium in the amniotic fluid is already a sign of a given degree of hypoxia (even if only temporary). An analysis of 176 cases with a positive amnioscopic finding prior to the onset of labour, in which the foetal blood pH was also tested, shows that the incidence of serious acidosis in these cases is very low, however:

pH 7.15 – 7.19 in 1.7% of cases of positive amnioscopy,
pH 7.2 – 7.24 in 6.8% of cases of positive amnioscopy.

It can thus be concluded that although amnioscopy is not a preventive method, it is a valuable way of diagnosing danger to the foetus if carried out in high risk pregnancies in the last days before labour.

AMNIOCENTESIS

This method was originally employed only in isolated cases, in the last trimester:

a) to obtain amniotic fluid samples for special tests in cases of Rh isoimmunization (Hofbauer 1956, Liley 1961, etc). With the steady increase in the range of amniotic fluid tests providing information on the state of the foetus (see the chapter on examination of the amniotic fluid), this method is acquiring an increasingly wider range of uses;

b) for exact recording of intraamniotic pressure during labour. This indication is practically unrecognized in Europe and is used by only a few institutions;

c) to collect amniotic fluid in the second trimester for an early diagnosis of congenital malformations, in connection with specific genetic examination (see the chapters on congenital anomalies and examination of the amniotic fluid). Although amniocentesis can already be performed in the 10th week of pregnancy in these cases, the optimal time is considered to be the 14th week, when the uterus already contains about 150 ml amniotic fluid. This indication is finding recognition in an increasing number of specialized institutions.

Main principles in the performace on amniocentesis: The operation is performed after objective localization of the placenta, under strict conditions of surgical asepsis and using local anaesthesia. The urinary bladder must first be emptied. If amniocentesis is carried out before the 37th week of pregnancy, substances inhibiting uterine contraction should be administered. The amniotic fluid is collected slowly, at a rate of about 7 ml/min, so as not to induce contractions.

If the above principles are strictly observed, the complications of amniocentesis are small. The most serious include injury to the mother's organs (bladder, intestine), peritonitis caused by introduction of an infection, the induction of premature contractions, the tranfer of foetal blood cells to the mother's blood stream, injury to the foetus (pneumothorax), exsanguination of the foetus caused by puncture of a large placental blood vessel. The indications for amniocentesis must therefore be defined very exactly (as the technique is improved it will be possible to extend them) and its performance must be confined to specialized institutions. Further workers should be trained in institutions which have already acquired some experience with this operation.

Diagnosis of an escape of amniotic fluid

The method described by Kittrich and Pospíšil (1956) for determining an escape of amniotic fluid is quick, simple and easy to evaluate, even for an inexperienced worker. A native vaginal smear is stained, without pre-fixing or drying, with aqueous 0.5% Nile blue sulphate solution. It is then covered with a cover-slip and, without further treatment, is evaluated immediately in a microscope. The presence of orange-stained non-nucleated cells or drops of vernix contrasting with the other blue-stained cellular elements is highly accurate evidence of an escape of amniotic fluid from the 32nd week of pregnancy. The reliability and advantages of this method have also been confirmed by other workers.

EXAMINATION OF THE AMNIOTIC FLUID

Bilirubin in the amniotic fluid

Spectrophotometric determination of the bilirubin concentration in the amniotic fluid (Liley 1961) is still one of the most reliable ways of diagnosing danger to the foetus from haemolytic disease. Optic density determined on a spectrophotometer in a 1-ml cuvette at 10 mμ intervals is expressed in extinction figures on a scale from 0 to 2 (the logarithms of absorbance values from 100% to 0%). The result is plotted on semilogarithmic paper. The points obtained at 365 and 550 mμ are joined by a straight line (slope) and over 450 mμ the difference between this slope and the actual curve is read on the ordinate (Fig. 14). The resultant figure is applied to a Liley empirical nomogram, with reference to the week of pregnancy (Fig. 15). The degree of danger to the foetus is evaluated from the zone of the nomogram into which the resultant value fits. The bottom zone is evidence of an intact foetus (the test

Fig. 14. Semilogarithmic paper. Abscissa: wavelengths in millimicrons. Ordinate: extinction values read on logarithmic scale of spectrophotometer. Bold curve: actual extinction values measured. Maximum above 450 mµ wavelength denotes presence of bilirubin in amniotic fluid.

Thin curve: course of extinction curve if amniotic fluid did not contain bilirubin. Difference between basal curve and actual curve measured at 450 mµ shown on ordinate. Difference read on Liley nomogram (see Fig. 9).

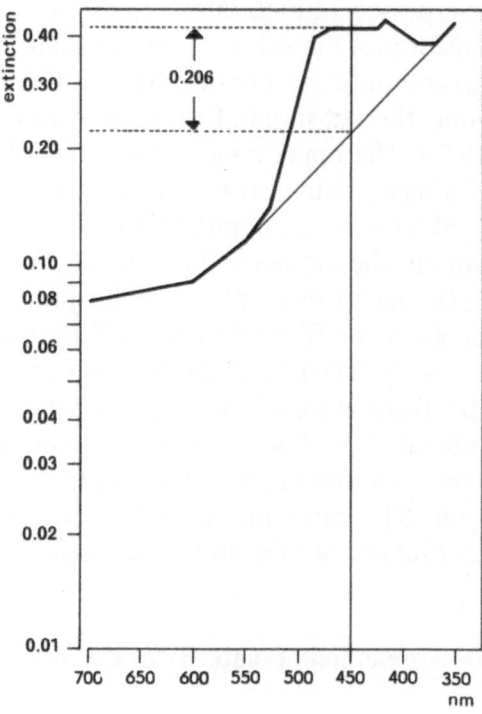

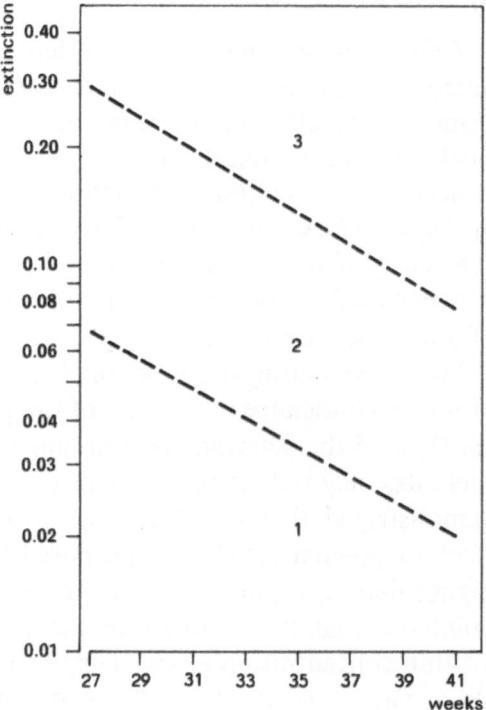

Fig. 15. Liley nomogram. Abscissa: weeks of pregnancy. Ordinate: extinction differences obtained by technique described in Fig. 14. Size of extinction difference (height of maximum on curve) evaluated with reference to week of pregnancy.

125

is repeated 14 days later). In the middle (intermediate) zone, the nearer the position of the value to the line dividing the middle and the upper zone, the greater the danger to the foetus. If the value lies in the lower half of the middle zone, the test should be repeated after 7 days (Schönfeld 1968, Poláček et al. 1970). The upper zone is indicative of acute danger to the foetus, or that it is already damaged by haemolytic disease.

Most important pitfalls in carrying out and evaluation: The tube containing the amniotic fluid should be wrapped immediately in black paper, as the yellow pigments are highly photo-labile. Before testing, the fluid should be spun, or filtered through Whatman filter paper, to remove any milky turbidity. The admixture of blood or meconium produces further maxima on the absorbance curve. A possibility of error also arises if term is wrongly estimated, so that the resultant values are wrongly plotted in the nomogram. Some authors improve the accuracy of the diagnosis of danger to the foetus from Rh isoimmunization by additionally determining proteins (Cherry et al. 1966) or oestriol in the amniotic fluid.

Determination of maturity of the foetus by analysis of the amniotic fluid

a) *Biochemical parameters*

Among the various tests for different substances or indicators of gas and energy metabolism (glucose, lactic acid, pyruvic acid, Po_2, Pco_2, BE, pH, osmolarity) in the amniotic fluid, the only one which has so far proved of practical value in perinatological diagnostics is determination of the creatinine concentration as a test of the maturity of the foetus (Woyton 1963, Pitkin et al. 1967). The creatinine level in the amniotic fluid rises during pregnancy (probably in association with foetal renal function) and after the 36th week it attains values of 1.8 to 2 mg%. Such a concentration is clear evidence of a mature foetus.

When evaluating the functional maturity of the foetus's lungs (which is of great significance in the case of imminent premature labour), Gluck et al. (1971) used the determination of phospholipids in the amniotic fluid (as surfactants, they reduce surface tension in the alveoli of the foetal lungs). He demonstrated that they suddenly rose (especially lecithin) from the 36th week of pregnancy. If their proposed lecithin/sphingomyelin (L/S) index is higher than 2, it indicates that the foetus's lungs are mature. Some authors point out that the maturity of the lung tissue can be estimated from the lecithin concentration alone. They consider 3.5 mg% to be the critical value (Bhagwanani et al. 1972). Clements et al. (1972) suggested a very simple

126

"foam test" for the determination of surfactants in the amniotic fluid. Its principle is the formation of persistent bubbles in tubes containing amniotic fluid in various dilutions, after shaking with ethanol. If foam is formed in all the first three tubes (i.e. up to at least 1 : 2 dilution), the test is positive, i.e. the foetus's lungs are mature. Foam in the first tube only testifies to their immaturity. The only special laboratory equipment required for this test is a shaker apparatus. The test is of very great orientative value.

b) *Cytology of the amniotic fluid*

The last weeks of pregnancy are characterized by an increase, in the amniotic fluid, of the number of cells stained orange by Nile blue sulphate (Kittrich et al. 1956). Brosens et al. (1966) utilized this to evolve a method determining the degree of maturity of the foetus:

$1-10\%$ orange cells = 34th to 37th week of pregnancy
$10-50\%$ orange cells = 38th to 40th week of pregnancy
$\geq 50\%$ orange cells = 40th week of pregnancy.

Some authors later pointed out that fewer than 10% orange-stained cells were sometimes found in the presence of a mature foetus (Chan et al. 1969) − a finding which somewhat detracts from the reliability of the method. Kittrich (1972) therefore suggested doing the cytological test first when determining the maturity of the foetus: if there are more than 10% orange-stained cells, the foetus can reliably be regarded as mature, if there are fewer than 10%, the diagnosis should be made more exact by testing the creatinine concentration in the amniotic fluid. Brosens and Gordon (1966) arrived at the same conclusion.

Cultivation of cellular elements from the amniotic fluid

After the 14th week of pregnancy, living foetal cells can be isolated from the $10-20$ ml amniotic fluid collected by amniocentesis and if these are then cultivated $2-5$ weeks, foetal chromosomes can be isolated. The resultant karyotypes allow the early diagnosis of certain developmental anomalies (see the chapter on developmental anomalies). In the same way, antenatal determination of the sex of the foetus is possible in cases in which the parents have a recessively sex-linked disease. This is a very exacting method, as regards both the correct collection technique and the cultivation technique, but the international literature shows that it is finding increasing application.

Oestriol in the amniotic fluid

The oestriol level in the amniotic fluid has recently come to be regarded as an even more exact criterion of foetoplacental dysfunction than the oestriol level in the mother's urine. The bottom critical limit concentration is said to be 100 µg/l, irrespective of the amount of amniotic fluid (Greene et al. 1965). Furthermore, although the diagnosis of danger to the foetus in Rh sensitization and diabetes by means of the urinary oestriol level is not very reliable, the determination of oestriol in the amniotic fluid is regarded as reliable from the 37th week of pregnancy.

LOCALIZATION OF THE PLACENTA

Objective localization of the placenta is carried out today for two main indications: a) before performing amniocentesis, b) in haemorrhage during the second and third trimester, after first stopping the haemorrhage, to exclude placenta praevia. X-ray examination has been replaced by other methods which are more reliable and which expose both the woman and the foetus to substantially smaller radiation doses.

Isotope placentography

The mother is injected i.v. with a labelled substance with a short half-life. Detection of the tracer 10 minutes later shows its accumulation in the placenta, which is a relatively large reservoir of maternal blood. The woman is examined in the supine position or lying on her side (for detection of a placenta localized on the dorsal wall of the uterus). Radiation is detected either by measuring activity at given points over the various parts of the abdominal wall, or scintigraphically, when the gamma-graph explorer meanders over the abdominal region and, row for row, progressively records the distribution of the radioactive substance. ^{24}Na and ^{131}I, which were used to label apyrogenic human serum albumin, were originally employed, but these were replaced by the more satisfactory short-lived isotope 99m-technetium. On administering 1 mc technetium, the whole body dose for mother and foetus is about 15 mrad, i.e. 100—300 times smaller than an X-ray radiation dose. 113 m-indium is even more satisfactory than technetium, because the preparation of the injection dose is less laborious, because it is readily available and because its activity over the urinary bladder does not interfere with the activity of a possible placenta praevia. Isotope placentography is almost 100% reliable.

Ultrasound detection of the placenta

This method is based on the principle of the Doppler effect, i.e. on the rebound of waves from a moving object (in the case of the placenta from the

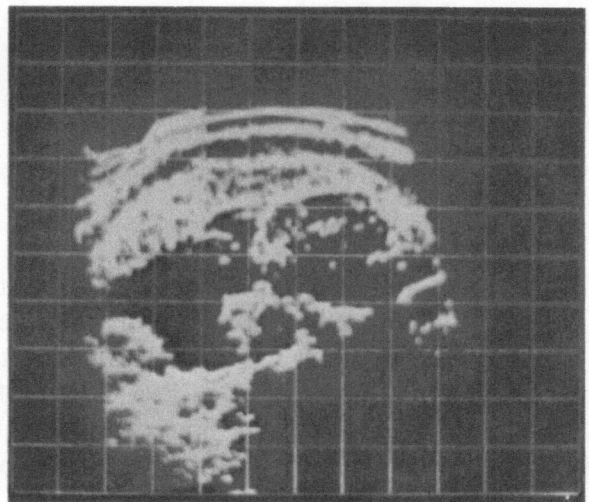

Fig. 16. Ultrasonic (B-scan) localization of placenta.
a) Original figure (transversal plane 2 fingers above umbilicus); placenta on left ventral wall, trunk of foetus on right.

b) Corresponding diagram

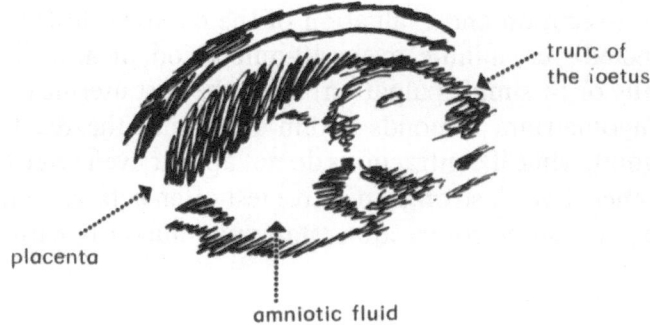

accumulated blood flow), since contact with this moving medium causes a change in ultrasonic wave frequency. The relief of parts of the foetus and the placenta is depicted on a screen with long persistence, so that the picture can be recorded photographically (Fig. 16a, b). Ultrasound placentography is an exact method (Donald and Brown 1961, Kratochwil 1975) and its advantage is that it obviates the radiation entailed in both X-ray and isotope radiography. Its disadvantage is the relatively high cost of the technical equipment.

Thermoplacentography

This method is based on the principle of direct colour exposure, of varying intensity, of a special metal foil applied to the woman's abdominal wall. Differences in exposure intensity are caused by minute temperature differences in the examination area, the maximum values being found in places with an accumulation of maternal blood (the placenta). The method is simple, requires no special apparatus and does not involve the risk of exposure to radiation.

THE OXYTOCIN TEST (SMYTH'S TEST)

The above author originally evolved this test as a method for determining the exact date for the onset of labour from the reaction of the myometrium to exogenous oxytocin (Smyth 1958). In this respect it did not come up to expectations, and was rightly criticized. If we employ this method to obtain information on the response of the myometrium with reference to the probable success of meditated induction of labour, however, it is of definite practical use. Its reliability in this respect is given in the Czechoslovak literature as 60%.

Execution and evaluation of the oxytocin test: 1 milliunit oxytocin is injected every minute, over a 10-min period, meanwhile recording (tocographically or by simple palpation) when the first uterine contractions appear. If the myometrium responds within 1—4 min, the reaction is evaluated as very good, while if contractions do not appear even after 10 milliunits, the reaction is negative. A strongly positive test often acts as "microinduction" of labour, e.g. if uterine contractions start spontaneously within 6—12 hours.

READINESS OF THE UTERINE CERVIX FOR LABOUR

In cases of protracted pregnancy, uncertain term and potential danger to the foetus, when we consider the possibility of inducing labour, palpation assessment of the readiness of the uterine cervix is a good auxiliary criterion. Today there are 5 recognized criteria of this examination method:

a) patency of the cervix, including the internal os;

b) the length of the cervix;

c) the position of the cervix, i.e. the direction of its axis (the more eccentric its position and the more dorsally it is directed, the smaller the degree of readiness);

d) the consistency of the cervical tissue;

e) the state of engagement of the presenting part of the foetus in relation to the pelvic orifice.

Various authors have confirmed the advantage of evaluating these individual criteria, especially if they are tested repeatedly, i.e. if the development of the readiness of the cervix is studied dynamically (Ulrich et al. 1959), thereby considerably increasing the reliability of the method. In an attempt to make this examination method as objective as possible, it was suggested that each of the five given criteria should first of all be evaluated separately by 0 to 2 points, according to how far advanced the finding is, so that the test as a whole has a range of 0 to 10 points (Niswander et al. 1967). The usefulness and advantages of this evaluation method were also confirmed in the Czech literature (Soukup et al. 1970). This method not only provides good information on the probable success of mediated induction of labour (Kronus et al. 1970), but it can also be employed for objective evaluation of changes taking place in the uterine cervix in the presence of imminent danger of premature labour (Štembera 1974).

ULTRASOUND DETERMINATION OF THE SIZE OF THE FOETUS

The size of the foetus needs to be determined in cases when the date of term is uncertain and in some pathological states when the size of the foetus does not correspond to its gestational age (inadequately compensated diabetes in the mother, a small-for-dates foetus). Even an experienced obstetrician, using simple palpation, can err by $\pm$ 500 g in 20% of the cases, and in 60% where the foetus is too small or over-large (Loeffler 1967). Ultrasound determination of the size of the foetus by measuring the biparietal diameter (BPD) of the foetus's head is based on the finding that the BPD increases proportionally with the gestational age or the weight of the foetus (Donald et al. 1961, Willock 1967). The actual BPD is measured reliably if the middle echo is shown on the screen in the middle of the head (scanner B, Fig. 17b), or if the echoes from the anterior and posterior parietal bone are of the same height

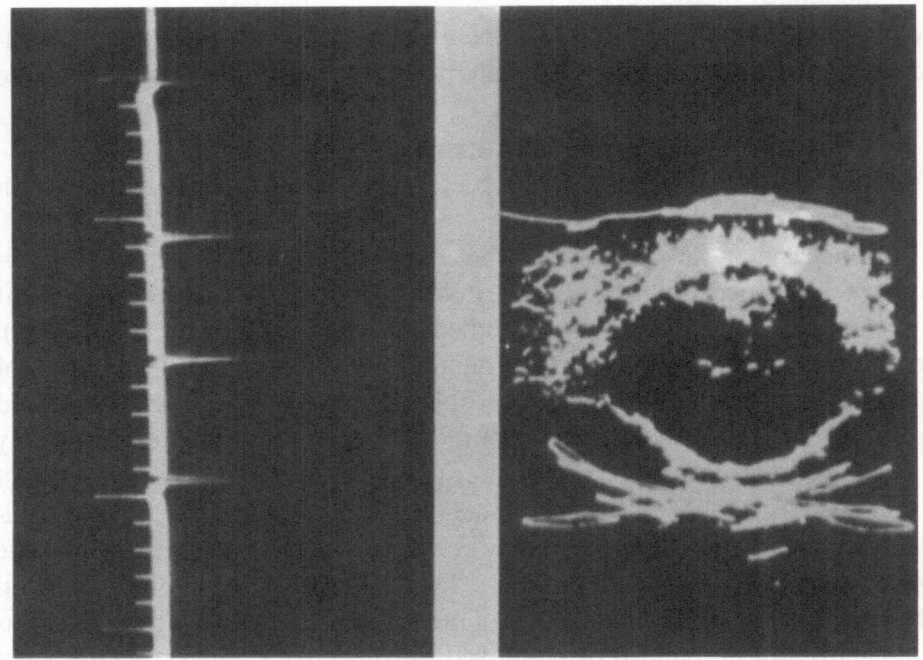

Fig. 17a. A-scan of head. First wave from top emitted signal, second and fourth correspond to rebound from parietal bones; distance between the two waves corresponds to biparietal diameter of foetal head. In middle: "middle echo" from falx cerebri.

Fig. 17b. B-scan of head. Detected in transversal plane, just above symphysis. The short, horizontal broken line is the middle echo (Kittrich, own material).

(scanner A, Fig. 17a). The BPD, measured on the screen with a millimeter rule, is inserted in correlation curves, one axis of which gives the size of the BPD in cm and the other the length of pregnancy or the weight of the foetus. There are differences between the correlation curves for physiological pregnancies and certain pathological states (poorly compensated diabetes, severe EPH gestosis) and even for different geographical regions (English and central European infants – Kittrich 1971).

The age of the foetus can be determined from the BPD with the greatest accuracy up to the 30th to 32nd week of pregnancy (Campbell and Newman 1971), as also confirmed by our own results (Kittrich 1973). The determination of foetal weight from the BPD in the last months of pregnancy is less accurate. According to the curve calculated for normal pregnancies from our own material, the weight of the foetus can be determined to within ± 300 g in only 67% of the cases; this corresponds to the best data in the literature.

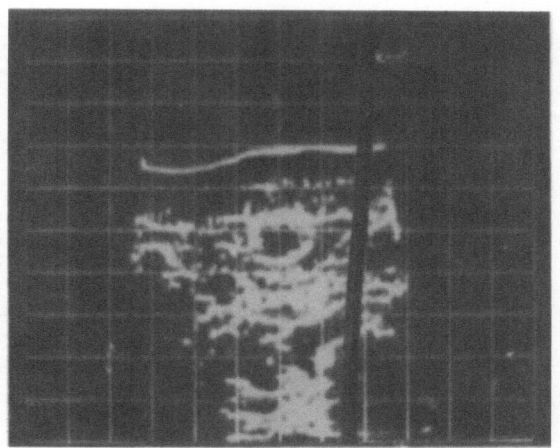

Fig. 18. Pregnancy on the 43rd day of amenorrhoea (transversal plane, just above symphysis). Circular shadow corrresponds to fertilized ovum (Kittrich, own material).

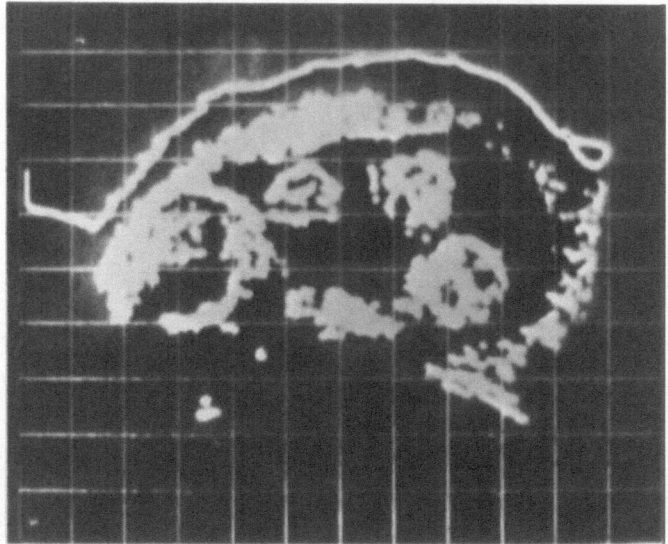

Fig. 19. Transverse position of the foetus (transversal plain at umbilical level). Section of head and all limbs (Kittrich, own material).

When determining the weight of the foetus, certain authors therefore now use thoracic and/or breech diameter, as well as the BPD. Some authors claim that diagnosis by means of the BPD is not possible in small-for-dates foetuses, while Willock et al. (1967) states that a weekly increase of 0.17 cm in the BPD precludes a small-for-dates diagnosis with 88% probability.

Further uses of ultrasound in obstetrics

In a number of cases, ultrasound can act as a substitute for X-ray examination. On a B-scanner, ultrasound can be used to demonstrate an early pregnancy (Fig. 18) and reliably determine the position of the foetus (Fig. 19),

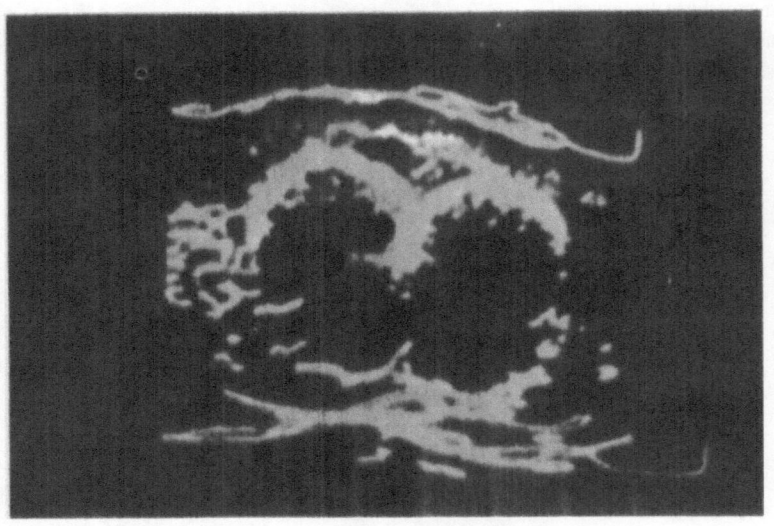

Fig. 20. Heads of twins in fundus uteri (transversal section of fundus) (Kittrich, own material).

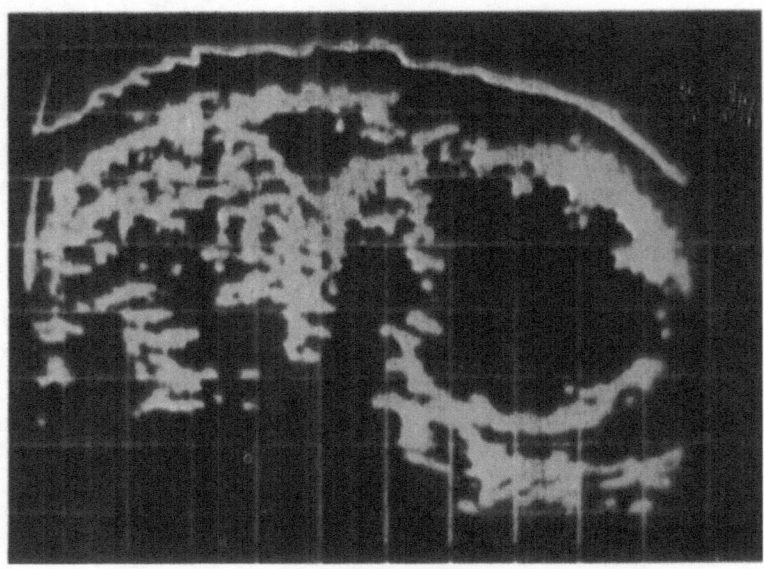

Fig. 21. Hydrocephaly (medial plane). Biparietal diameter of head 12.2 cm (measured by A-scan) (Kittrich, own material).

a multiple pregnancy (Fig. 20), hydrocephaly (Fig. 21), hydrops foetalis and myomas during pregnancy (Fig. 22), Simple, small portable instruments (Dopton, Sonicaid, Udop, Hewlett-Packard) are replacing the old method of auscultation of the foetal heard sounds with a wooden or metal stethoscope; the directly audible sound emitted by the apparatus after applying the detector to the woman's abdomen is useful both for instruction purposes and also, in many cases, for keeping the woman calm. The character of the sound displays differences typical for the foetal heart sounds and the umbilical and placental blood vessels. The past few years have seen rapid development of new ultrasonic equipment for the B-scanner, which functions on the principle of the visualization of different tissues in 10 shades of grey or in different colours. These instruments allow very detailed evaluation of the shape and structure of various foetal organs and it will be possible to use them to diagnose a number of congenital developmental anomalies of the foetus.

PROSPECTS FOR THE DIAGNOSTICS OF PLACENTAL DYSFUNCTION AND DANGER TO THE FOETUS

The rapid development of medical electronics and biochemistry and the use of tracers has greatly advanced the diagnostics of high risk pregnancy in recent years. We can already tell, from some studies, the direction which this progress is going to take.

Automatic processing of data on different biological parameters

The number, frequency and intensity of different changes in the rate and oscillation of monitored foetal heart sounds, the intensity, frequency, duration and total number of uterine contractions during the whole of labour and the reciprocal relationship between these two constantly changing factors and their influence on the foetus represent so many variable data that their rapid evaluation during labour will continue to be virtually impossible without the aid of an automatic computer. The same applies to evaluation of the foetal ECG.

Telemetric transmission of biological parameters

The detection of biological parameters in the foetus (by phonocardiography or ECG) and their direct transmission to the recording instruments greatly

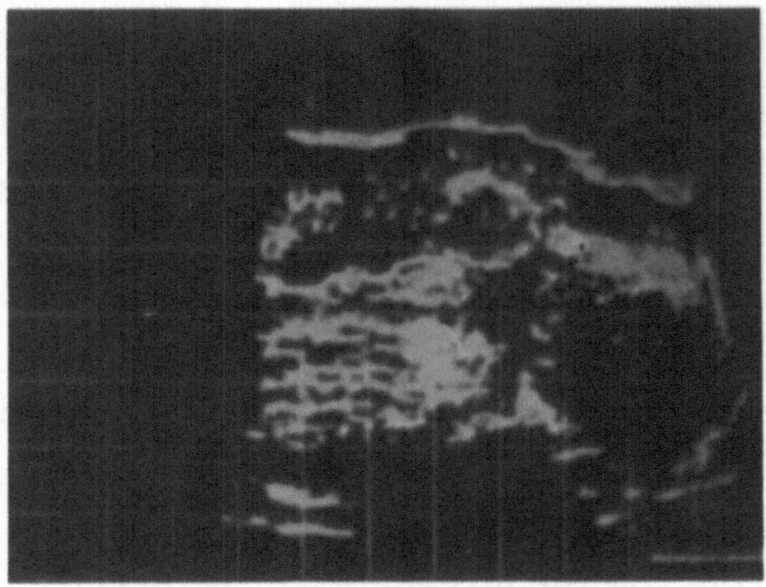

Fig. 22. Pregnancy, 18th week, with myoma praevia filling lesser pelvis. Head proximally, in centre of the picture, trunk of foetus to left of head (medial plane) (Kittrich, own material).

limits the woman's movements and requires the presence of the apparatus and the staff who service it directly in the labour ward (delivery theatre). The telemetric transmission of these data does away with both the above drawbacks. Microtelemetric systems for monitoring the FHR, whose pick-ups weigh only a few grammes and whose transmitter weighs only a few decagrams, have been constructed. The data can be transmitted over a distance of 100 meters and are received by a conventional radio-television receiver.

Foetal electroencephalography

Although the first successful F-EEG recording was made in 1942, and this method was not seriously elaborated until the 1950's, at the end of the 1960's authors were still saying that foetal bioelectrical activity of the brain displayed typical changes in correlation to the uterine contractions, but that it was difficult to find a satisfactory explanation for them. In recent years, typical waves were described between the contractions, in contractions of different intensities, in rupture of the amniotic sac, in Dip I and II, while epileptic activity was described in ischaemia of the brain, etc. The problem of the numerous artefacts caused by the maternal pulse and respiration and the movements of the foetus, etc. is still unresolved, however, and remains an obstacle to the production of commercially available instruments for the practical utilization of this method.

Other prospective methods for diagnosing the placental dysfunction

Methods which could mean a new lead in the diagnostics of placental dysfunction and danger to the foetus in the near future undoubtedly include:

Transcutaneous monitoring of oxygen tension, using a Clark type of oxygen electrode which could be applied to the foetus's head (Huch and Huch 1973).

The administration of certain labelled substances to the mother (e.g. ^{75}Se-methionin, with study of their movement from the maternal to the foetal blood stream and evaluation of their placental transfer within 30 min, as a test of placental function (Garrow 1970).

Further substances in the amniotic fluid, which could contribute to the diagnosis of certain pathological states, are also being sought.

SUMMING-UP OF THE METHODS

From the last 10 years' development of methods diagnosing danger to the foetus or placental dysfunction, we can draw the following basic conclusions:

(1) The long-recognized dividing line between the physiological and the pathological is gradually changing, in that the pathological sphere is widening at the expense of what was formerly regarded as the physiological sphere.

(2) Increasing efforts are being made to objectify and quantify this dividing line, so as to allow the comparison of individual cases and thus facilitate both reciprocal communication between workers and mass processing of these data. It is a principle of this sector of perinatal medicine also that we do not know and understand a given phenomenon until we are able to express it numerically.

(3) There is no sole, universal method for the reliable diagnosis of every type of intrauterine danger to the foetus. Many authors therefore tend to use a combination of several of these methods (Gaál et al. 1967, Michalkiewicz et al. 1967, Štembera et al. 1967, Kubli et al. 1971).

(4) All this, however, means an accumulation of data which the individual finds it very difficult to evaluate. At the present stage, this problem is resolved, for the time being, by drawing up different indexes and coding systems. If however, we want to prevent the situation from getting out of hand, thereby making our work useless, we shall not be able to dispense with the aid of automatic computers in this field.

PREVENTION AND THERAPY
OF THE HIGH RISK FOETUS

Genuine prevention of a high risk foetus presenting the hazard of perinatal mortality or morbidity consists in the prevention or treatment of the pathological state causing danger to the foetus. Prevention and therapy in this sense are discussed in the chapters on the pathological states in question. Although it does not obviate the primary cause, properly indicated induction of labour can, to some extent, be a very effective way of preventing perinatal injury. Conservative therapy is at present unfortunately confined to the last minutes or hours preceding birth and its purpose is to see the endangered foetus safely through the change from intrauterine to extrauterine life. When this is not successful, the only other choice is prompt surgical termination of labour (surgical therapy).

INDUCTION OF LABOUR

Our approach to induced labour, as to surgical delivery, should always be a very responsible one. In the first place, this operation ought to have its indications, its contraindications and its conditions, although their range will no doubt still be discussed and revised for a long time to come, not only owing to rapid technical development of the diagnosis of foetal risk and of the induction technique itself, but also on the basis of the results of long-term morbidity studies of children from high risk pregnancies.

Indications for induced labour: The first group, which includes diabetes, Rh isoimmunization, the finding of turbid amniotic fiuid in amnioscopy and an interval of over 24 hours following an escape of amniotic fluid after the 37th week of pregnancy, is almost universally recognized today. The indications in these high risk states are discussed in the relevant separate chapters. Most workers regard protracted pregnancy, toxaemia and an unfavourable history as the second most important group of indications, but their views on when, and under what circumstances, these high risk pregnancies become an indication for induced labour differ. In principle, it can be claimed that they do so when the use of different examination methods shows the presence of danger for the foetus (see methods).

Induced labour is **contraindicated** in cases in which it is clear that delivery by the vaginal route would constitute a danger to the foetus (and possibly the mother also) (cephalopelvic disproportion, transverse position, placenta praevia centralis, presentation of cord).

The **condition** for induced labour ought to be objectively demonstrated by the readiness of the organism for labour (see methods). This condition cannot always be met, however, e.g. if amnioscopy demonstrates turbidity of the amniotic fluid, or the results of spectrophotometric tests of the amniotic fluid in Rh isoimmunization are positive, and the maternal organism is not yet ready for labour. In this case, if we do not want to terminate pregnancy immediately by primary Caesarian section, we induce labour, bearing in mind that the hopes of successful induction are lower than normal and that if we fail, we shall still have to undertake Caesarian section.

The induction incidence cited by different authors depends upon the concentration of high risk pregnancies in the given institution, as well as on the range of recognized indications. Omitting those (nowadays isolated) authors who hardly perform induction at all, institutions can be divided, according to induction frequency, into three groups (Tab. 42):

Table 42. Comparison of induced labour frequency and intra- and postnatal mortality in these cases in different maternity institutions

Group	Author (institution)		Induction frequency (%)	Intra- and postnatal mortality (per mille)
I	Láska et al.	1970	1	
	Magát	1970	1.7	
	Kronus et al.	1970	1.8	0
II	ICMC (Podolí)	1970 – 1971	8.2	0
	Gazárek et al.	1970	· 11.7	8.5
III	Turnbull et al.	1968	30 – 35	17.3

The induction of labour in every third pregnancy (often only at the request of the woman herself) is fundamentally at variance with efforts to ensure the largest number of physiological births possible. We believe, however, that, with "active prevention of perinatal morbidity", 2% of inductions in a normal population sample is the absolute minimum and, on the other hand, 8 – 10%

in institutions where there is a concentration of high risk pregnancies is not exaggerated radicalism.

When evaluating perinatal mortality and morbidity in induced labour, we must not forget:

a) that this evaluation does not include cases in which antenatal death of the foetus was the indication for induction,

b) that the reason for which we induce labour is precisely a high risk foetus, so that we cannot place the blame for any morbidity in these cases solely on induction, which cannot always prevent the consequences of previous intrauterine injury.

Unsuccessful induced labour: Apart from perinatal mortality and morbidity, the following could also be regarded as failures:

a) a raised incidence of postnatal depression of the infant or of signs of intranatal hypoxia (unconfirmed — Horský et al. 1969);

b) an increase in the frequency of Caesarian sections (unconfirmed — Hudcovič et al. 1969);

c) if induction does not lead to delivery within 24 hours, or if uterine contractions do not appear at all. This type of failure depends upon various factors (the readiness of the organism for labour, the week of pregnancy, the indications for induction, the induction method, etc.) and is therefore **estima**ted differently by different authors (5–20%).

The induction method is an important factor in the success of induction. It would be wrong to claim that any one method is the most satisfactory for every case. Of the different methods employed today we can only point out their advantages and disadvantages, their special merits and the frequency with which they are used.

(1) *Pre-induction preparation:* Oestrogens, vitamin B — nowadays their advantages are stressed less than in the past.

(2) Induction is usually initiated by *rupturing the foetal membranes*. Some authors actually consider it wrong not to do this; it is only occasionally carried out during induction by oxytocics. The interval between rupture (which is followed by about 2 hours diminution of the uteroplacental blood flow) and the initiation of infusion is very important if we are to avoid potentiated deterioration of the foetal oxygen supply.

(3) *Oxytocics.* Only synthetic oxytocin is used today. Differences exist solely in the administration method:

a) intramuscular administration (repeated) is used less and less. Its disadvantage is sudden stimulation of uterine activity, associated in 30% of the cases with adverse changes in the foetal heart rate (demonstrated by monitoring);

140

b) i. v. drip (1 IU/100 ml infusion solution), formerly the commonest method;

c) i. v. drip (1 IU/400 ml infusion solution $= 2\,\mu IU/ml/min$). This method is gaining increasing support (Gazárek et al. 1970, Magát et al. 1970);

d) oral administration of Syntocionon or ODA-914 (deamino-oxytocin). The advantage of this method is its simplicity for both the nursing staff and the patient. Its disadvantage is that it is often associated with a raise incidence of surgical termination of labour owing to foetal hypoxia and frequent failure of induction because of unreadiness of the cervix.

(4) *Prostaglandins*. F_2 and E_1 are used out of 14 isolated compounds. So far we have not enough experiences with it in Czechoslovakia. Its advantage is said to be its efficacy in any week of pregnancy.

STIMULATION OF UTERINE ACTIVITY DURING LABOUR

This chapter is not intended to be a recapitulation of the one on induced labour, although repetition of certain principles will be unavoidable.

Rupture of the foetal membranes during the first phase of labour sucessfully stimulates uterine activity, but temporarily reduces the uteroplacental blood flow, as demonstrated by a higher subsequent incidence of Dip I (see methods), especially in high risk cases. Oxytocics ought also to be administered during indicated stimulation of uterine activity, both for therapeutic reasons (protraction of labour stages I and II, dystocia) and to prevent protracted labour in the presence of weak uterine activity and raised risk for the foetus (either owing to a high risk pregnancy or for signs of intranatal hypoxia). Their i. m. administration should be kept to a minimum. On the other hand, the infusion of 1 IU/400 ml 5% glucose is gaining even more support for stimulation of the contractions than for induction (Raffai et al. 1970, Brutar 1970, Kronus et al. 1970). Although this method greatly reduces the danger of foetal overdosing, very frequent and careful control of the size of the infusion, the foetal heart beats and uterine activity is nevertheless a categorical necessity until we are able, in all these cases, to monitor the foetal heart rate and uterine activity continuously and to regulate the size of the infusion by micropumps. Such objective recording will reduce the percentage of cases in which the stimulation of uterine activity fails owing to underdosing. We must not forget that, with this low concentration, the dose of oxytocin must be increased during the second stage of labour.

Methyloxytocin (MTO) is excellent, particularly in high risk cases. Its vascular effects are smaller than those of oxytocin (Jungmannová 1947, Šula et al. 1970), so that it has a better secondary effect on foetal metabolism, chiefly during hypoxia (Hodr et al. 1970, 1974). Consequently, it is being used by more and more maternity institutions, both in Czechoslovakia and elsewhere (Bärtschi et al. 1972). Suitable combination of oxytocics with spasmolytics or ataractics is important. Frequent, but timely stimulation of uterine activity can play a significant role in the prevention of protracted labour or the control of dystocia, and hence in reducing the frequency of surgical delivery owing to foetal hypoxia, as well as the incidence of serious intranatal hypoxia itself.

As with induced labour, it is hard to estimate the optimum mean percentage of cases in which uterine activity needs to be stimulated. Ten per cent in a normal population sample and up to 30% in institutions with a high concentration of high risk cases do not seem to us to be exaggerated estimates.

INHIBITION OF UTERINE ACTIVITY DURING LABOUR

Like the stimulation of uterine activity, its inhibition, in given cases, can be a preventive or a therapeutic measure. These comparatively rare cases include not only tetanic contractions or precipitate labour with very intensive contractions, but also specific arrest of uterine activity prior to performing Caesarian section indicated for acute intranatal foetal hypoxia. Intensive contractions reduce the uteroplacental blood flow and thereby further potentiate hypoxia in an already hypoxic foetus. If 6% of all infants delivered by Caesarian section die after birth (perinatal mortality for Bohemia and Moravia, 1969), it is largely due to failure to restore their severely impaired acid-base balance. If we improve the uteroplacental circulation by stopping the contractions, we give the foetus a chance of coping with its acidosis while still in utero. This transplacental intrauterine correction is a far better and more physiological way for the foetus than postnatal correction (Caldeyro--Barcia et al. 1969, Štembera et al. 1973). Substances of the beta-adrenergic group are today the most satisfactory for suppressing uterine contractions (see the chapter on premature labour).

CAESARIAN SECTION

The range of indications for Caesarian section and its frequency have gradually increased in the past decade, chiefly with respect to the foetal indications, while the figures for the maternal indications $(1-5\%)$ have hardly altered. There are now only one or two instituons, in a few countries, which cling to the old, conservative point of view and do not perform more than 1% Caesarian sections.

If we try to draw up a modern list of the indications for Caesarian section (a difficult feat because of the high incidence of combined indications), the following occupy first place, on an equal footing: foetal hypoxia (alteration of the foetal heart rate), abnormal posture and presentation of the foetus and non-progression of labour (irregular uterine activity), i.e. mainly foetal indications. Only then come placenta praevia (and premature abruption of the placenta) and toxaemia. When extending the indications and frequency of Caesarian section, we must bear in mind that, like any other operation, it represents a given danger for the mother. It carries a 10 times higher maternal death rate than other forms of delivery, but an anlysis of 74 women who died in association with Caesarian section in Czechoslovakia in 1964−1968 (Kotásek et al. 1970) shows that disease of the mother was the main cause of death. This is demonstrated by the completely different sequence of the indications in these cases. The first two places are taken by 12 cases of toxaemia (including 9 of eclampsia) and 12 of placenta praevia, i.e. all maternal indications. Combined indications (mainly dystocia) come third, post-mortem Caesarian section fourth and alteration of the foetal heart rate, in a single case, only fifth. Although foetal indications for Caesarian section are the most numerous, they account for only a very small percentage of maternal deaths.

If Caesarian section is to be effective against hypoxia or in preventing perinatal morbidity, it must be performed in time. Unfortunately, it is here that the commonest mistakes are made, in an effort to conduct labour with a hypoxic foetus until the conditions are ripe for vaginal termination of labour. In the case of failure, this means performing Caesarian section at the last minute. In a nation-wide analysis of intra- and postnatal foetus and infant deaths, we find that 8% were Caesarian deliveries. This figure contrasts sharply with the results of long-term studies of infants delivered by Caesarian section in good time, which show that perinatal morbidity among these infants is lower than after a difficult vaginal delivery (Zoltan et al. 1960), or even after a protracted labour (Bolte 1968).

Analyses by leading Czechoslovak institutions, discussed at a conference on Caesarian section in 1970, show that $2-3\%$ Caesarian sections answer modern requirements for the timely prevention of perinatal mortality and morbidity in a normal population sample (with good antenatal care) and 4 – 5% in institutions with a concentration of high risk pregnancies. The high figures given by some western authors are partly associated with differences in the organization of care of the pregnant woman during the antenatal period and labour.

FORCEPS AND THE VACUUM EXTRACTOR

Forceps should be a therapeutic and preventive "medium" for the prompt and safe termination of labour in acute foetal hypoxia, and not (however rarely) a traumatizing instrument. For this reason, the use of high forceps was virtually abandoned in obstetrics in Czechoslovakia years ago and the indications for Caesarian section were extended instead. Despite this, in the annual national analysis we still find 13 infants lost through the use of high forceps. The other indication sphere for forceps is the prevention of protraction of the second stage of labour, which is a high risk factor. In both indication spheres, therefore, the question of time plays a decisive role. If mid and low forceps in the hand or under the supervision of an experienced obstetrician carry only a minimum risk of mechanical injury, the loss of 52 infants every year in Bohemia and Moravia on using these forceps must be due primarily to their late employment. The results of retrospective studies of perinatal mortality after the use of forceps are characterized by widely differing data (from 0 to 13%). The only thing which can throw light on this question are long-term prospective studies which will make it possible to differentiate not only the type, the method and the indication for the use of forceps, but also all the other high risk factors participating in this form of surgical delivery.

Many of the above remarks also apply to use of the vacuum extractor, whose chief merits compared with forceps (the possibility of using it even when the head is high up in the pelvis and the simpler technique both in application to the head and in traction) have often proved fatal to the infant in the hands of an inexperienced operator or if too loosely indicated. The first optimism with which the vacuum extractor was sometimes hailed, both in Czechoslovakia and elsewhere, was succeeded by the realization that it can also be a traumatizing instrument, especially in high risk cases. For instance, it ought never to be used in hypoxia and diabetes. On the other hand, if the second stage of labour is not progressing, but the head is already largely engaged and there are no other risks, use of the vacuum extractor is warranted. Intra- and postnatal mortality is put at about 43 per mille and perinatal morbidity at up to 10%. As in the case of forceps, we are at present unable to distinguish the part played in these data by the actual operation and the part played by the primary risk for which the operation was indicated.

CONSERVATIVE THERAPY

Because of its limited scope, this chapter cannot be either a therapeutic guide or a detailed bibliographic survey of how to proceed in different foetal risk situations. All it can do is to draw attention to modern, proven lines of therapy and their main principles and to give the reasons for them.

Inhalation of oxygen by the mother is one of the oldest ways of treating foetal hypoxia. The historical development of this treatment, successive changes in views on it and its effect on foetal energy metabolism and the foetal circulation were reviewed, up to 1965, in the monograph "Foetal Hypoxia" (Štembera 1967). Two authors (Saling 1963 and Koleta 1968) expressed doubts as to the efficacy of this treatment and provoked a discussion in which most of their objections were convincingly refuted, however. Detailed studies have demonstrated that the inhalation of oxygen by the mother has the following effects on the foetus:

a) it raises a low Po_2 in the foetal blood (Mendéz-Bauer et al. 1967, Newman et al. 1967, Rorke et al. 1968, Štembera et al. 1969, Takeda et al. 1969, Chamberlain 1970, Wood 1970) and the foetal tissues (Caldeyro-Barcia et al. 1966), which is of decisive importance for assuring cellular metabolism;

b) it reduces a raised Pco_2 in the foetal blood (Newman et al. 1967), thereby preventing further deterioration of foetal respiratory acidosis;

c) it reduces the foetal blood lactate level (Štembera et al. 1969, Jacobson 1970) and thus prevents deterioration of metabolic acidosis;

d) it reduces the incidence of Dip II (Mendéz-Bauer et al. 1967), as an expression of improved foetal heart metabolism (see methods).

The question of the uteroplacental circulation is still open (Finnilä et al., 1971, found that it fell after O_2 inhalation) and so is the question of the pH in the foetal blood; some authors found that the pH fell after O_2 (Saling 1963, Davey 1969, Finnilä et al. 1971), while others found no change in it (Mendéz--Bauer et al. 1967, Štembera et al. 1969, Jacobson 1970). It was this which drew attention to the circulation.

Influencing the uteroplacental circulation means blocking undesirable vaso-constriction, which can occur not only after inhaling oxygen, but also as a result of various pathological states (toxaemia) or intranatal stress. Saling (1963) recommended supplementing oxygen inhalation by the administration of Theophyllin. The positive effect of ATP on both the uteroplacental blood flow and foetal gas metabolism and acid-base balance (Horská et al. 1970) led to its being used to supplement oxygen inhalation (Horská et al. 1972). A similar beneficial effect was obtained by combining the administration of Complamine with oxygen inhalation (Finnilä et al. 1971).

The administration of glucose to the mother as treatment of an endangered foetus, which was first used over 70 years ago, is likewise discussed in detail from the clinical and the metabolic aspect in the monograph "Foetal Hypoxia" (Štembera 1967). The latest studies have simply confirmed earlier conclusions, cited in this monograph, on the positive effect of glucose administered to the mother as an i. v. drip on the hypoxis foetus, in which it replenishes depleted energy reserves and helps to restore acid-base balance to normal.

Just as pediatricians, for some years past, have been able to treat neonatal acidosis, obstetricians now attempt to **treat foetal acidosis by administering sodium bicarbonate or THAM (organic buffer) to the mother,** often together with glucose (Rooth 1964, Persianinov et al. 1968, Chiladze et al. 1970, Gazárek et al. 1969). The results of this therapy are not at present conclusive. In the mother, acid-base balance improved mainly in cases in which she had already displayed signs of acidosis (protracted labour). An increase in the pH was also demonstrated in foetal blood microsamples obtained from the skin of the head (Newman et al. 1967, Jacobson 1970), mainly after THAM. These positive changes were only temporary, however, in both mother and foetus (Jacobson et al. 1967). The maternal pH does not seem to influence metabolic acidosis in the hypoxic foetus directly (Wood 1970). The latest, very promising, results to be described were obtained with Dipyridanol (Michel 1970).

The finding that fibrinolytic activity (which is always higher in foetal than in maternal blood) rises markedly during foetal hypoxia presents an entirely new aspect of the prevention of postnatal injury to the infant. It forms the basis of the treatment of foetal hypoxia with ε-aminocaproic acid (50 – 100 mg/kg) or Trasylol (1,000 – 2,000 KI units/kg), administered to the mother in the form of a 10 minutes' infusion about 20 minutes before delivery (Ludwig 1968).

146

CARE OF THE „HIGH RISK"
NEWBORN INFANT

COOPERATION BETWEEN OBSTETRICIAN AND
PAEDIATRICIAN

Close cooperation between the obstetrician and the paediatrician in the perinatal period is a comparatively recent innovation. Not so long ago, the care of the newborn infant during the first days of life was the province of the obstetrician, who assessed the infant's state primarily from the angle of the immediate birth results. Its further care was entrusted almost entirely to the female staff, on the assumption that at least 90% of newborn infants are normal and healthy and did not require special medical attention.

The care of newborn infants requiring active medical care was resolved by calling in the paediatrician as a consultant, or by transferring the infant to the children's department of a hospital. Systematic preventive examination of all newborn infants was rare, so that the choice of patients for examination by a specialist depended chiefly on the experience of the paramedical staff and their assessment of the situation. This naturally meant that the less obvious anomalies were often overlooked.

After the Second World War, this situation was felt to be generally unsatisfactory. The rapid decrease in total infantile mortality which occurred in all the more advanced countries turned attention to mortality in the first days of life, where the drop was relatively small. It also became increasingly clear that the majority of permanent disorders, particularly in the neuro-mental sphere, originate during the perinatal period. These quantitative and qualitative reverses promoted an immense interest in theoretical and practical infant problems in the perinatal period. One direct outcome of this interest was a rapid increase in new data on the physiology and pathology of the foetus and the newborn infant and, in the clinical sphere, the elaboration of better and more sophisticated diagnostic and therapeutic methods. As care of the newborn infant became more exacting and effective, the responsibility of physicians for prompt and correct application of the new methods naturally increased. A typical example of this is the diagnosis and treatment of severe forms of icterus neonatorum, which, in a very short time, became an important and responsible part of the work of neonatal departments.

This trend inevitably required a new approach mainly in the form of intensified cooperation with paediatricians, for whom care of the newborn infant meant extension and enrichment of their traditional diagnostic and therapeutic methods. Over the past 25 years, paediatricians in most countries have taken over the responsibility for medical care in the neonatal departments of maternity hospitals and preventive examination of all newborn infants has become the rule even in small maternity homes. This allows the timely detection of less obvious or incipient anomalies which do not directly endanger life, but which require early initiation of treatment, e.g. orthopaedic defects, minor anomalies, etc.

The care of healthy and term infants was accompanied by development and intensification of the activity of units for newborn infants needing active care, originally mainly for infants with a low birthweight. These units were at first attached almost entirely to children's clinics and departments and it was only later that some of the larger maternity hospitals were completed by them. From relatively simply operated centres aimed chiefly at improving the physical environmental conditions, they developed in time into intensive care centres with expensive and complicated equipment and a highly specialized staff.

It is now customary, all over the world, for the newborn infant leaving the delivery room, after primary adaptation, to be placed under continuous paediatric care. The role of the paediatrician in primary care, in the delivery room, has been less conclusively resolved. In Czechoslovakia, in about 1950, obstetricians and paediatricians agreed on the principle that the paediatrician should take over full responsibility for the care of the newborn infant at the time of birth. This "symbiosis" of obstetricians and paediatricians was pioneered by Prof. Trapl, the director of a maternity clinic in Prague, who can be regarded as one of the first perinatologists. In the spirit of this principle, paediatricians are called in to attend the birth of all infants born after a high risk pregnancy or labour, or if unexpected complications develop. This system has basically proved its worth, one reason being that it allows the obstetrician to give the mother his undivided attention, which is very important particularly in high risk births. The weakness of the system may be that, in small and remote maternity homes, the paediatrician cannot be reached out of working hours, or only after some delay. In this situation, the postnatal care of the newborn infant, including resuscitation, is undertaken by the obstetrician, according to agreed principles. The objection that the obstetrician is better able to evaluate the infant's state after delivery, because he possesses continous and detailed information on all the risk factors of the pregnancy and labour, need not be taken very seriously. In our experience, the summing up and handing over of the basic details to the paediatrician in the delivery theatre does not, in an individual case, present any real problems. Furthermore, prenatal risks merely constitute a probable danger for the infant and the decisive factor for determining the form of care is the infant's condition after delivery.

In some institutions, the anaesthetist, if present at the birth, is responsible for the first care or treatment of the newborn infant. He is doubtless fully qualified to assure adaptation of respiration and circulation, but is less competent to give a complex evaluation of any pathological changes outside this sphere.

The last phase of care of the newborn infant, i.e. its discharge into extra-institutional care and arrangements for follow up, or, in the case of high risk infants, for rehabilitation, is purely the paediatrician's affair. Obstetricians have every right to be kept informed of the long-term results of their work, but a complete system for this "feedback" has so far not been elaborated.

Exact determination of the time when responsibility for the care of a new individual passes from the obstetrician to the paediatrician is obviously necessary both from the administrative and the forensic aspect. On the other hand, the moment of transfer ought not to set a limit to the specialist interests of the two fields of medicine. The great majority of pathological and abnormal situations found in infants after birth are caused by risk factors acting during pregnancy or labour. Primary prevention of neonatal pathology (if it can be foreseen) is the obstetrician's duty, while the paediatrician who receives the newborn infant from the hands of the obstetrician logically has more of a curative task, since he has the job of remedying existing disturbances by appropriate treatment. Daily experience shows that the results of postnatal therapeutic effort depend largely on the degree of success of the obstetrician's preventive activity. For instance, every week by which he can prolong pregnancy in a woman showing signs of imminent premature labour increases the chances of survival for the premature infant, and the same applies to the prevention of hypoxia, perinatal trauma, diabetic foetopathies, etc. This close association between prenatal and postnatal pathology and the resultant practical consequences naturally require a good knowledge and reciprocal understanding of the problems of the other field. In our opinion, in serious cases the paediatrician-neonatologist ought to have a say when considering the best steps to be taken in the prenatal period, while the obstetrician should cooperate with the paediatrician in resolving certain situations developing after birth. The combination of prenatal prevention of risk to the foetus and postnatal therapy of the newborn infant forms the main content of the joint field of perinatology.

Such a close cooperation between a chiefly surgical and a chiefly medical field obviously brings problems which may impair the smooth course and the results of care of the infant in the perinatal period, from differences of opinion or inadequate personal relationships. These snags can be obviated by a clear division of responsibility, reciprocal agreement on methods and especially by a high standard of work from each of the partners concerned, thus creating an atmosphere of mutual confidence and respect.

THE NEONATAL UNIT IN THE DELIVERY THEATRE

The neonatal unit in the delivery theatre, or "paediatric corner", is the place where the newborn infant receives attention after delivery and, where necessary, treatment ensuring vitally important adaptation to the extrauterine environment, with special reference to respiratory and circulatory function. The infant is here also first classified according to its degree of development (see next chapter), organic and functional anomalies are determined and the ward where the infant is to be placed and its further care are decided.

Uniform and adequate heating, ventilation and illumination are general requirements for the neonatal unit in the delivery theatre. It should be isolated from the rest of the delivery theatre and should be large enough to hold the necesary equipment and allow 2 – 3 workers to attend to 2 infants simultaneously in comfort.

The room must have two tables with a washable surface, cupboard space for a stock of infant linen, a cupboard or shelf for equipment, a table with a balance and a slotted length gauge and a drawer in the table for writing materials (records). The lights over the examination tables should not be situated directly above the infant. While the infant is being treated, auxiliary heating elements directed towards the examination table from a height of about 150 cm should always be switched on.

For weighing the infant we recommend an automatic or semiautomatic balance for up to 10 kg. The mobile incubator must be pre-heated to 33 °C prior to the anticipated birth of a low birthweight infant and must be switched on while initiating resuscitation of an asphyxiated infant.

The oxygen resuscitator must have a locking device preventing the pressure from exceeding the safety limit during inflation; a water valve allowing regulation within limits of 15 – 30 cm H_2O is perfectly reliable. Oxygen is supplied from a central distribution system, which is safer than the use of compressed oxygen cylinders. An adequate number of oral aspirators, with a Pipka flask and catheters of various sizes, must always be available. It is important for the aspirator catheters to have one central opening at the rounded tip and to be kept in a dry, sterile vessel. An aspirator allowing the regulation of negative pressure is an advantage.

For infants, the laryngoscope must be specially constructed with a straight spoon, and must be supplemented by endotracheal tubes (No. 3.5, 4, 4.5 and 5). All these components should be kept in sterile vessels.

Along with regular control of the insufflator, oxygen cylinders and aspirators, the source of light of the laryngoscope should also be checked and care should be taken that all resuscitation aids are always in readiness and are not used for other purposes.

The neonatal resuscitation box should be equipped with a large stop-watch to determine the precise time of birth and record the Apgar score after exactly one, five and ten minutes.

Small aids necessary for the first postnatal care of the infant can be included in the following five groups:

(1) Sterile aids kept in 2 per mille aqueous Septonex*) solution (hypodermic syringes, beaded exploring needles, forceps. Pean forceps, scissors, a scalpel, high speed thermometers).

(2) A sterile vessel with packs for the newborn infant (tape, gauze squares, a cottonwool brush for marking the infant and − if Créde's silver nitrate is used − a dropper).

(3) Solutions, clearly marked: 1% Septonex tincture for disinfecting the umbilical stump, in an economical dropper bottle. Two per mille aqueous Septonex solution for routine disinfection of aids. Ophthalmoseptonex in original pack, with dropper, used for Créde's prophylaxis (solution is thermostable), or 1% silver nitrate, which must be changed every 3 days (thermolabile). Benzine for wiping skin before marking infant and dye solution for marking.

(4) Drugs: 10% glucose (10 ml in sterile ampules), 4.2% sodium bicabonate, medical oxygen, vitamin C in ampoules.

(5) Other materials: phonendoscope, wall thermometer, receivers for vomit, linen container, rubbish bin with pedal. A wash-basin, foot-operated and paper towels, at least in the delivery theatre, would be an advantage. Two per mille Septonex solution for disinfecting hands. Small aids include tubes for taking blood samples, lancet for collecting capillary blood and sterile cellulose. For records: printed forms sent with infant to department or other institution.

The remarks made in connection with basic aids indicate some of the principles of care of the newborn infant in the delivery theatre. In large hospitals, the first care is allocated to a children's nurse, but in most cases it is carried out by the midwife. The first operation is usually determination of the Apgar

*) Quaternary ammonium salt commonly used in Czechoslovakia for external disinfection.

score 1 minute after complete delivery (if necessary, also 5 and 10 minutes after). The nurse cleans out the air passages, treats the skin and the umbilical stump, disinfects the eyes, measures and weighs the infant and marks it for identification. If the infant needs special care, in particular resuscitation, these procedures are postponed until its state improves. In the case of low birth-weight infants, some of these operations are likewise postponed, if necessary, until the infant has been transferred to the ward.

A paediatrician is called in to the delivery of infants exposed to a high risk pregnancy or labour, or after delivery if any unexpected abnormality is found. He examines the infant and initiates the proper treatment, the primary aim of which is to ensure normal respiration. Resuscitation methods are described in the chapter on the asphyxiated newborn infant.

POSTNATAL CLASSIFICATION OF NEONATES

Findings made in recent years have shown that the widely used system of classifying neonates according to birthweight is inadequate for differentiating basic categories of neonates with different clinical problems and different short- and long-term prognosis. The newborn infant must therefore be evaluated from the length of gestation and from the stage of somatic development, which is determined from birthweight and other parameters of intrauterine growth.

According to the length of gestation, newborn infants are classified as:
(1) pre-term (born at 37 weeks or earlier)
(2) term (born at 38 to 41 weeks), and
(3) post-term (born at 42 weeks or later).

Calculated gestational age is computed as the time elapsing from the first day of the last menstrual period to delivery and is commonly expressed in completed weeks. Where the date of the last menstrual period is not reliably known, the estimated gestational age is given (determined from the first movements, the foetal heart sounds, the size of the uterus and postnatal examination of the infant).

According to the rate of foetal growth, newborn infants are classified as:
(1) small-for-gestational age (with a birthweight below the 5th percentile of the foetal growth curve),
(2) appropriate-for-gestational age (with a weight between the 5th and 95th percentile), and
(3) large-for-gestational age, with a weight over the 95th percentile.

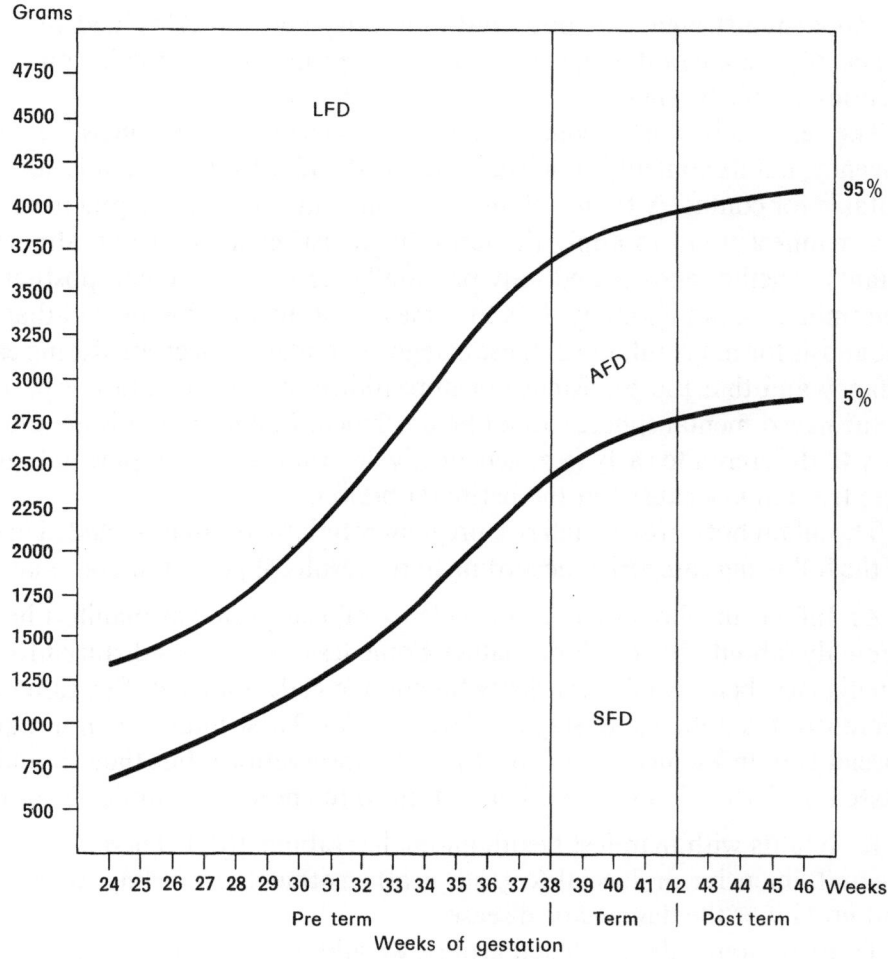

Fig. 23. Postnatal newborn classification by birthweight and gestational age. SFD — small-for dates. AFD — appropriate-for-dates. LFD — large-for-dates.

Most countries have their own tables and curves for normal foetal growth; the tables for the Czech population are given on p. 199 and 200. Some authors give the 10th and 90th percentile as the dividing lines between normal and altered foetal growth.

Simultaneous use of the time and growth criterion allows the newborn population to be divided into 9 main categories (Fig. 23).

In practice, it is most important to differentiate between pre-term and small-for-gestational age neonates. The proportion of post-term or large-for--gestational age infants in the newborn population is small.

Only term neonates with an appropriate weight are developmentally "normal"; the other categories are born with a greater or lesser degree of risk.

It was demonstrated that postnatal morbidity and mortality and the incidence of permanent damage were in inverse proportion to the length of gestation and birthweight.

The term "high risk neonate" caught on because of its conciseness and cogency, but its content is not exactly defined and, furthermore, it is not very suitable for contact with the infant's environment. In perinatal practice there is a manifest trend to apply the term "high risk neonate" to all abnormal infants, whether endangered only prenatally, or with an actual, postnatally determined health anomaly. It is to some extent justified by the fact that the prognosis for many infants in these categories remains uncertain during early infancy and that the persistence or appearance of abnormalities, especially in the neuro-mental sphere cannot be precluded. In addition, it is not always easy to differentiate early (e.g. genetically determined) developmental disorders from injury caused in the perinatal period.

The infant born after a high risk pregnancy or labour can be included in one of the following categories, according to the results of postnatal examination:

A. Infants in whom there is no evidence of a suspected or manifest health anomaly (about 20% of all neonates). Some lesions, such as disturbances of intelligence, behaviour and sensory function (e.g. deafness), or fits, cannot be demonstrated until a later stage of development. These infants do not require special care in the neonatal ward (or only observation), but they should be passed on for further care, with attention to the need for long-term control.

B. Infants with manifest health anomalies (about 10%). These require increased, intensive or special (e.g. surgical) treatment, according to the type and gravity of the damage or disease.

To these prenatally predicted groups we add, after birth:

C. Infants with postnatally found pathological conditions after pregnancy or birth not associated with a determinable risk for the foetus. They include the majority of congenital developmental defects, certain types of small foetuses, prenatal infections and haemolytic disease outside the Rh system, etc.

D. Infants in whom a pathological condition develops after birth. This small, and today less significant group mainly includes infections contracted after birth, haemorrhagic conditions, chance traumata, etc.

The main clinical types of neonates requiring exceptional care or further follow-up and treatment are:

Asphyxiated infants
Traumatized infants
Pre-term infants
Small-for-dates infants

154

Post-term infants
Infants with haemolytic disease
Infants of a diabetic mother
Infected infants
Anaemic and plethoric infants
Genetically stigmatized infants

WARDS OF THE NEONATAL DEPARTMENT

According to the results of postnatal evaluation of their stage of development or the gravity of any pathological changes, newborn infants are transferred from the delivery room to the relevant neonatal unit.

(1) **The ward for physiological neonates** is an essential part of the maternity hospital and takes all term infants free from determinable pathological conditions or serious risk (about 90% of all neonates). Every neonatal ward should have an observation unit, which has a dual purpose:

a) It allows closer control of infants in whom the postnatal examination leaves doubts as to whether they will need active therapeutic care in the ward for pathological neonates, or whether they can be placed among the physiological infants. There are two main groups of such neonates — infants born with minimum or inconclusive findings after a high risk pregnancy and cases with mild perinatal complications (e.g. low Apgar scores up to 5 minutes), which are only transient and show a tendency to rapid improvement. A final decision can usually be made within 24 hours after birth, only seldom later. In some hospitals, all infants are subjected to active observation for the first 24 hours after birth, to enable prompt detection of any unforeseen alteration in their condition.

b) In hospitals not possessing a ward for neonatal pathology it provides the basic essential care for infants in need of treatment elsewhere until the time of their transfer. Even with the best organized transportation services there may be a delay of several hours, and to neglect essential care in the first hours (hypothermia, hypoxia, starvation) could have serious consequences.

(2) **The ward for pathological neonates** takes infants requiring active therapeutic care, either directly from the delivery room or from the observation unit (if the infant's condition deteriorates). The central part of the ward is the neonatal intensive care unit, which ensures continuous personal and instrumental control of the infant's condition and a constant medical emergency

155

service. It admits infants in an adaptation crisis, who are in danger of death or permanent injury, irrespective of the degree of development at birth. The IC units are very expensively equipped and their operation requires a highly qualified staff, so that they can be established only in large institutions.

The neonatal pathology ward does not normally take contagious diseases. Any cases of infection, especially of the skin and the gastrointestinal and respiratory tract, are isolated in the isolation unit of the maternity department or are transferred to the paediatric department, according to their severity and the available facilities. Some IC units leave serious cases of infection among the other neonates, in the supposition that modern incubators provide adequate protection against cross infection.

(3) **The ward for low birthweight neonates** is sometimes separated from the ward for pathological neonates, or may be in another institution altogether. It admits the infants with a birthweight of less than 2,500 g who have not had. or have got over, an adaptation crisis, i.e. mainly cases of mild and moderate prematurity or retarded growth. All what these infants need is a modification of their daily regimen and a longer than normal stay in hospital. To leave them in the ward for physiological neonates would greatly encumber the running of this ward.

The field organization and cooperation of the individual units of neonatal departments is resolved in different ways. The ideal solution is a large maternity hospital equipped for all forms of care of the newborn infants (both physiological and pathological) and combining, under one roof, every type of prenatal, perinatal and postnatal infant care. In most countries, these comprehensive institutions are rather the exception. Owing to the present system of hospital building, we more often find, even in large regional hospitals, that healthy term infants are left in the neonatal ward (or observation unit) of the maternity hospital, while infants in need of active therapeutic care are transferred to the ward for sick neonates in the children's hospital. The disadvantages of this separation obviously increase with the distance between the two hospitals.

The wards for pathological neonates in children's therapeutic institutions are very diversely organized and equipped. In the past, they were used mainly for the large group of low birthweight infants, who were looked after there from the first hours of life until they attained a satisfactory weight (usually about 2,500 g) and could be discharged home. The present trend of intensive care units, with high diagnostic and therapeutic standards, inevitably leads to the concentration of all serious cases of neonatal pathology in a single department.

For small maternity departments, the only possible solution is to transfer a premature or sick infant to the relevant department of a cooperating larger institution. The infants are transferred in a special ambulance with a portable incubator, which provides the most essential environmental conditions (warmth, oxygen) and thus largely reduces the danger of the infant's suffering from the journey.

THE OBSERVATION BOX OF THE NEONATAL DEPARTMENT

The observation unit is a separate part of the neonatal ward, or a room in the neonatal department, where infants requiring quick transport to a special intensive care unit, or needing active observation in the first hours after birth, are brought from the delivery theatre. Every maternity hospital should be equipped with an observation unit.

An infant requiring transport should be removed 2−4 hours after birth in a portable incubator with oxygen. During transport, the nurse checks the environmental temperature and clears the upper airways and stomach by aspiration. She takes detailed records with her of all anamnestic, pregnancy and postnatal data and of previous treatment and care.

The indications for **rapid transfer** of the infant are:

(1) a birthweight of 2,000 g or less;

(2) a low Apgar score after 10 minutes and persistence of other pathological signs 1 hour after birth;

(3) development of a pneumopathy (increasing tachypnoea, retraction of the sternum, groaning expiration, cyanosis or pallor);

(4) attacks of apnoea with cyanosis in an oxygen environment, repeated vomiting, signs of CNS irritation (excitability, convulsions);

(5) an infant of a diabetic mother, an infant born before the 37th week of pregnancy to a mother with latent diabetes, a post-term infant born after the 42nd week with signs of intranatal hypoxia;

(6) an infant with a serious malformation, with signs of prenatal infection and with a confirmed haemolytic disease.

The indications for **active observation** during the first hours of life are:

(1) an infant with a birthweight of 2,000 to 2,500 g, with a normal Apgar score and good vitality and free from any signs of incipient respiratory disturbances; the infant may be premature, or, more probably, small-for-dates;

(2) an infant born after the 37th week of pregnancy to a mother with latent diabetes;

(3) an infant with a low Apgar score after 1 and 5 minutes, but of 10 points after 10 minutes;

(4) infants born to toxaemic mothers or after a prolonged pregnancy, with signs of intranatal hypoxia, and surgically delivered infants strongly affected by the drugs administered to the mother;

(5) mild cases of the haemolytic disease, requiring only the control of the bilirubin level;

(6) an infant born after a high risk pregnancy and labour, or a genetically endangered infant displaying no pathological signs at birth.

All other infants free from any clinically detectable risk are placed in cots for physiological neonates.

According to its development in the observation unit during the first 24 hours, the infant is either transferred to a special intensive care unit, or to the normal neonatal ward. The necessity for simultaneously handing over written records, with data on the time of appearance and the duration of observed anomalies, must be emphasized, since the time factor is the basic prognostic criterion for the infant's further care.

The observation unit of the neonatal department has room for 1 infant in an incubator and for $3-4$ in cots. It can be estimated that about 8% of newborn infants will need this temporary care. The proportion of infants requiring intensive care after observation will vary in the region of 5%, according to the concentration of women with high risk pregnancy. With increasing transfer of high risk infants in utero to central maternity hospitals in every region, the number of high risk infants transferred in an incubator will decrease.

The equipment of the observation unit is fairly simple and is largely the same as in the normal neonatal department. In addition, it has one incubator allowing oxygen to be supplied, an insufflator, an aspirator and permanent stomach tubes. The normal records are extended by data on the respiration and pulse rate after at least every feed or, if necessary, more frequently.

A future requirement for these units are monitors of the infant's functions, analysis of the oxygen in the incubator and permitting at least daily the testing of blood sugar, electrolytes, bilirubin and acid-base balance.

In preventive and active therapy in the observation unit we observe the following principles:

(1) early initiation of $5-10\%$ glucose feeding with an indwelling stomach tube from the 3rd hour of life;

(2) oxygen therapy for cyanosis;

(3) antibiotics if strictly indicated by the findings in mother and foetus;

(4) correction of acidosis is not repeated if this was done in the resuscitation

box in the delivery theatre and the infant was brought in within the stipulated 2 – 4 hours; if the infant was brought in later, it can be repeated automatically, using the same method.

THE INTENSIVE CARE UNIT

This comprises the neonatal pathology and low birthweights' wards. As the 2,500 g weight limit has receded into the background in the intensive care sphere, so has receded the significance of infections complicating the adaptation period. It was even found better to leave contaminated infants in the intensive care unit in an incubator. With proper isolation and antibiotic therapy, the danger of contamination for other infants in the unit is very slight. With postnatal infections contracted after the adaptation period the situation is quite different and it would be very wrong, for example, to leave a 2-week-old neonate with infectious gastroenterocolitis or otitis, etc. in a special ward for high risk neonates.

Organizational linkage of the neonatal intensive care unit (NICU) to the whole system of obstetric and paediatric perinatal care significantly influences neonatal mortality. The comparison of the neonatal mortality (in the 1st week) between Canadian hospitals with and without a NICU shows that the best results are achieved when intensive obstetric and paediatric care are concentrated organizationally in the same hospital.

	Neonatal mortality per 1,000 live births	
	Year 1967	Year 1968
(1) Quebec hospital with obstetric and neonatal ICU	6,3	6.42
(2) Quebec hospital with obstetric ICU and affiliated to external neonatal ICU	8.48	6.46
(3) Quebec hospital with obstetric ICU but not affiliated to neonatal ICU	10.2	9.64
(4) Hospital aoutside Quebec not affiliated to neonatal ICU	13.69	—

The above data come from hospitals with over 1,000 births a year. They do not include neonates with a birthweight of < 1,000 g.

According to the experiences of large centres, long-range calculation of the number of beds and nursing staff is possible. If the bed in a neonatal intensive care units is defined as one which allows monitoring and treatment by means of special life-saving apparatus, then the bed: specialized nurse ratio is 1 : 1 (maximum 1 : 2). The newborn infant is treated for an average of 6 days in the intensive care unit, so the number of patients per bed per year is about 60.

The number of intensive care beds for a given region is calculated from the number of live births and neonatal mortality:

$$\frac{\text{neonatal mortality in region} \times 3}{60} \times \text{number of live births in region in thousands.}$$

In Czechoslovakia this would work out roughly as follows:

$$\frac{13.8 \times 3}{60} \times 220 = \frac{41.4}{60} \times 220 = 911 : 6 = 152, \text{ i.e. } 152 \text{ IC beds}$$

would cover neonatal intensive care requirements in Czechoslovakia.

Only isolated examples of this system, i.e. based on the above calculations, are to be found at present. As already mentioned, both in Czechoslovakia and in other European countries, in the paediatric part of intensive care we are more likely to encounter, for the time being, the development of intensive care sections forming part of the premature infant's ward, although the method described above would probably be more satisfactory. At the same time, some premature infant's wards will evidently not be able to treat newborn infants with adaptation disturbances requiring intensive care at all, but only infants with a low birthweight, until they are ready for discharge as physiological neonates.

In 1970, the Czechoslovak perinatal commission recommended the places (mostly regional towns) where high risk pregnancy care ought to be concentrated, and which therefore should also have in the same building the best possibly equipped obstetric and paediatric intensive care units. How soon this plan can be put into operation is a matter of time, financial resources and adequate staffing. At present, as regards the paediatric part of intensive care, it seems likely that special rooms (intensive care sections) will be set aside in selected wards and that the infants, after overcoming adaptation difficulties, will continue to receive normal care in the same ward until they are discharged home. The reason for this is mainly that if the intensive care unit were completely separate from the ward where their care is completed, it would entail considerable shifts of the nursing staff.

According to experiences in Czechoslovakia, wards which have intensive care rooms (1 − 2) and also cater for low birthweight neonates and all infants given intensive care until they are discharged home, ought to have about 20 (but not more than 35) beds, including 5 – 10 incubators. Such wards ought to have 1 ward sister and 12 nurses working in 3 shifts, so that there are always 3 nurses on duty simultaneously. The doctor assigned to this ward would not work, or have any duties, anywhere else.

In the optimum situation, i.e. if high risk pregnancies, births and the intensive care unit are all under one roof, the problem of transfer does not arise. Where transfer is necessary, the best means of transport, for our requirements, is a portable incubator, a special ambulance and the attendance of a trained nurse who can provide the most essential care during the journey. The incubator must have a thermoregulation, an oxygen supply, facilities for aspiration, and must allow easy observation of the infant. In indicated cases, the infant must be transferred in the first hours after birth, as otherwise it could die before intensive care can even be started. This implies that transfer must also be possible at night and during holidays.

Technical progress is steadily raising the level of care, but is also making it more expensive. For instance, 1 day's treatment in an IC unit costs about 200 dollars (U.S.A.), or a full course about 7,000 francs (Switzerland), in Czechoslovakia up to 20,000 crowns. As already stated, the IC unit should therefore be planned, organized and equipped with the greatest deliberation, so as to ensure that it will be utilized with the maximum efficiency.

From the building aspect, an area of 4.5 m² must be allowed for one incubator or bed. It is best to concentrate the actual ICU in one large room (or at most two) containing all the incubators and apparatus (monitors, respirators, perfusors, etc.). In the other sections (the normal part of the ward), it is best to have 2 – 4 infants to a room. Apart from the patient's rooms, the IC centre must include a room for blood replacement transfusions and minor operations, a small laboratory (Astrup), an X-ray room (straight radiograms are sufficient), a kitchen for preparing feeds, a nurses' room, a room for the doctor, a bedroom for mothers (4 – 6 beds), a mothers' dining-room, a discharge room, a social room (lounge), 2 lavatories, a shower for staff and mothers, a small dressing-room and a room for dirty linen and cleaning materials. If the centre is used as a training (postgraduate, post-diploma) centre for para-medical personnel, medical students and doctors (perinatalogists), it ought also to have a study and a small lecture room. The NICU should be on the same floor as the labour ward, directly next to the labour room and near the section for physiological neonates and infants under observation.

At present, there are only a few such perinatal centres in existence, although experience shows that it is the most economical way of utilizing IC. In Czechoslovakia, we shall presumably try to arrive at this ideal solution by adapting existing departments and by making full use of the above pattern when building new hospitals.

Equipment

The concentration of intensive care in one room means that the necessary equipment must be organized differently from the usual pattern, if the nursing staff are to put their working time to the best possible uses for the care of the patient. All daily supplies are kept directly in the room in storage wall containing normal and special linen, sterile packs with instruments for all operations, drugs, disinfectants, gloves, etc., in short, everything needed for the infant's care and treatment. With this organization, the space in which the nurse moves while on duty is reduced to a minimum, so that her performance is twice that stained in a traditionally organized ward.

The supply of oxygen, compressed air, suction and electric current for the apparatus is also resolved in an entirely new manner. Incubators, respirators, monitors and infusion pumps require many various inlet tubes and cables. With the traditional wall outlets, this means horizontal inlets, which hamper movement round the incubators. A modern solution was therefore evolved, in which oxygen, electric current, etc. are supplied from special mobile modules vertically from the ceiling. The modules are either rods attached to the ceiling by a hinge, with tubes or cables and with terminals or sockets at the end, or have the form of retractable cylinders, again containing all outlets, suction vessels, etc. In Czechoslovakia, we now endeavour to persuade firms authorized to build the central oxygen supply, for instance, to accept this modern concept, which saves time and facilitates the work of the nursing staff.

Since the incubator and diagnostic and therapeutic equipment keep the infant in contact with given forms of electric current for a long time, exceptional safety demands are made on their instalation, e.g. separation of the electricity sources for monitors from apparatus with greater current requirements (incubator, heating circuits, lamps, etc.). Insulation transformers and current detectors prevent the transmission of induced current from power sources and equipment (incubators, infusion pumps) to the infant. The use of low-voltage battery apparatus and automatic switches, which function when the current reaching the infant approaches danger intensity, is of advantage.

Fluorescent tubes are used for lighting, although they have the disadvantage of not showing the true colouring of the skin. This can be counteracted by using special colours on the walls (beige is the best). When dealing with the infant directly, the illumination can be improved by the use of standard lamps providing both white and warm yellow light.

Air conditioning for controlling any air-borne infections is regarded as a normal part of the equipment of the ICU. Equipment which changes the air 16–18 times an hour is recommended. Today these traditional installations are criticized because irregular, eddying currents develop, especially round incubators, people, etc. This defect can be counteracted by aerotechnical equipment constructed on the laminar flow principle, in which the air is driven and flows vertically through a large number of holes from the ceiling to the floor, where it is drawn off. This method is supposed to give air with maximum freedom from infection.

A room for replacement transfussions, which can also be a small laboratory, forms parts of the NICU. This room also has a storage wall and a supply of electricity, O_2, etc., led from the ceiling.

It is beneficial if parents can watch their infants — and the care they receive — from a glass-walled corridor. In some wards, these visits are permitted all day and they seem to provide a better solution than verbal information given outside a strictly closed ward. As a special feature, we may add that the parents can actually take their child, in the incubator, into their arms. One wall of the incubator is incorporated into the glass wall of the corridor and is fitted with two large rubber gloves leading from the corridor. The mother is allowed into the ward as soon as the infant's state permits, to feed and tend it — though only, of course, in the pre-discharge room, where normal care is given. Before being admitted, the mother must undergo bacteriological tests (nose, throat, stools).

Every IC has its own X-ray room (the apparatus can be movable). Direct radiograms, with the infant suspended, are very valuable for quick determination of basic diagnoses (non-patency of the alimentary tract, cardiac malformations, pneumopathies). The most modern units have a "magnifying" X-ray apparatus, which gives a radiogram in which the X-rayed site (e.g. part of the chest) is 9 times larger than on standard film.

The main item of equipment in the ICU is still the incubator, the chief function of which is to protect the newborn infant against heat losses. The modern incubator must also allow the patient to be observed from all sides, have an oxygen supply and optimum humidity and suitably situated apertures for the hands of the medical and nursing staff, permitting the infant to be examined, treated and fed within the incubator. The temperature of the air circulating in the incubator is kept at a constant level by thermostatic control. The latest incubators have a device based on the servomechanism principle, which, again by means of a thermostat, makes the incubator temperature dependent on the infant's rectal or skin temperature. Its purpose is to avoid sudden changes in body temperature, and the danger of apnoeic pauses after such changes. The maximum attainable temperature in the incubator (usually 37 °C) is ensured by two functionally separate systems. Filters ensure bacteriological purity of the indrawn air and remove coarse dust particles; in this respect they are not 100% perfect, however, and further improvement of the filtration systems is under consideration. On the other hand, it is claimed that a laminar flow device makes individual filtration more or less superfluous. The incubator should have a separate opening giving access to the infant's head, to facilitate laryngoscopy, intubation and care of the infant's respiration in general without removing the infant from the incubator. In the wall of the incubator there should also be openings for a suction tube, cables to the monitors and tubes for parenteral or peroral nutrition. Modern incubators allow weighing of the infant inside them (the surface on which the infant lies is actually a part of the scales). The position of the bed and of the infant can be altered as required. Further parts of the incubator are an apparatus for aspirating secretory matter from the infant's air passages and stomach, and a special oxygen input terminating in a small mask; small tents for the infant's head, only made of transparent material, or a compressor with a nebulizer (performance 4 – 10 l/min), are also used. The humidity of the inflowing air can be altered as desired. Facilities for X-raying the infant directly in the incubator have also not been forgotten, as the plate can be slipped directly into the floor. The incubator is also fitted with a retractable stand for infusion bottles, a folding shelf for a monitor or an infusion pump and its own reflector. The openings for the hands of the staff have easily operated doors and are not of the iris type, since doors are easier to clean and disinfect.

Immediately after birth, while still in the delivery room, or if taken from the incubator for examination or treatment the infant is kept warm by means of infrared tubes about 1.5 m from its body. Heat losses can also be prevented by wrapping the infant in thin aluminium foil. Cooling caused by the administration of cold solutions or blood (e.g. in replacement transfusions) should likewise be avoided and the solution (or blood) passed through a heater to raise its temperature to 35.5 °C. New diagnostic apparatus and equipment for monitoring the main body functions have made an important contribution to intensive care of the newborn infant. In IC of adults, central monitoring units save the nurses a great deal of time, but in IC of the newborn, the nurse must stay constantly with the infant. Small portable electronic apparatus is therefore the best for IC of the newborn.

At present, monitors determining respiratory function are the commonest. "Apnoea detectors" and respiration monitors merely record respiratory movements and respiration frequency, and signal, by sound and light, any variation in the number of breaths in excess of a given, selected limit. They thus cannot detect, in an infant with chest and abdominal movements of a respiratory type, whether the glottis is occluded, or whether obturation of the main air passages has occurred, with arrest of respiratory gas exchange. The fact that such episodes quickly lead to bradycardia − which is detected by the heart monitor − gave rise to the opinion that heart monitors ought possibly to be given precedence in the monitor equipment of the ICU. The monitoring of respiration by means of impedance plethysmography, which records blood and gas volume changes in the lungs, has spread considerably in recent years. The measurement of changes in flow resistance between two electrodes on either side of the chest, on the transthoracic impedance principle, is still being developed. Its purpose is to measure the amount of fluid (blood, lymph) in the chest in relation to the amount of air, and the development of this ratio from the moment of birth. This type of monitoring produces technical problems related to the number of electrodes and is prone to defects from too poor adhesion of the electrodes to the skin and (in the smallest infants) to inadequate flat surface, for attaching the electrodes to the chest, where the intercostal depressions and skinfolds cause interference, resulting in poor conduction from the space between skin and electrode. It requires a great deal of experience and skill on the part of the staff to maintain proper conductivity of the electrodes for the necessary hours and days without producing false alarms, or interruption of the signals. The needle electrodes used in electroencephalography possess excellent conductivity, but they carry the danger of skin infections. The cheapest monitors registering body movements (mainly respiratory) record air pressure changes in the mattress (composed of large numbers of air-filled compartments) on which the infant lies.

Heart monitors record the heart rate (beat to beat), or integrate the individual beats or show the ECG curve on an oscilloscope. A change in respiration frequency is a valuable sign, not only of diminishing ventilation, but also of the development of cardiovascular disturbances. The onset of many forms of cardiac arrhythmia (e.g. ventricular fibrillation) can be detected only by an oscilloscope, which must be observed continuously. Units which can choose only one form of monitoring are recommended to use a heart monitor rather than a respiratory monitor, since respiratory disturbances (particularly apnoea) are manifested as a drop in the heart rate within 30 seconds. On both the heart and the respiratory monitor we can set an upper and a lower limit, which, if exceeded, sound an acoustic warming signal.

Monitoring of the peripheral pulse and blood pressure has limited uses for diagnostic purposes. The equipment is constructed on different lines and most of them record only systolic pressure reliably.

Continuous measurement of the oxygen concentration in the air of the incubator is considered to be important. Apparatus using a Clark oxygen electrode have proved to be the most satisfactory. The oxygen supply should be regulated according to the blood gas values (Po_2 and Pco_2) found in the infant's arterial blood. Since catheterization of the umbilical artery and prolonged arterial intubation are relatively frequently accompanied by complications, the measurements are usually done in capillary blood. An Astrup type apparatus was found to be the best for measuring blood gas values.

Determination of the microhaematocrit and blood sugar level ought to be possible in the ICU itself. There should also be a portable X-ray apparatus in the unit, for taking X-rays for diagnostic purposes. The unit should have a small dark room where transillumination of the skull and ophthalmological examinations can be carried out. In cases of necessity the incubator or bed can be covered with a dark "tent" during the examination.

The use of continuous positive airway pressure equipment (Gregory box) and of resuscitation and artificial respiration apparatus in IC units has grown considerably. Oxygen and pressure equipment (usually for respiration through a mask, with intermittent, limited overpressure) are normally employed in the delivery room to revive newborn infants in acute hypoxia, while in the actual ICU we constantly find new, more complicated and, of course, more expensive, equipment. Volume and timed respirators exist, as well as pressure respirators. Today, volume apparatus is mainly used for long-term respiration (chiefly for very immature neonates). The infant is usually intubated. Suitable overpressure, underpressure and frequency values can be set on these respirators and the percentual oxygen supply ($21 - 100\%$) can naturally be altered. The best equipment takes into account the state of the infant's respiratory centre. If the patient starts to breathe independently, the apparatus changes from controlled to assisted respiration. Artificial respiration units with negative pressure also exist. They are actually a type of iron lung and their advantage is that they facilitate venous return to the heart and do not require intubation, which is a frequent source of complications. So far, however, there have been difficulties with the construction of such respirators for infants with a birthweight of under 1,200 g (the problem being the sealing of the negative pressure space). The question of nurses and doctors is an inseparable part of the respirator problem. They must be able to service the respirator perfectly and must be utterly dedicated to their task — otherwise even the best technical equipment will fail to achieve therapeutic success.

Infusion pumps (perfusors) relieve the work of the nurses and allow a continuous, accurately dosed supply of fluids, nutrients and salts. They also reduce the incidence of complications (e.g. embolisms and infections), especially since the advent of millipore filters, which can be introduced into the pump $\rightarrow$ patient lead. Drip systems are falling into disuse, despite improvement by the incorporation of a fine needle allowing 1 ml to be divided into 100 drops. Another improvement was the division of the infusion solution among a series of separate chambers, which were emptied in turn. It is claimed that pumps, for the first time, allow for example good control of the blood sugar level and correction of acidosis. A further virtue of the perfusion technique is that it does away with the blocking of catheters, tubes and needles by clotted blood, refluxed when the infant cried. In Europe, perfusors with changeable syringes are the commonest, while in America, perfusors using peristaltic, external pressure on the infusion tube, thereby making it unnecessary to handle the sterile infusion solution, are more frequent. If the perfusor motor stops, a buzzer sounds or a light comes on. The nurses' main task, when setting up an i.v. infusion, is to see that it is not administered paravenously.

The storage wall in the IC room ought to contain all the necessary diagnostic and therapeutic materials in adequate amounts, in single-use packs or sterile packets, e.g. feeding tubes, umbilical catheters, infusion tubes with fine, plastic-winged needles (for fixation), a set of laryngoscopes, endotracheal tubes, etc. The unit should naturally always be well stocked, in case of a sudden influx of patients.

The ICU must also be equipped for phototherapy (see section on hyperbilirubinaemia).

We are aware that the IC requirements enumerated above are, at present, maximalistic, but, after all, this is one of the main ways of ensuring a non-handicapped population.

INFUSION THERAPY AND ADMINISTRATION OF ANTIBIOTICS

Infusion therapy

The composition and amount of the infusion fluid must be close to the newborn infant's requirements as regards the supply of calories, water and electrolytes, which depend on body stocks and the rate of their release. When administering fluids, certain specific features of the neonatal period should be taken into account:

The state of water and electrolyte balance immediately after birth varies, even in infants with the same birthweight. Differences in the length of gestation, placental function, amniotic fluid turnover (swallowing and excretion by the foetus) and the size of placental transfusion produce differences in body composition and particularly in the water content. With advancing maturity, the water content per kg body weight falls. The greater amount of water in the body of immature neonates does not mean that they are better protected against dehydration, however.

In the newborn infant, the excretory function of the placenta is taken over by the kidney, whose complex mechanisms keep the volume and composition of the extracellular fluid relatively stable. Although various comparisons with older infants are unfavourable to the function of the neonatal kidney, under normal conditions it is entirely adequate. The small, and postnatally improving, renal blood supply and changes in its distribution in the kidney seem to be a no less significant factor in the explanation of the partial functional imperfection of the kidney after birth than its formerly emphasized morphological immaturity (e.g. the thickness of the glomerular epithelium, the shortness of Henle's loop, etc.).

Water and electrolytes are lost both via the kidney and extrarenally, in the latter case primarily by insensible perspiration. After birth, extrarenal water losses are more important and, according to our findings, on the first two days of life they are about 5 times higher than renal losses. On subsequent days they amount to over 20 ml/kg/24 hours. Urinary sodium excretion is low in this phase and usually does not exceed $0.5-1$ mEq/kg/24 hours.

The diluting capacity of the kidneys is good, but excretion of a single oral water load is limited, especially on the first three days of life. If isotonic glucose is administered in a dose of 3% body weight, only about 10% is excreted in 2 hours. This capacity rapidly improves and by the end of the first week it equals that at one month. The administration route also plays a role, since diuresis is somewhat greater after intravenous than after oral administration. Slow infusion is tolerated better and the newborn infant is able to excrete a dose as much as 200 ml/kg/24 hours.

The newborn infant's concentrating capacity, with different dehydration methods, attains values of $600-800$ m Osm/l; this is lower than in older infants, but the newborn infant, in normal circumstances, does not need such a fully maximum concentrating capacity. During the first days, water losses are mainly extrarenal, so that even the most efficient concentrating capacity would mean the saving of only a little water. Catabolism places greater osmolar load on the kidneys and a larger amount of water is thus needed for excretion; at the same time, the influence of growth, which helps to maintain a steady state through raised incorporation of proteins and electrolytes, is absent.

The ability of the kidneys to excrete a salt load is another important aspect. Raised salt intake tests showed that the neonatal kidney assures better salt retention than excretion. A raised sodium intake leads to expansion of the extracellular fluid, with a sudden weight increment and often manifest oedema. A rapid infusion of hypotonic saline and, in particular, the infusion of hyperosmolar solutions ($NaHCO_3$ or amino acid solutions) also causes expansion of the extracellular fluid in the newborn infant. This is followed by natriuresis, for whose mechanism no entirely satisfactory explanation has so far been found (Fig. 24).

Attempts to induce acute sodium loss, with diminution of extracellular fluid volume, by means of the diuretic Fursemide showed that the newborn infant

168

is unable to compensate these losses by raised sodium retention as rapidly as infants over the age of one month. The newborn infant seems to be protected against an abnormal increase in the amount of extracellular fluid better

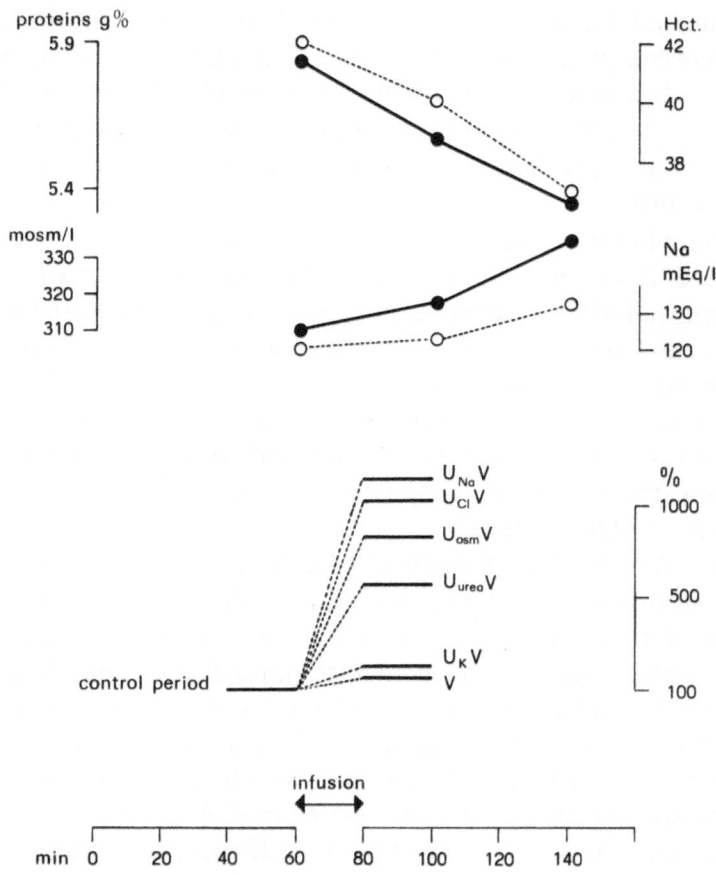

Fig. 24. Changes in protein and sodium concentration, haematocrit and osmolarity of serum after infusing a single dosis 10 ml/kg of amino acids (top part of the Figure). Changes in urine flow and in Na, Cl and urea excretion ($U_{Na}V$, $U_{Cl}V$, $U_{urea}V$) and osmolarity ($U_{osm}V$) are compared with control period.

than against a decrease. It should be emphasized that the kidney's primary task is to excrete surplus water, electrolytes and other substances and that intake mechanisms must exist for coping with the resultant deficiency. The reabsorptive, conserving function of the kidney can slow down the rate of dehydration, but it cannot lead to rehydration (Janovský et al. 1970).

In pathological states in which, for various reasons, the infant cannot be fed via the gastrointestinal tract, we use today permanent intravenous infusion by means of an infusion pump. Its purpose is to maintain or rectify impaired water-electrolyte balance in the milieu intérieur and provide caloric requirements, at least in part. From the above specific features of the maintenance of a water and salt steady state in the newborn infant, we can derive certain general rules for the administration of fluids during this period.

(1) In the first days of life there is no need to maintain an absolutely steady balance between water and electrolyte intake and loss and we need only prevent manifest biochemical and clinical signs of dehydration. Except for a decrease in circulating blood volume, when the administration of plasma or blood is indicated, there is no need for rapid correction and attainment of normal values.

(2) Sodium losses on the first days after birth are negligible and need not be compensated. Abnormally high losses in the gastrointestinal secretions during vomiting and diarrhoea and urinary losses in the "salt-losing syndrome" are exceptions. Even the physiological newborn infant has a negative sodium balance during the first days of life.

(3) The composition of the solution is today dictated by the desire to cover the newborn infant's energy requirements and to reduce catabolism by the early administration of $10-15\%$ glucose, rather than to maintain exact water and electrolyte balance.

The amount of fluid and the rate of its administration are modified to suit the newborn infant's condition; although, with slow infusion, a newborn infant with intact circulatory and renal function can tolerate relatively large doses, we do not consider it expedient to administer more fluid than 100 ml/kg per 24 hours. In the first day of life, half that amount is sufficient.

During the first three days, therefore, all we need do is replace water and calories by administering $10-15\%$ glucose. $NaHCO_3$ is added only to correct severe acidosis. On subsequent days we must replace salt losses, which for sodium, chlorides and potassium amount, under normal conditions, to 0.5 to 2 mEq/kg/24 hours. We recommend administering sodium and potassium in a concentration of 2 mEq/100 ml glucose solution.

(4) Care should be taken when using solutions with a high osmolar concentration, since they can cause sudden water shifts associated with the danger of cerebral haemorrhage. The chief amongst these are $NaHCO_3$ and amino acid solutions, whose osmolarity is about 6 times greater than that of plasma.

(5) In pathological states of the newborn infant, a low urine flow is usually due to poor renal blood flow from circulatory failure. In these infants, we must reckon with narrowing of the range between the minimum and maximum toleration limit for electrolytes and water. Compensation of circulatory failure is accompanied by improvement of renal function. The kidney condition is

thus secondary and does not, as a rule, require specific treatment (diuretics, osmotically active solutions).

(6) It is a good thing to try placing the newborn infant on oral nutrition as soon as possible. The regulative influence of the diet has also a beneficial effect on the acid-base balance. If parenteral nutrition is still necessary after the first week of life, it is best to administer the infusion into a large vein through an indwelling catheter and to modify the composition of the solution.

Usual infant management cannot be used for the newborn infant, especially as regards rehydration therapy for infantile diarrhoea. We cannot draw up a scheme for the parenteral administration of fluids which would be valid for all pathological newborn infants, who differ in respect of their body composition, body water content, metabolism and magnitude of losses caused by the basic disease.

The simplest aid for evaluating hydration during an infusion is to weigh the infant regularly and supplement this by urine collection. The composition and rate of the infusion are modified according to the amount and composition of the urine and weight changes. The administration of an excess amount of fluid is avoided by following weight and the urine flow, together with circulatory function and the state of hydration of the subcutaneous tissues. Monitoring of serum electrolytes and osmolarity is a valuable aid.

When administering fluids to newborn infants intravenously, we must always proceed individually and keep a sensitive balance between the two extreme states endangering the newborn infant, i.e. dehydration and an excess supply of fluids, with expansion of the extracellular fluid, an overloaded circulation and even water intoxication. Experience shows the latter situation (the danger of over-hydration) to be the commoner. We must rid ourselves of the idea that the administration of an excess amount of fluids can improve the viability and prognosis for the jeopardised newborn infant.

Administration of antibiotics

Parenteral fluid administration can also be utilized for treating infections, by giving antibiotics with the infusion.

For prevention (which we now restrict as far as possible) and for instituting treatment until the results of the bacteriological tests are known, the following antibiotics are today the most suitable:

(1) Ampiclox neonatal, 1 vial (containing 50 mg ampicillin and 25 mg cloxacillin) i.v. or i.m. 4–6 times daily, or

(2) Kanamycin, 7.5 mg/kg twice daily together with ampicillin (50 to 100 mg/kg/day) or with crystalline penicillin (150,000 – 300,000 units daily)

in three doses. The disadvantage of the latter combination is that kanamycin cannot be given intravenously. The isolated use of ampicillin does not protect newborn infants against *Staphylococcus aureus* infections.

In a demonstrated *S. aureus* infection, Ampiclox treatment can be succeeded by cloxacillin in the same dose. Among anti-staphylococcal antibiotics, lincomycin (10 mg/kg/day in 2 doses, i.m. or i.v.) and cephalosporins are very effective. About 80% of *S. aureus* strains are still sensitive to erythromycin.

In Gram-negative bacterial infections, which are the commonest today in the neonatal period (about 2/3 of all infections), ampicillin is relatively effective and the least toxic (it does not act on *Pseudomonas aeruginosa*, most *Proteus* strains and about 50% of *E. coli* strains). For more serious infections we can use Polymyxin E (Colistin, Colimycin) 2−4 mg/kg, twice daily, i.m.), for *Pseudomonas aeruginosa* infections carbenicillin (Pyopen) (100−300 mg/kg/day, 3−4 doses daily), or the wide spectrum antibiotic gentamicin (2−6 mg/kg/day, 2 doses daily), which is relatively the most toxic of all the antibiotics named here.

A combination of carbenicillin and gentamicin is sometimes satisfactory for *Pseudomonas aeruginosa* infections, while gentamicin combined with cephalosporins has the widest antibacterial spectrum. At present we have no experience with the administration of tobramycin in newborn infants.

When administering antibiotics in the neonatal period we must observe certain principles:

(1) Their prophylactic administration should be avoided as far as possible and they should be used only after careful deliberation.

(2) When administering them intravenously with an infusion pump, we should always, first of all, give a priming dose by i.v. (or i.m.) injection to form a high antibiotic level rapidly in the body fluids.

(3) We must reckon with slower degradation and excretion of the antibiotic, particularly in the following newborn infants: extremely immature, with a circulatory disturbance, in shock, with a low urine flow. In these cases it is sufficient to administer antibiotics (especially semisynthetic penicillins only twice daily.

(4) When treating infections, the choice of antibiotics must always be based on the results of bacteriological tests, particularly tests of bacterial sensitivity to antibiotics.

DIAGNOSTIC VALUES AND THERAPEUTIC DOSES

Tables 43a,b and c give the values of the most important indexes for auxiliary diagnostic purposes in the first hours of the infant's life. The values of the indexes 1 – 12 and 22 – 29 come from the laboratories of the Institute for Care of Mother and Child, Podolí, Prague. The values of the indexes 13 and 14 are taken from Usher et al. (Acta paediat. scand. *52*, 497, 1963), 15 – 21 from Achary and Payne (Arch. Dis. Child. *40*, 430, 1965) and 40 – 47 from Wolff and Goodfellows (Paediatrics *16*, 753, 1955).

In the survey of therapeutic doses for newborn infants, we have given only the most important in practice and most commonly used drugs, omitting antibiotics, which were discussed in the preceding chapter ("Infusion therapy and antibiotics"). A detailed pharmacopoeia of the neonatal period will be found in the 3rd edition of Schaffer and Avery's textbook "Diseases of the newborn", published by the Saunders Co., Philadelphia, London, Toronto, 1971.

Therapeutic doses for newborn infants

ACTH i.m., 3 – 5 units/kg/day in 4 doses.

ADRENALINE s.c., 1 : 1,000 aqueous solution, 0.01/kg, if necessary repeat dose after 2 – 3 hours.

ALBUMIN i.v., 1 g/kg, slowly. Danger of hypervolaemia.

BLOOD, whole, i.v., 10 ml/kg, red cells i.v., 5 ml/kg.

CALCIUM GLUCONATE i.v., 0.5 – 1 g/kg/day in 3 doses. 10% solution. Danger of bradycardia if administered quickly. P.o., 0.5 – 1 g 2 – 4 times daily as 5% solution.

CORTISONE p.o., 0.5–2 mg/kg/day in 4 doses. Danger of spread of infection.

DARAPRIM i.v., 0.05 mg/kg/day, together with folic acid (10 mg i.m.) because of toxicity.

DIGITOXIN p.o., i.v., 0.025 mg (25 µg)/kg in 3 – 6 doses at 6-hour intervals.

SILVER NITRATE as 1% solution for disinfecting eyes. Solution in delivery theatre should be changed for fresh every 3 days.

FIBRINOGEN i.v., 50 mg/kg. Repeat only after checking clotting time.

GAMMA GLOBULIN i.m., preventively 0.22 ml/kg. For agammaglobulinaemia 1 ml/kg every 2 – 4 weeks.

GENTIAN VIOLET locally, as 1% aqueous solution.

GLUCAGONE i.m., i.v., 100 – 300 µg/kg, repeat after 6 – 12 hours.

HEPARIN i.v., 40 units/kg, maintaining dose 100 units/kg every 4 hours, with check of clotting time. Danger of haemorrhage.

HYDROCORTISONE p.o., 3 – 10 mg/kg/day in 4 doses. I.m. or i.v., 25 to 50 mg every 6 hours.

METHYLENE BLUE for methaemoglobinaemia, 0.1 – 0.2 ml/kg of 1% solution, slowly.

MYCOSTATIN p.o., 100 – 200 thousand units every 6 hours; locally, 2% solution 3 – 4 times daily.

NALLINE (Nalorphine) i.m., i.v., 0.1 – 0.2 mg/kg per dose.

OPHTHALMOSEPTONEX for disinfecting eyes, 1 drop into each eye; 10 ml bottle can be used in delivery theatre until empty.

PHENOBARBITAL p.o., i.m., 8 – 12 mg/kg/day in 4 – 6 doses.

PLASMA i.v., 20 ml/kg.

PREDNISONE p.o., 1 – 3 mg/kg/day in 4 doses.

PROSTIGMINE i.m., 0.5 – 1 mg every 4 – 6 hours. P.o., 1 – 5 mg every 4 – 8 hours.

SEPTONEX for general and biological disinfection as 2 per mille aqueous solution. Stock solution in neonatal department in 1% concentration (10 g powder/1 l water).

SODIUM BICARBONATE for correcting acidosis, 8.4% solution. For dosage see p. 196.

THAM, 0.3 molar solution in dose of 1 ml/kg for every 0.1 pH unit below 7.4. I.v., 1 ml/min.

Vitamin A p.o., preventively, 600 – 1,000 units/day.

Vitamin B_1 (thiamine), preventively 0.5 – 1 mg p.o., therapeutically 10 mg every 6 – 8 hours i.m.

Vitamin B_6 (pyridoxine), preventively 100 μg/1 l feed p.o., therapeutically 2 – 5 mg/day p.o.

Vitamin B complex, 1 ml into i.v. drip or i.m., premature infants 3 × 2 drops daily.

Vitamin C (ascorbic acid), preventively 25 – 50 – 100 mg/day p.o., therapeutically 100 mg i.m. every 4 hours.

Vitamin D, preventively 400 units/day p.o.

Vitamin K_1, preventively 1 – 2 mg i.m. (1 dose only), therapeutically 2.5 – 5 mg i.m. every 6 – 12 hours, checking prothrombin time.

Table 43a. Diagnostic test values. A: Normal values in capillary blood of term neonates

No.	Index	Symbol	Umbilical		1 hour	12 hours	24 hours	48 hours	72 hours	7 days
			vein	artery						
1	Glucose (enzymatically) mg%	G	67 ±22		26 ±16		35 ±15	42 ±14	48 ±17	
2	Lactate mg%	L	26 m = 1.9	27 m = 1.8	30 m = 1.3	27 m = 0.8	26 m = 2.1	23 m = 0.8	22 m = 0.5	23 m = 0.9
3	Pyruvate mg%	P	1.7 m = 0.16	1.7 m = 0.19	2.6 m = 0.07	2.4 m = 0.08	2.3 m = 0.09	2.2 m = 0.04	2.2 m = 0.04	2.2 m = 0.05
4	L/P quotient	L/P	15.4	15.4	11.3	11.5	11	10.5	10	10.2
5	Excess lactate mg%	XL			4 m = 0.7	3.5 m = 0.8	3.7 m = 1.2	1.9 m = 0.5	0.5 m = 0.2	1.3 m = 0.3
6	Bilirubin mg%		1.69				4.7	5.9	7.8	
7	pH	pH	7.27 m = 0.04	7.23 m = 0.01	7.33 m = 0.09	7.38 m = 0.01	7.38 m = 0.009	7.39 m = 0.06	7.41 m = 0.007	7.41 m = 0.04
8	P_{CO_2} tension mmHg	P_{CO_2}	33.6	40.5	39.7 m = 1.9	35.2 m = 1.5	33.3 m = 1.1	32.2 m = 1.1	31 m = 2.3	34.3 m = 1.4
9	Negative base excess mEq/l	BE	–10.1	–10.3	–5.5 m = 0.4	–3.5 m = 0.4	–4.1 m = 0.4	–4.2 m = 0.5	–3.2 m = 0.6	–2.5 m = 0.5
10	Stand. bicarbonate mEq/l	st. bic.	16.5	16.9	19.7 m = 0.3	21.4 m = 0.4	20.7 m = 0.3	20.7 m = 0.4	21.5 m = 0.5	21.9 m = 0.4
11	Non-esterified fatty acids mEq/l	NEFA	0.26 m = 0.04		0.73 m = 0.08	1.24 m = 0.08	1.05 m = 0.09			
12	Haemoglobin g%	Hgb	15.2	15.3	19.4 m = 0.3	19 m = 0.6	17.4 m = 0.5	18.8 m = 0.4	18.7 m = 0.3	17.3 m = 0.4

No.	Index	Symbol	Umbilical vein	Umbilical artery	1 hour	12 hours	24 hours	48 hours	72 hours	7 days
13	Haematocrit after clamping cord immediately %	Htc	after 30 min: after 4 hours:		47.3 + 2 47.9 ± 2.3		43.6 ±2		43.8 ±1.3	
14	Haematocrit after clamping cord after 5 minutes %	Htc	after 30 min: after 4 hours:		59.2 ± 1.5 64.1 ± 1.5		61.5 ±1.5		60.3 ±1.4	

Table 43a (cont.)

No.	Index	Symbol	Umbilical blood	1 – 12 hours	12 – 24 hours	24 – 48 hours	48 – 72 hours
15	Sodium mEq/l	Na	147 126 – 166	143 124 – 156	145 132 – 159	148 134 – 160	149 139 – 162
16	Potassium mEq/l	K	7.8	6.4 5.6 – 12	6.3 5.3 – 7.3	6 5.2 – 7.3	5.9 5 – 7.7
17	Chloride mEq/l	Cl	103 98 – 110	100.7 90 – 111	103 87 – 114	102 92 – 114	103 93 – 112
18	Calcium mg%	Ca	9.3 8.2 – 11.1	8.4 7.3 – 9.2	7.8 6.9 – 9.4	8 6.1 – 9.9	7.9 5.9 – 9.7
19	Phosphorus mg%	P	5.6 3.7 – 8.1	6.1 3.5 – 8.6.	5.7 2.9 – 8.1	5.9 3 – 8.7	5.8 2.8 – 7.6
20	Urea mg%	Ur	29 21 – 40	27 8 – 34	33 9 – 63	32 14 – 77	31 13 – 68
21	Total protein mg%	Prot.	6.1 4.8 – 7.3	6.6 5.6 – 8.5	6.6 5.8 – 8.2	6.9 5.9 – 8.2	7.2 6 – 8.5

Table 43b. B. Normal ventilation values and BP in term neonates

No.	Index	Symbol	1 hour	12 hours	24 hours	48 hours	72 hours	7 days
22	O_2 consumption, ml/kg/min	$\dot{V}_{O_2}$	6.3 m = 0.46	6 m = 0.42	7.3 m = 0.51	6.6 m = 0.4	9.2 m = 1.14	8 m = 0.71
23	CO_2 output, ml/kg/min	$\dot{V}_{CO_2}$	4.6 m = 0.33	4.5 m = 0.27	5.5 m = 0.33	5 m = 0.28	6.4 m = 0.87	6.3 m = 0.49
24	Respiratory quotient	RQ	0.75 m = 0.03	0.76 m = 0.03	0.75 m = 0.02	0.75 m = 0.02	0.68 m = 0.01	0.81 m = 0.03
25	Vol. per cent oxygen	vol.% O_2	17 m = 0.9	16 m = 0.8	17 m = 0.9	18 m = 0.5	19 m = 0.6	19 m = 0.7
26	Minute ventilation, ml/min	MV	808 m = 51	751 m = 31	903 m = 59	907 m = 56	834 m = 81	995 m = 66
27	Tidal volume, ml	TV	13 m = 0.9	14 m = 0.7	17 m = 1.2	15 m = 1.1	17 m = 1.6	17 m = 1.6
28	Respiration frequency	f/min	63 m = 2.3	55 m = 2.7	56 m = 1.9	56 m = 2.2	51 m = 2.2	53 m = 1.4
29	Systolic blood pressure, mmHg	BP	79 68 – 110		78 64 – 102		82 66 – 106	97 72 – 120

Table 43c. Haematological values: (1) in neonates with birthweight of less than 1,200 g

No.	Index	Symbol	1 – 3 days	4 – 7 days	2 weeks	4 weeks	6 weeks	8 weeks
30	Haemoglobin	Hgb	15.6	16.4	15.5	11.3	8.5	7.8
31	Reticulocytes	Rtc	8.4	3.9	1.9	4.1	5.4	6.1
32	Thrombocytes	Thr	148 th.	163 th.	162 th.	158 th.	210 th.	212 th.
33	Leucocytes	Le	14.8 th.	12.2 th.	15.8 th.	13.2 th.	10.8 th.	9.9 th.
34	Segments	Se	46	32	41	28	23	23
35	Band cells	BC	10.7	9.7	8	5.9	5.8	4.4
36	Lymphocytes	Ly	32	43	39	55	61	65
37	Monocytes	Mo	5	7	5	4	6	3
38	Eosinophils	Eo	0.4	6.2	1	3.7	2	3.8

Table 43c (cont.) (2) in neonates with birthweight of 1,200 – 1,500 g

No.	Index	Symbol	1 – 3 days	4 – 7 days	2 weeks	4 weeks	6 weeks	8 weeks
39	Haemoglobin	Hgb	20.2	18	17.1	12	9.1	8.3
40	Reticulocytes	Rtc	2.7	1.2	0.9	1	2.2	2.7
41	Thrombocytes	Thr	151 th.	134 th.	153 th.	198 th.	212 th.	244 th.
42	Leucocytes	Le	10.8 th.	8.9 th.	14.3 th.	11 th.	10.5 th.	9.1 th.
43	Segments	Se	47	31	33	26	20	25
44	Band cells	BC	11.9	10.5	5.9	3	1.4	2.1
45	Lymphocytes	Ly	34	48	52	59	69	64
46	Monocytes	Mo	3	6	3	4	5	5
47	Eosinophils	Eo	1.3	2.2	2.5	5.1	2.6	2.3

179

PROGNOSIS FOR "HIGH RISK" NEONATES

The outcome of perinatal risk for the newborn infant can be:

(1) death of the foetus or newborn infant (perinatal mortality),

(2) survival with a permanent injury or developmental disorder (perinatal morbidity),

(3) survival with normal development.

Perinatal mortality has long been studied as an important index of the level of mother and child care, but it is only relatively recently that the great health and economic significance of permanent defects acquired in the perinatal period has been recognized and analysed. Developmental disturbances originating in the early stages of pregnancy, which include the vast majority of congenital developmental defects, can involve any organ or function, while in perinatal injury it is almost always the central nervous system which is affected. The reason for this is the exceptionally high susceptibility of nervous tissue to a deficiency of energy obtained by the oxidation of carbohydrates, on which the main pathogenic factors of the perinatal period − hypoxia, acidosis, hypoglycaemia and hyperbilirubinaemia − have a negative effect. The injury is thus mainly metabolic, at cell level, and seldom of mechanical or infectious origin. Furthermore, the regenerative capacity of nervous tissue in the postnatal period is very limited and structural changes tend to be permanent. In subsequent development, the afflicted children can display signs forming a syndrome usually defined as a perinatal encephalopathy or, in milder cases, as mild cerebral dysfunction. In such cases we may find the following anomalies:

(1) locomotor disturbances (hypotonic, hypertonic, extrapyramidal syndrome),

(2) subnormal intelligence,

(3) behaviour disturbances,

(4) disturbances of sensory function (deafness, retinopathies, refraction defects),

(5) convulsions.

The extent and gravity of all these defects vary from borderline states to severe disability and may be combined in varying ways. Injury to other organs (kidneys, gastrointestinal tract, liver) can also occur in the perinatal period, but its role in the child's subsequent development is far less important. Long-term retardation of body growth was demonstrated in some infants with a low birthweight (Poláček and Syrovátka 1976).

Numerous recent follow-up studies have given more accurate insight into the importance of perinatal pathogenic factors for long-term development, but estimation of the individual prognosis while the infant is in hospital remains difficult. We take into account primarily the following three of prenatal data:

(1) the mother's history, including the result of previous pregnancies,

(2) risk factors during pregnancy, and

(3) labour-induced stress.

We also pay attention to

(4) evaluation of the infant's state immediately after birth (usually expressed as the Apgar score). A low score after 1 minute may by an expression of temporary depression in the last phase of expulsion and if it does not persist, its prognostic significance is but small. A marked drop in the score (below 7 points) after 5, and especially 10, minutes can be associated with permanent changes in nervous activity.

The evaluation of prenatal risk and the Apgar score gives only the statistical probability of permanent lesions and does not allow exact conclusions in individual cases. More reliable in this respect is

(5) study of the clinical, and particularly the neurological findings in the infant during the first days or weeks of life. The gravidity and persistence of anomalies are an important, though not absolutely reliable, guide for individual evaluation of the infant's later development. Mild and evidently functional involvement of the central nervous system is manifested after birth as temporary depression of nervous activity. In more serious cases, depression is followed by manifest pathological signs:

(1) disturbances of muscular tone (hypotonia, hypertonia, spasms),

(2) reactivity disorders (hyperexcitability to gross tremor, or, conversely, apathy and, in the severest cases, a comatose state, with the disappearance of any response to external stimuli).

In addition we may find disturbances of automatic functions, lung ventilation, sucking, swallowing or sleep, which can be a cause of death.

The longer the persistence of acute signs after birth, the greater the probability that they are an expression of structural and irreparable damage to nervous tissue. If the findings become normal within 24 hours, the prognosis is usually good. Persistence for three days may be associated with signs of delayed motor development in subsequent months, although these generally tend to improve. The persistence of neurological findings for more than 7 – 10 days is very serious and is evidence of permanent lesions. These conclusions apply chiefly to term neonates born with signs of damage and are less reliable for premature infants.

The prognosis for infants born to mothers with diabetes mellitus depends primarily on the level of antenatel care and less on the quality of postnatal care. If the mother's diabetes is well compensated, the duration of pregnancy need not be significantly shortened and diabetic foetopathies do not develop.

In these cases, the prognosis is not different from the prognosis for term neonates in general and it can be evaluated by the same criteria, i.e. by a drop in the Apgar score (especially after 10 min) and by the persistence of neurological anomalies in the first postnatal days. The prognosis for infants born prematurely to mothers with diabetes is uncertain and the proportion of cases of motor retardation and permanent injury is high.

The prognosis for infants with acute signs of nuclear jaundice is fundamentally poor, because destruction of the nerve cells is irreversible. A latent phase is followed by signs of retarded motor development with mainly extrapyramidal features (especially choreoathetosis). The extent of the trauma varies considerably, from mild locomotor lesions to complete locomotor incapacitation. Its gravity can be estimated only approximately in the postnatal period and, in particular, it is impossible to detect injury of the nucleus of the VIIIth nerve and resultant hearing disorder.

Evaluation of the prognosis for low birthweight infants in the postnatal period is even more difficult than for term infants. Apart from risk factors acting during pregnancy and labour, their postnatal state can be complicated by an adaptation crisis in which they are negatively influenced by hypoxia, acidosis, hyperbilirubinaemia and, last but not least, starvation. These postnatal adverse factors can undoubtedly be a primary cause of central nervous system injury, or can aggravate existing lesions. It has been generally demonstrated that the statistical probability of central nervous injury increases with shortening of pregnancy and with lower birthweight, even on separate evaluation of the two criteria. In a group of children with a birthweight of 1,500 g and under, born in our institute, at the age of 3 years we found a perinatal encephalopathy in 20%; in some series, the proportion of injured children is significantly higher (40 – 50%). It is virtually impossible to estimate the individual prognosis during the postnatal adaptation phase, but during subsequent weeks, while the premature infant is still in the department, neurological lesions of a permanent character (mainly disturbances of muscular tone) can be determined in afflicted infants. Particularly unfavourable results are found in premature infants with a low-for-gestational-age birthweight, in whom adverse prenatal and postnatal factors potentiate each other.

In summing up, it can be claimed that the possibilities of estimating the later development of nervous and mental functions in high risk infants in the neonatal period are limited. Persistence of the above neurological signs 1 to 2 weeks after birth in term infants, or their appearance within 2 – 3 months in low birthweight infants, is almost always a sign of a perinatal encephalopathy. On the other hand, findings of minor muscular tone and postural reflex anomalies, or mild degrees of motor retardation, as a rule, tend largely to improve in later months.

182

Subtle mental and behavioural disorders and disturbances of sensory functions cannot be foreseen in newborn infants. This means that the neurological and psychological development of high risk infants must be followed up, since reliable conclusions cannot be reached for 2 – 3 years and sometimes not until the child is of school age. The best time, frequency and methods for this control of high risk children in field practice is still under discussion, and likewise the question of rehabilitation methods is not completely settled.

CATEGORIES OF „HIGH RISK" NEONATES

THE ASPHYXIATED NEWBORN INFANT

Asphyxia neonatorum is a traditional, though not absolutely accurate, term applied to respiratory disorders at birth, associated with hypoxaemia (cyanosis) and hypoxia manifested mainly in depression of nervous functions (atonia, areflexia). A newborn infant who fails to make respiratory efforts within 30 seconds, or to breathe rhythmically within 90 seconds, can be described as asphyxiated.

Asphyxia neonatorum is a syndrome having various causes. It can be divided into two main groups:

I. central, i.e. primary depression of respiratory centres in the medulla oblongata, resulting from

(1) by far the most frequently, intrauterine hypoxia of the fetus, of varying gravity and duration,

(2) anaesthesia or analgesia during labour,

(3) rarely, trauma affecting the CNS.

II. peripheral, i.e. postnatal impairment of the brain oxygen supply, which can be caused by

(1) impaired pulmonary aeration and ventilation (obstruction of the air passages and lungs, congenital developmental defects of the lungs and chest, diaphragmatic hernia, pleural exudate, etc.),

(2) cardiovascular dysfunction (congenital cardiac defects, shock),

(3) haematogenic factors (severe anaemia of the foetus).

Each of these factors can cause a delay in, or inadequacy or absence of, the onset of breathing and, moreover, several can operate simultaneously. Whatever the primary cause, the result is always a decrease in the blood oxygen content and the development of respiratory and metabolic acidosis. These changes aggravate the depression of respiratory centres, with further deterioration of pulmonary ventilation. If the resultant vicious circle is not broken, the infant dies.

Clinical gravity is today estimated almost solely by a scoring system (usually Apgar's) evaluating five clinical features (heart rate, respiratory effort, muscle tone, reflex response and skin colour) 1, 5 and 10 minutes after complete delivery (Tab. 44).

Table 44. Apgar scoring

Sign	0	Evaluation		Minutes		
		1	2	1	5	10
Heart rate	Absent	Below 100	Over 100			
Respiratory effort	Absent	Slow, irregular	Good, crying			
Muscle tone	Limp	Flexion of extremities	Active motion			
Response to catheter	No response	Grimace	Crying, cough			
Colour	Blue, pale	Extremities blue	Pink			
			Sum			

The most important of these five features is the heart rate and respiratory effort. The absence of cardiac activity denotes clinical death, a drop in the heart rate below 100/min is a reliable sign of asphyxia, while an increase to over 100/min is usually the first sign of recovery. The evaluation of respiratory effort is less conclusive; if the infant does not breathe, we often cannot tell whether it is suffering from primary or secondary apnoea, the prognosis for which is very different. The three remaining features complete the picture, but they may be due to other factors, such as cold, sedation or immaturity. The score at 1 minute is an index of asphyxia and of the need for an active approach; the score at 5 or 10 minutes is more reliable as an index of likely death or permanent damage.

The clinical picture of postnatal asphyxia, of any origin, is dominated by disturbances of pulmonary ventilation, which can vary from a mild delay in the onset of breathing to the picture of clinical death. An experienced assessment may nevertheless reveal subtle differences in its course, allowing the detection of less common causes of respiratory failure.

Asphyxia neonatorum is by far most frequently a continuation of intra-uterine hypoxia, which, in turn, may be the result of a whole series of obstetrical complications. Acute hypoxia has four phases. The first is raised respiratory activity, often terminating in convulsive movements. This is followed by relatively brief respiratory arrest, i.e. primary apnoea, during which the infant may recover without active assistance. The third phase is gasping, very different in appearance from normal, rhythmical breathing and lasting about 10 minutes. The last phase is terminal respiratory arrest, or, "secondary" apnoea, which ends with the cessation of heart action if effective treatment is not undertaken. The heart rate, and then the blood pressure, fall during primary apnoea.

It can be definitely assumed that these findings in experimental animals are capable of general application, although the clinical circumstances in human infants are more complex. The appearance or duration of the individual phases of hypoxia is strongly influenced by a number of subsidiary factors, e.g. the duration and depth of prenatal hypoxia, the development of maturity and general health of the infant, medication of the mother, etc. Individually, the infant's clinical state after birth is determined by the phase of hypoxia in which delivery is completed. Secondary apnoea is particularly serious; the longer its duration after the last gasp, the longer the time needed for recovery, and hence the greater the risk of injury.

The influence of general anaesthesia and analgesia of the mother is manifested, in the newborn infant, in prolongation of primary apnoea and the onset of rapid, very superficial and barely perceptible breathing. Muscle hypotonia is another characteristic, especially if the mother has been given relaxants. Pharmacological inhibition of respiration must, of course, be born in mind in surgical delivery with general anaesthesia; this is often indicated in cases complicated by foetal hypoxia and it may be difficult to distinguish between the two causes of respiratory failure.

Inhibited respiration caused by mechanical trauma in the form of cerebral haemorrhage or spinal cord injury is now very rare. It should be considered if, after a difficult labour, the infant is delivered in a state of shock, with superficial and irregular breathing which is not improved by active resuscitation. These infants often die despite transitory establishment of pulmonary ventilation.

If respiratory failure is more peripheral in origin, some degree of pulmonary ventilation is usually established, but gaseous exchange in the lungs is inadequate and signs of general hypoxia persist.

Obturation of the airways and aspiration of the amniotic sac contents into the lungs can cause respiratory embarrassment, but the real importance of these factors is hard to evaluate and is probably overestimated. During delivery, the fluid is expelled from the airways by compression of the thorax in the birth canal and is replaced by air during recoil of the thorax after birth. Moreover, the viscosity of the amniotic fluid is many times greater than that of air and very long respiratory effort in the liquid medium is needed before the fluid reaches the lungs.

Rarely, congenital malformations of the lungs or thorax are a cause of respiratory failure, the commonest being diaphragmatic hernia. In severe cases, extrauterine life cannot be maintained even when gasping continues for some time, but milder cases can be saved by operation.

Congenital heart diseases, such as transposition of the large blood vessels and other severe anomalies, may cause respiratory disturbances. Respiration can usually be established, but signs of inadequate oxygenation of the blood persist or intensify and further examination will reveal underlying pathological conditions.

Severe anaemia at birth may be due to advanced haemolysis of foetal red cells through the action of maternal antibodies. Where isoimmunization was ascertained during pregnancy, the diagnosis is easy. Severe blood losses caused by different types of haemorrhage are rare, but they are dangerous and require early treatment (blood transfusion). In a pale newborn infant it may be difficult to distinguish between severe anaemia and asphyxia with shock; with the former, breathing usually starts adequately, but the signs of life are feeble and the condition deteriorates.

The prevention of intrauterine asphyxia is a basic obstetrical problem in which considerable successes have been achieved in recent years, largely owing to technical progress. The results of postnatal care of the asphyxiated newborn infant depend in large measure on the level of prenatal care of the endangered foetus.

Resuscitation of the newborn infant is indicated if it does not display inspiratory effort within 30 seconds of birth, or does not breathe regularly within 1 – 2 minutes. As prenatally a drop in the heart rate below 100/min is a reliable sign of asphyxia requiring active resuscitation and continuing bradycardia a sign of continued danger. Modern resuscitation methods are simple and relatively effective but they should, of course, be applied as sparingly as possible.

Patent airways are maintained by suction clearance of the mouth, pharynx and nose (and if need be the stomach), using a suction flask or other suitable instrument. Clearing the airways is logically the first step in postnatal care and is a routine measure for practically every newborn infant, although in our opinion its importance is sometimes overestimated. The onset of the respiratory movements often observed after aspiration clearance of the upper air passages is rather the result of intensive reflex stimulation and failure of this manoeuvre is actually a sign of inhibition of nerve reflexes and a reason for continuing resuscitation.

Intubation of the trachea is indicated only when laryngoscopy shows that it is blocked by semi-solid or viscous matter. In our experience it is required in exceptional circumstances only, especially if the level of obstetrical care is good.

The administration of oxygen is the method of choice for treating asphyxia. Its aim is to raise the P_{O_2} in the arterial blood and tissues, with a simultaneous decrease in pulmonary vascular resistance. In the presence of some respiratory movements, oxygen can simply be inhaled through a mask, but the effectiveness of this technique obviously depends on spontaneous respiratory capacity.

With apnoeic infants, positive pressure ventilation must be instituted by means of a resuscitation apparatus ensuring that intraalveolar pressure does not exceed the safety limit. The initial pressure required to expend the lungs is relatively high, i.e. $30-35$ cm H_2O, but after the first inflation it can be reduced. Pure oxygen, which has been shown to be harmless over a short period, is generally employed, but some hospitals use a mixture containing $40-60\%$ oxygen, with equally good results. The surest way to inflate the lungs is by intubation of the upper trachea, but in our experience a well-fitting mask is almost always sufficient. The optimum inflation rate is about 40/min, with a short break after each minute to assess the infant's response. The most satisfactory duration of one inflation is about 1 second. The effect of resuscitation should be controlled from the chest movements and the change in skin colour.

Infusion of alkali. The use of positive pressure ventilation is usually effective in raising the P_{O_2} in the blood, but CO_2 elimination and the restoration of a normal pH after severe asphyxia are rather slow. Correction of the blood pH by the infusion of a base and glucose can greatly improve the infant's condition, particularly during secondary apnoea. If the infant's respiratory effort does not improve within 5 minutes at most, and especially if the heart rate stays below 100/min, $3-4$ ml/kg body weight 8.4% sodium bicarbonate solution, with an equal amount of glucose, should be administered via the umbilical cord, normally through a blunt-ended cannula. This sometimes produces immediate and surprising improvement.

Cardiac massage is carried out if an asphyxiated foetus has been delivered late and the heart has stopped beating. In exceptional cases, cardiac arrest may occur suddenly and unexpectedly. In massage, the left of the sternum is pressed rhytmically to a depth of about 2 cm with two fingers, at a rate of $60-80$/min. It is less commonly known that cardiac massage can be an effective aid when heart action is normal, but arterial pressure is too low and positive pressure ventilation alone has not lead to rapid improvement.

The administration of analeptics such as lobeline or nikethamide has now virtually been abandoned. They have some effect during primary apnoea, in which various other stimuli are also effective, however, and they are explicitly harmful in secondary apnoea, when a positive effect could be most desirable. It is more logical to administer an antidote inhibiting the anaesthetic.

The other techniques and apparatuses recommended or formerly employed are not used, because they are ineffective or actually dangerous.

The infant must be protected against chill during resuscitation, since this increases energy losses. The body temperature of all infants falls slightly after birth, but in protracted resuscitation of a naked, wet infant, it can drop dangerously low. The infant should be dried, covered with heated napkins and warmed by supplementary heaters placed obliquely above the examination table.

As soon as regular respiration has been established, the infant is moved to the pathological neonatal ward, or at least to the observation unit. It is placed in a heated incubator and given oxygen as required. Frequent control of its temperature, its skin blood supply, the number and quality of its breaths and its manifestations of life is essential. The airways produce more secretion after asphyxia and must be frequently cleared by aspiration. The presence and persistence of neurological anomalies are of considerable significance for the long-term prognosis.

THE TRAUMATIZED NEONATE

With the development of obstetrics, gross mechanical traumatization of the newborn infant is declining and in well run institutions it is now very rare.

The mildest forms of trauma include skin injuries, with the possible danger of secondary infection. Subcutaneous haematomas sometimes occur during delivery — most frequently in breech deliveries and premature infants. In extremely immature infants they can culminate in a crush syndrome. As the incidence of protracted births diminishes, transitory pressure deformities of the contact parts of the foetus are disappearing. Necrotic processes in the subcutaneous fat (adiponecrosis subcutanea), subconjunctival or retinal haemorrhages, injury of the sternocleidomastoid (torticollis) and fissures or fractures of the skull are now rare.

Peripheral nerve pareses most often involve the facial nerve and the brachial plexus and less frequently the radial nerve. Involvement of the 5th to 6th cervical nerve root gives rise to upper arm paralysis (Erb-Duchenne), while injury of the 7th to 8th root causes paralysis of the small muscles of the hand and fingers (Klumpke's paralysis). Brachial plexus paralyses can also be associated with diaphragmatic nerve paralyses, in which the diaphragm on the affected side is elevated and immobile.

Peripheral traumata include mechanical injuries of the blood vessels, liver, kidneys, adrenals and spleen and rare mechanical injuries of the heart and lungs. Likewise the organs of respiration can be injured by unsparing resuscitation.

A serious, and usually fatal, form of trauma is intracranial haemorrhage – subdural, subarachnoid, intraventricular (haemocephalus) or into the spinal cord tissue (haemorachis). Intranatal pressure changes can lead to cerebral oedema. Subependymal haemorrhage may not be manifested until rupture into the ventricules occurs; usually this is a complication with infants of a very low birthweight.

Apart from the usual signs of the asphyxia syndrome, marked central signs are also apparent, e.g. restlessness, excitability, spasms and convulsions, or apathy, somnolence and unconsciousness, hypotonia, hypertonia or alternation of these, pallor, cyanosis and intermediate forms, hypothermia and hyperthermia. In severe cases in addition to these disturbances of central regulation, we may find pronounced optic signs, e.g. anisocoria, nystagmus, strabismus, flaccidity of the eyelids, Graefe's sign. The face usually has a mask-like expression and the anterior fontanelle is bulging, spongy and pulsating. Moro's reflex is always impaired and the basic primitive reflexes (sucking, swallowing, grasp) are commonly distinctly abnormal.

In the differential diagnosis we should take tetanus neonatorum, Oppenheim's amyotonia congenita and other congenital CNS defects into account. The treatment is symptomatic and corresponds to resuscitation techniques for asphyxia, with the usual auxiliary examination. Where the neurological signs are unilateral, transillumination of the skull and subdural puncture are indicated.

The use of the vacuum extractor, which has largely replaced forceps in some hospitals, merits special attention. Views on the use of this instrument are very varied and it is hard to make an objective comparison of the advantages and disadvantages of the two methods. The high incidence of local trauma at the site of application of the extractor is generally not regarded as dangerous, although even these minor traumata are liable to secondary infection. Fissures and fractures of the skull, retinal haemorrhages and abnormal EEG recordings have also been described after vacuum extractor delivery. Some workers consider that the incidence of these disturbances is no higher than in forceps delivery, while others prefer properly applied forceps.

190

THE PREMATURE NEONATE

From the time aspect, the criterion of prematurity is birth in the 37th week of gestation or earlier, and from the weight aspect, a birthweight of under 2,500 grammes.

The anatomical and morphological characters and functional maturity of the infant depend mainly on the stage of pregnancy. Body weight and length are less significant when evaluating the degree of maturity. Today it is comparatively easy to distinguish premature from small-for-dates neonates, who, with the same birthweight, are more mature. We are all acquainted with the anatomical signs of immaturity, which include a relatively large, dolicho-cephalic head (about $^1/_3$ the length of the body), fine hair less than 1 cm long, diastasis of the abdominal muscles, a shift in the insertion of the umbilical cord towards the symphysis, a poorly developed subcutaneous fat layer, marked erythema, abundant lanugo, subcutaneous oedema, soft auricular, nasal and cranial cartilages, soft nails not reaching the fingertips, protruding eyes, small nipples, too few sweat glands, undeveloped plantar creases, too few creases on the scrotum, non-descent of the testes in boys and the labia minora not covered by the labia majora in girls.

The signs giving the best correlation with maturity are shown in Table 45 (Usher et al. 1963).

Table 45. Developmental signs of a newborn infant

Lenght of pregnancy in weeks	Up to 36	37 — 38	39 and over
Plantar creases	some transverse in anterior third only	some transverse in anterior two thirds	numerous, over entirety of the sole
Diameter of nipple + areola (mm)	<2	2—4	>4
Hair	fine, downy	fine	rougher, straight
Pinnae	flexible, cartilage not evident	cartilage discernible	tough, cartilage clearly palpable
Testes	in inferior part of canal	just descending	fully descended
Scrotum	small, with few creases	larger, with more creases	large with numerous creases

Functional maturity of organs also correlates with the number of weeks of pregnancy. The presence of vitally important reflexes (sucking, swallowing, cough) and various other functions, e.g. respiration, thermoregulation, depends on the degree of maturity of the CNS. A basal type of respiration (Cheyne-Stokes, gasping) is more common in premature infants. Respiration is further impaired by the immaturity of the lungs themselves (too few alveoli, an incomplete alveolar capillary network, cuboidal epithelium of the alveoli). The intercostal muscles and the diaphragm are underdeveloped and the bones of the chest are soft. Premature infants often have a respiratory distress syndrome, to which persistence of the ductus arteriosus and foramen ovale, a deficient enzymatic apparatus (e.g. carboanhydrase) and absence of the anti-atelectatic factor in the alveoli also contribute. Inadequate O_2 and CO_2 exchange leads to impaired acid-base balance (respiratory acidosis), with accumulation of organic acids (metabolic acidosis). Thermoregulation is very imperfect. In addition to immaturity of central thermoregulation, the imperfect peripheral component of thermoregulation also plays a role (reduced energy supplies, low mucular acitivity, inability to sweat, a thin skin, etc.). The circulatory and blood systems are likewise immature. The capillaries are more permeable and fragile and form a sparse network. The heart is often overloaded. The level of blood-clotting factors (e.g. vitamin K) is also low in premature infants and they have a different response to stress with regards to hormone production and release (e.g. insulin). The RBC count tends to be raised on the first days, from poor hydration (a raised haematocrit), and a raised erythroblast count, anisocytosis, reticulocytosis and polychromasia (caused by immaturity and hypoxia) are more frequently found. The leucocyte count is usually 10,000 – 25,000. The blood protein concentration is lower than in mature neonates.

Low functional capacity of the alimentary tract is manifested in poor sucking and swallowing, regurgitation and subileose states. These are determined by the reflex insufficiency mentioned above and also anatomically (the cardiac sphincter is less developed than the pyloric sphincter, the wall of the stomach and intestine is less muscular and the gastric and intestinal mucosa contain few glands). Premature infants retain less nitrogen and fat from their food than mature and small-for-dates neonates. Immaturity of the liver (mainly enzymatic) is manifested chiefly in frequent and prolonged jaundice and a low blood sugar and prothrombin level, etc. For renal function, see the chapter "Notes on drip therapy".

We still keep to weight distribution when evaluating the therapeutic results of the department for low-birthweight neonates. We generally employ 250 g divisions up to 2,500 g (or 2,499 g), usually without a lower limit in the under 1,000 g (999 g) group, and without distinguishing between premature and small-for-dates infants and twins. In mortality analyses, deaths within the first 7 days (strict neonatal mortality) or up to the age of 1 month (28 days) (broad neonatal mortality) are counted.

In the care of the premature infant we repeat the principle which applies to the labour room, i.e. all care which is not vitally essential is postponed after primary adaptation of the infant (1 – 3 hours after birth). The maximum attention is given to handling the infant sparingly, to cleaning out its upper air passages and to ensuring an adequate environmental temperature.

The premature infant's diagnostic programme must begin as soon after birth as possible, since the greatest physiological and biological reverses and adaptation pathologies occur between the first breath and the 12th hour of life. The infant should be clinically controlled as often as possible, especially in the first 12 hours. The purpose of the records made during this time is to give a clear survey of the infant's condition and to encumber the staff as little as possible. In our institute we use two special case sheets for neonates treated in the intensive care unit – one filled in by the physician (Tab. 46) and the other by the nursing staff (Tab. 47). Respiration, the action of heart and the rectal or skin temperature are preferably checked continously by means of monitors, or at intervals of 15, 30 or 60 minutes. Some departments employ Silverman's method of evaluating respiratory function, in which the results of clinical examination are expressed by a points system. The exclusion of malformations (of the gastrointestinal tract, heart and diaphragm) needing urgent operation and objectivization of the respiratory distress syndrome (RDS) require a prompt X-ray (a straight radiogram with the infant suspended). If the RDS deteriorates, another X-ray should be taken after the 4th hour of life. The acid-base balance of the newborn infant should be tested within the first hour (Astrup), preferably in arterial blood. Today it is generally tested in arterialized capillary blood obtained by pricking the warmed skin of the heel, or in blood taken from the infant's radial or temporal artery. The use of blood from the umbilical artery is now discouraged. because of the danger of complications. In the near future, measurement by means of transcutaneous oxygen electrodes will evidently become the most popular method. In newborns with signs of hypoxaemia, P_{O_2} < 50 mm Hg, cyanosis and apnoeic spels, an oxygen test in recommended. If the infant's Pa_{O_2}, after administering pure oxygen, is less than 50 mmHg a special respiratory therapy is indicated. If only the P_{CO_2} value in capillary blood is available, values of over 70 – 80 mm or increase of Pa_{CO_2} of 10 mmHg in one hour are an indication for the use of assisted ventilation. The blood sugar level, ionized calcium, the osmolarity of the blood (or Na, K, Cl), the microhaematocrit and the urine (with special reference to possible infections of the renal tract) are also investigated. The Er, Hb and Leu values must be determined and a differential leucocyte count

Table 46. Physician's record

	Infant's name ....
	....
Finding at (time) on (date):	
Blood supply, skin:	pink, erythema, pale, grey, acrocyanosis, icterus ...., diffuse cyanosis, stagnation cyanosis ...., petechiae ...., suffusion ...., tox. exanthema ...., special findings: ....
Oedema:	diffuse, UE, LE, feet, head, eyelids
Respiration:	frequency ..../min, abdominal, thoratic, mixed, shallow, gasping, Cheyene-Stokes, grunting, apnoea ...., on ausculation:
Heart:	rate ..../min, sounds....................
Neurological:	quiet, apathetic, excitable, normotonia, hypotonia, hypertonia, opisthotonia, Moro's reflex................, grasp r. LE ...., UE ...., sucking r...................., convulsions (tonic, clonic, asymmetrical) tremor, other findings ....
Head:	wide fontanelle ...., cranial sutures................, mouth ...., nose ....,
Abdomen:	liver ...., spleen...................., umbilicus...................., special findings ....
Other findings:	....
Classification in weight scheme:	normal ...., less than 10.5 percentile
	Signature:

must be done. Some departments also determine the total blood protein or the protein fractions. These tests should also be performed within the 1st hour of life, then again after 4 hours and after that according to the course of adaptation and the results of the tests. If an infection is suspected, blood (2 ml) should be taken for culture and this, together with the results of nasal, throat and stool smears, with the differential leucocyte and thrombocyte count, is the decisive factor in the administration and choice of antibiotics.

Early postnatal therapy is based on the results of a comprehensive, continuous and examination control of the newborn infant. To some extent it is rather schematic. In principle, it means combating hypoxia, acidosis, hypoglycaemia and hypothermia, which give rise to further disturbances of homeostasis. The use of an incubator is still the main element of treatment. The newborn infant's body temperature can be linked to regulation of the incubator temperature, thereby protecting it against fluctuation. The oxygen supply is regulated according to the blood gas values. Pa_{O_2} should by maintained between $80-100$ mmHg. The inspired oxygen concentration can be raised

Table 47. Nurses' record

Date:							Infant's name:			
Time in hours Incubator temperature Infant's temperature										
Skin	pink pale grey acrocyanosis cyanosis icterus									
Respiration	frequency/min thoracic abdominal gasping apneustic grunting apnoea (min)									
Neurological	excitability hypertonia opisthotonus convulsions hypotonia									
	sucking of gastric content vomiting micturation stools infusion in ml									

(Further details on back of sheat)

Nurse's name:

to 100 % by the use of miniature tents over the infant's head, administration through a funnel. The oxygen is moistened and preheated. The use of continous positive airway pressure (e. g. Gregory box) or of respirators represents a new chapter in RDS therapy. It must be stressed that the respirator should be used for as short time as possible only and that the initiation of independent respiration should be respected. It has recently been recommended that inspiration and expiration should take place in the positive pressure zone. Respirators with negative pressure spread out in the last period. Vasodilators (acetylcholine, Perphyllon), phospholipid aerosols and substances promoting fibrinolysis have not assured the results of treatment of pneumopathies to much.

As regards the administration of oxygen, and particularly the question of when to withhold it, the capillary blood Pa_{O_2} or P_{CO_2} is an objective criterion. As soon as these values return to normal, we stop supplying oxygen. If these tests cannot be carried out, we stop as soon as the clinical signs disappear (oxygen must usually be added for $3-7$ days).

The use of $NaHCO_3$ is a very common way of correcting metabolic acidosis. The amount is calculated by the formula BE (base excess) $\times$ 0.3 of the infant's b.w. (kg) $=$ mEq/l $NaHCO_3$ $=$ ml 8.4% $NaHCO_3$. In most departments, $^1/_3$ to $^1/_2$ of the calculated amount is administered i.v. together with glucose (1 : 1) in a single dose over $15-20$ min, adding the rest to the drip mixture. The influence of correction must be studied by repeated testing after Astrup. Bicarbonate represents a considerable osmotic load which can have negative side effects, while overdosing leads to alkalosis. Respiratory acidosis is much harder to correct. Organic buffers (Tris buffers, THAM) are now not very often used, for fear of their toxic effect on neonatal liver and brain tissue, so that the respirator and oxygen are still the main media. The amount of THAM used for correction is calculated by the formula BE $\times$ kg $=$ ml 0.3 mol THAM (always together with glucose). The 24-hour dosage should not exceed 12 ml THAM/kg b.w.

The question of supplying the energy sources for the premature infant is becoming increasingly important, since hypoglycaemia has been demonstrated relatively frequently in these neonates in the first days of life.

The endogenous carbohydrate and fat reserves of very immature and small--for-dates neonates are negligible. Neonates with respiratory disorders have raised energy requirements. In these groups, therefore we start nutrition in the first hours after birth − the reverse of the method normal $10-15$ years ago. In the above groups we begin administering $5-10$ % glucose through an indwelling plastic tube, in amounts of $1-3$ ml and usually at 1- to 3-hour intervals.

We can determine whether the alimentary tract is capable of functioning by intubating the stomach (calibration: glabella-xyphoid process distance + + 2 cm) and then using withdrawal into a syringe before administering each dose to see whether the stomach is empty. If nutrient solution (coloured yellow or green) is withdrawn from the stomach, the next dose is not administered. If oral administration proves impossible or inadequate, or if the infant's clinical condition is serious, i.v. nutrition is employed, preferably into peripheral veins ($5-15$% glucose) or via the umbilical vein. The catheter can be introduced for a distance of only $1-2$ cm, when deeper we must check whether it actually leads towards, or directly into the vena cava. The blood glucose level must be controlled. Hyperglycaemia is indicative of an overdose, or low utilization of glucose, while hypoglycaemia is a sign that the supply of glucose is inadequate, or that the rate of its utilization is high. If hypoglycaemia, or very low values, are found repeatedly, carbohydrate reserves can be mobilized, with good effect, by glucagone (0.3 mg/kg b.w.) or adrenaline (0.03 ml aqueous solution, 1 : 1,000).

If oral nutrition is impossible, fat can be administered i.v. from the 2nd day in the form of single doses (1 − 2 g/kg/24 hours over 15 − 20 min) or a permanent drip (4 g/kg/24 hours). Amino acids are also used (i.v.), mainly because of their presumed protective effect on brain tissue. In a situation of raised energy consumption they are also catabolized, however, and act as a source of energy, thereby stimulating and placing a strain on renal excretory function. The supply of energy source should at least cover the infant's basal metabolic requirements (30 − 40 Cal/kg/24 hours). This, of course, also concerns the infusion volume and the nutrient solution concentration. In practice, 40 to 80 ml/kg/day is generally given on the 1st and 2nd day.

The use of antibiotics is warranted for a demonstrated adnatal or postnatal infection. Their preventive use is being abandoned. Wide spectrum antibiotics are employed. Today, the main pathogens are Gram-negative bacteria, which often settle permanently in respirators, wash-basins and air-conditioning apparatus, especially in departments where antibiotics are used too freely. Experimental studies on the inhibitory effect of antibiotics on mitochondrial activity may propose a review of their use, particularly as regards premature infants.

The need for a raised vitamin supply is also generally recognized − vitamins C, B complex and K (the last only for signs of haemorrhagic disease) from the 1st day of life and A and D from the 7th.

Plasma and blood (5 − 10 ml/kg/24 hours) are administered for various reasons. The most actual is that they supply factors preventing excessive bleeding due to a metabolic coagulopathy. Experience with heparin is still deficient and its administration requires tests of clotting factors (factors II, V, VII, IX and X, a platelet count, fibrinogen). Electrolytes are also administered together with plasma and blood (see the chapter "Notes on drip therapy").

A number of aetiopathogenetic problems related to the premature infant still remain unresolved, especially in the field of circulation and respiration (closure of circulatory shunts, the role of surfactants in the development of pneumopathies), haematology (intravascular disseminated metabolic coagulopathies), metabolism and endocrinology.

Present-day therapy consequently tends to polypragmatism or schematism and is largely symptomatic. An active therapeutic approach is justified, however, since early removal (abolition) of the basic dangers, in the presence of structural immaturity of the organism, is at present the most effective way of preventing permanent sequelae in the development of premature infants.

THE SMALL-FOR-DATES NEONATE

A newborn infant is described as "small-for-dates" (syn: prenatally dys-trophic, dysmature, retardation of foetal growth, foetal malnutrition, light-for-dates) if its birthweight — and other growth parameters (length, head and chest circumference, etc.) — are below the range limit of those relevant to the week of gestation in which the infant was born. Such infants do not form an aetiologically and pathogenetically homogeneous group and, from the causal aspect, two main groups can be differentiated:

(1) Growth disturbances starting in the early stages of pregnancy and caused by genetic information changes (18 or D_1 trisomia, Down's syndrome) or infection of the embryo (rubella syndrome), so that delayed growth accompanies, or is the equivalent of, a congenital developmental defect.

(2) Foetal nutrition disturbances in the second half of pregnancy, which account for the vast majority of small-for-dates neonates and can be caused by various mechanism, e.g. poor nourishment of the mother and utero-placental and foetoplacental circulatory disorders, including a pathological placenta. Prenatal malnutrition endangers the foetus in women with toxaemia and hypertension and also in multiple pregnancies, but in many cases no pathological condition is found in the mother and a small-for-dates diagnosis is not made until the infant is actually born.

A small-for-dates diagnosis is determined objectively on the discrepancy between growth parameters and the length of pregnancy. It can be evaluated exactly (especially in the case of premature infants) only by means of tables or graphs for normal foetal growth. Czech tables of weights and lengths are given separately for either sex in Tables 48 – 51 (Poláček 1971).

The most important criterion is the birthweight, which is low in all small--for-dates foetuses, while body length and head circumference may not vary much from normal. Of the organs, growth of the lungs, liver and thymus is the most retarded, the heart and spleen are less affected and the brain suffers the least. Neonates whose birthweight is below the 5th percentile of the appended tables are regarded as small-for-dates; a smaller body length or head circumference is of supplementary significance. The length of pregnancy should be determined with the maximum possible reliability, but we must reckon with an error of at least ± 1 week. Gross errors, e.g. of a whole menstrual cycle, can be rectified by evaluating minor details of somatic development, e.g. the grooves in the soles, the size of the nipples and the state of the hair and the auricular cartilage, and by neurological and EEG examination.

The postpartal adaptation of small-for-dates neonates is proportional to their gestational age and not to their birthweight, so that infants born after

Table 48. Birthweights – boys

Week of pregnancy	5%	10%	25%	x̄	75%	90%	95%
24.	639.42	708.79	824.96	953.75	1082.54	1198.71	1268.08
25.	738.59	803.77	912.93	1033.95	1154.97	1264.13	1329.31
26.	846.28	903.35	998.35	1104.92	1210.89	1306.49	1363.56
27.	990.97	1041.17	1125.26	1218.47	1311.68	1395.77	1445.97
28.	1097.08	1147.13	1230.96	1323.88	1416.80	1500.63	1550.68
29.	1221.71	1274.84	1363.84	1462.50	1561.16	1650.16	1703.29
30.	1330.89	1393.72	1498.97	1615.65	1732.33	1837.58	1900.41
31.	1523.58	1594.66	1713.72	1845.70	1977.68	2096.74	2167.82
32.	1656.36	1734.75	1866.05	2011.61	2157.17	2288.47	2366.86
33.	1790.76	1874.68	2015.24	2171.05	2326.86	2467.42	2551.34
34.	1927.88	2026.92	2192.82	2376.73	2560.64	2726.54	2825.58
35.	2048.11	2165.14	2361.16	2578.46	2795.76	2991.78	3108.81
36.	2183.11	2313.26	2531.24	2772.89	3014.54	3232.52	3362.67
37.	2385.73	2524.25	2756.26	3013.46	3270.66	3502.67	3641.19
38.	2568.25	2710.72	2949.35	3213.88	3478.41	3717.04	3859.51
39.	2676.74	2829.24	3084.65	3367.79	3650.93	3906.34	4058.84
40.	2738.16	2889.90	3144.07	3425.83	3707.59	3961.76	4113.50
41.	2813.01	2968.03	3227.68	3515.51	3803.34	4062.99	4218.01

Table 49. Birthweights – girls

Week of pregnancy	5%	10%	25%	x̄	75%	90%	95%
24.	628.01	675.68	755.54	844.06	932.58	1012.44	1060.11
25.	679.62	727.64	808.08	897.25	986.42	1066.86	1114.88
26.	793.22	842.64	925.43	1017.20	1108.97	1191.76	1241.18
27.	911.60	965.41	1055.55	1155.47	1255.39	1345.53	1399.34
28.	1002.99	1059.31	1153.64	1258.20	1362.76	1457.09	1513.41
29.	1111.75	1168.51	1263.59	1368.98	1474.37	1569.45	1626.21
30.	1276.92	1339.31	1443.81	1559.65	1675.49	1779.99	1842.38
31.	1392.20	1470.65	1602.06	1747.73	1893.40	2024.81	2103.26
32.	1559.23	1644.72	1787.91	1946.64	2105.37	2248.56	2334.05
33.	1671.52	1770.97	1937.55	2122.20	2306.85	2473.43	2572.88
34.	1840.79	1946.20	2122.76	2318.48	2314.20	2690.76	2796.17
35.	1979.28	2094.84	2288.39	2502.96	2717.53	2911.08	3026.64
36.	2111.78	2241.35	2458.38	2698.96	2939.54	3156.57	3286.14
37.	2246.08	2394.34	2642.67	2917.95	3193.23	3441.56	3589.82
38.	2273.47	2443.83	2729.17	3045.48	3361.79	3647.13	3817.49
39.	2326.04	2500.15	2791.76	3115.03	3438.30	3729.91	3904.02
40.	2370.78	2542.58	2830.33	3149.32	3468.31	3756.06	3927.86
41.	2502.22	2662.89	2931.99	3230.30	3528.61	3797.71	3958.38

the 35th week of pregnancy are not, as a rule, subject to the respiratory complications typical for preterm infants of the same weight. The main danger for light-for-dates neonates is considered to be the development of hypoglycaemia, i.e. a drop in the blood sugar level below 30 or 20 mg%. This tendency to hypoglycaemia is probably due to rapid exhaustion of their

Table 50. Lenght on the 5th day — boys

Week of pregnancy	5%	10%	25%	$\bar{x}$	75%	90%	95%
24.	31.35	32.17	33.55	35.08	36.61	37.99	38.81
25.	31.45	32.39	33.98	35.74	37.50	39.09	40.03
26.	32.41	33.37	34.97	36.75	38.53	40.13	41.09
27.	33.36	34.31	35.91	37.67	39.43	41.03	41.98
28.	35.34	36.15	37.51	39.01	40.51	41.87	42.68
29.	36.19	37.00	38.36	39.86	41.36	42.72	43.53
30.	37.72	38.48	39.76	41.17	42.58	43.86	44.62
31.	39.87	40.60	41.81	43.16	44.51	45.72	46.45
32.	41.50	42.11	43.14	44.28	45.42	46.45	47.06
33.	42.64	43.20	44.15	45.19	46.23	47.18	47.74
34.	43.45	44.04	45.03	46.13	47.23	48.22	48.81
35.	44.08	44.70	45.74	46.89	48.04	49.08	49.70
36.	45.25	45.79	46.71	47.73	48.75	49.67	50.21
37.	45.90	46.53	47.58	48.75	49.92	50.97	51.60
38.	47.16	47.75	48.73	49.81	50.89	51.87	52.46
39.	48.14	48.70	49.63	50.67	51.71	52.64	53.20
40.	48.53	49.08	50.01	51.03	52.05	52.98	53.53
41.	49.95	50.30	50.88	51.53	52.18	52.76	53.11

Table 51. Lenght on the 5th day — girls

Week of pregnancy	5%	10%	25%	$\bar{x}$	75%	90%	95%
24.	30.47	31.22	32.48	33.87	35.26	36.52	37.27
25.	29.32	30.34	32.05	33.95	35.85	37.56	38.58
26.	31.05	32.13	33.93	35.92	37.91	39.71	40.79
27.	32.79	33.75	35.35	37.13	38.91	40.51	41.47
28.	34.83	35.65	37.01	38.53	40.05	41.41	42.23
29.	35.05	36.01	37.63	39.42	41.21	42.83	43.79
30.	37.18	38.10	39.65	41.37	43.09	44.64	45.56
31.	39.07	39.89	41.27	42.80	44.33	45.71	46.53
32.	41.13	41.75	42.80	43.97	45.14	46.19	46.81
33.	42.06	42.66	43.66	44.76	45.86	46.86	47.46
34.	43.02	43.58	44.53	45.57	46.61	47.56	48.12
35.	43.83	44.40	45.35	46.41	47.47	48.42	48.99
36.	44.52	45.14	46.18	47.33	48.48	49.52	50.14
37.	45.54	46.19	47.27	48.47	49.67	50.75	51.40
38.	45.83	46.55	47.74	49.07	50.40	51.29	52.31
39.	46.24	46.94	48.12	49.43	50.74	51.92	52.62
40.	46.57	47.25	48.38	49.63	50.88	52.01	52.69
41.	47.40	47.99	48.98	50.08	51.18	52.17	52.76

limited carbohydrate reserves, especially if combined with inclement environmental factors, such as starvation, hypothermia, tachypnoea, etc. It is remarkable that most neonates, as distinct from older infants tolerate a low blood sugar level without any manifest signs. In "symptomatic" hypoglycaemia they develop nonspecific signs, such as apathy, hypotonia, shivering, cyanosis and apnoeic attacks, which disappear after a small dose of hypertonic glucose, thereby confirming the diagnosis. Hypoglycaemia with clinical signs is associated with the possibility of permanent CNS damage. In our experience, if the proper treatment is used, i.e. prevention of hypothermia and the institution of glucose solution nutrition in the first hour after birth, clinically manifest forms of hypoglycaemia are a very rare complication. If the peroral administration of glucose fails to prevent a serious drop in the blood sugar level, it must be given in the form of an intravenous drip (60 – 90 ml/kg/24 hours).

The prognosis for small-for-dates neonates is uncertain. The proportion of stillbirths is higher than normal, because foetal malnutrition can readily turn to acute intrauterine asphyxia. Newborn infants with a less severe degree of malnutrition are often very active after birth, take their food well and soon catch up on weight. Severe forms are characterized by raised neonatal mortality. The long-term development of small-for-dates is a serious problem. It has been demonstrated that about one third display retarded growth later in childhood, and sometimes nervous and mental disorders. Delayed somatic and mental development was found to be particularly frequent and serious in preterm infants with a subnormal birthweight.

The treatment of serious cases among small-for-dates neonates is virtually the same as for premature infants with the same birthweight and is based on the infant's actual condition. The possibilities of correcting disturbances of prenatal growth and development are at present very limited.

THE POST-TERM NEONATE

With increasing timely induction of labour, the number of post-term infants is declining. The clinical manifestations of postmaturity are in a given correlation to the number of weeks by which term is exceeded. The reliability of postnatal classification depends on the accuracy of the estimated term. Postmaturity is primarily a problem of older primiparas.

Some post-term infants give the impression of having benefited by their prolonged stay in the uterus. Because this group is so large (60 – 70 % of all post-term neonates), some obstetricians do not acknowledge postmaturity to be a risk factor at all.

Protraction of pregnancy beyond calculated term may give rise, in the infant, simply to over-weight and macrosomia, but it can also result in true hypermaturity, dysmaturity or malnutrition owing to placental dysfunction and chronic deficiency of the nutrients and oxygen supply to the post-term foetus. Placental dysfunction can likewise occur some time before term, however, and premature infants can also display dysmaturity.

High birthweight post-term infants in whom placental function remains intact beyond term run the risk of perinatal CNS and peripheral trauma. If this does not occur, they usually develop normally (some of them actually prosper extremely well). If the infant displays no signs of being over or under normal size, and if no risk factors are detected either prenatally or postnatally, it must be assumed that term was wrongly calculated, or that any anomalies were minimal and clinically imperceptible.

In our material, we were able to differentiate 3 groups of post-term infants, characterized as follows:

(1) Active, small weight loss, skin fresh, good turgor, small, common anomalies on first days, further progress good to excellent. Large proportion with high weight (over 4,000 g).

(2) Lower than term weight, size bordering on small, dehydration and exfoliation of skin, maceration of palms, soles and scrotum. Respiratory disturbances lasting not more than 24 hours. Prognosis good.

(3) Small-for-dates by less than 5 percentiles of correlative curve, "old" expression, signs of aspiration of turbid amniotic fluid, circulatory and respiratory disturbances lasting over 24 hours, disturbances of thermoregulation (hypothermia), dehydration, and of sugar regulation (hypoglycaemia). Prognosis less promising.

Preventive and therapeutic measures are the same as for premature and asphyxiated infants. In group 3, we emphasize that the triad: postmaturity — small size for dates — aspiration of turbid amniotic fluid is an indication for the administration of wide-spectrum antibiotics and long-term follow-up.

THE NEWBORN INFANT WITH HAEMOLYTIC DISEASE (ERYTHROBLASTOSIS FOETALIS)

The basic condition for the development of haemolytic disease is blood incompatibility between mother and foetus, i.e. the presence of antibodies against certain foetal red cell antigens in the maternal plasma. Immune type maternal antibodies reach the foetus via the placenta, are bound to the red blood cells and cause their premature destruction. Blood incompatibility can be manifested in any of the red cell antigen systems, but in actual practice only incompatibility in the ABO and Rhesus systems is important.

a) **Haemolytic disease in the Rhesus system.** Abnormal destruction of the red blood cells starts about half-way through pregnancy, so that the full picture of haemolytic disease can develop with a prenatal component, i.e. with progressive haemolytic anaemia of the foetus, terminating in severe cases in intrauterine death or in the birth of a moribund, hydropic infant, and with a postnatal component, i.e. the development of severe hyperbilirubinaemia, which can terminate in death or permanent CNS injury, as sequelae of nuclear jaundice (kernicterus).

The condition can be anticipated if the mother is rh negative and the father Rh positive, if anti-Rh antibodies are detected during pregnancy and in multiparas who have already had a child with haemolytic disease. A paediatrician should be present at the birth; if labour needs to be induced prematurely, the optimum time should be chosen by agreement. Transfusion of the placental blood is **contraindicated.**

After delivery, umbilical blood is collected, as follows:

(1) coagulable blood for serological tests (blood group, Rh factor, direct Coombs test) or for matching with donor blood for a replacement transfusion,

(2) coagulable blood for determining the serum bilirubin level,

(3) 1−2 ml non-clotting blood, into dry heparin (recommended for determining the Hb level and the red cell and reticulocyte count).

Coagulable venous blood from the mother is also sent for serological tests. A diagnosis of haemolytic disease in the Rh system is based on a positive direct Coombs test in neonatal blood which is also taken as decisive in all controversial cases, e.g. if the mother was not examined during pregnancy.

Clinical examination and treatment of the infant:
Three clinical degrees of haemolytic disease can be differentiated, each being directly correlated to the degree of foetal anaemia.

I. Hydrops foetus universalis. In addition to characteristic oedema and ascites we find pallor, extreme anaemia (Hb less than 4 g%) and extreme hepato- and splenomegaly. Many hydropic foetuses are stillborn, while the rest are mostly moribund and die soon after birth. Some cases can be saved by the following treatments:

(1) Immediate reduction of blood volume by up to 50 ml to lower venous pressure and prevent pulmonary oedema, later followed by ligation of the umbilical cord.

(2) Tapping of the ascites above the symphysis or the left inguinal ligament.

(3) The intramuscular administration of 3−5 mg prednisone.

(4) A replacement transfusion of concentrated group O, rh negative, blood as soon as possible, without matching, by alternate removal and slow injection

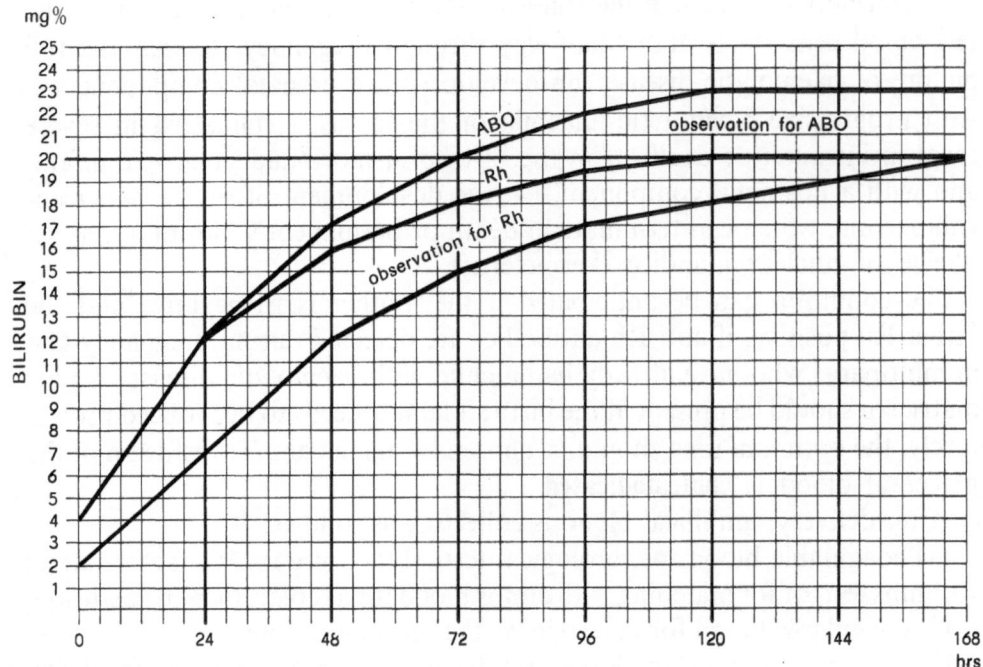

Fig. 25. Bilirubin indication curve after Poláček; in zone above Rh and ABO curve replacement transfusion necessary (Poláček 1965).

of the concentrated blood in amounts of 5 – 10 ml, through a catheter introduced into the umbilical vein, up to a total of 50 – 60 ml.

(5) Placing the infant in a heated incubator, with a high oxygen supply and/or assisted respiration, in the intensive care unit.

(6) A replacement trasfusion (after the infant's condition has improved).

II. Haemolytic disease with severe anaemia (the "intermediate" form). The infant is in a manifestly grave condition, with extreme pallor, Hb less than 7 – 8 g%, oedema, marked hepatosplenomegaly, haemorrhagic diathesis and feeble vitality. Unless treated promptly and adequately, these infants die of anaemia before jaundice develops. They must be placed at once in a heated incubator with an oxygen supply and their blood must be changed as soon as possible.

III. Haemolytic disease with mild or moderate anaemia (the commonest form). As a rule, these infants are viable and they sometimes do not appear ill at all. In more severe cases they are subicteric, with a yellowish umbilical cord and mild to moderate hepato- and splenomegaly, but display normal vitality. During the first 24 hours they become increasingly jaundiced and in severe cases kernicterus may develop within 16 – 20 hours.

Treatment in the labour room (group II and III) consists in early ligation of the umbilical cord and collecting blood samples from mother and child.

204

The infant is then trasferred to the intensive care unit and laboratory tests are carried out.

The basis form of therapy is blood exchange, the need for which is decided by the rate of increase in the bilirubin level and its final value. Poláček's indication graph (Fig. 25) can be used as a guide. If the bilirubin level is in the absolute indication zone, replacement is performed at once (it can, if necessary, be safely postponed for up to 12 hours after birth). If the bilirubin level is in the observation zone, it is checked at 24- or 12-hour intervals and replacement is performed if there is danger of its exceeding the 20 mg% limit. The simultaneous presence of anaemia of less than 12 g% is a relative, and of less than 10 g% an absolute, indication for replacement, even if the bilirubin level is in the observation zone. With premature infants, early replacement is preferable. The usual amount of blood to be exchanged is $160-170$ ml/kg.

With severely anaemic infants (group II), the blood must be changed as soon as possible, using initial reduction of the blood volume, i.e. the removal of two and the injection of one syringe-full of concentrated blood until the venous pressure drops below 10 cm H_2O (this can be measured with a perpendicular cannula introduced into the umbilical vein). Further exchange is carried out in a negative balance, which is not compensated at the end of the operation. In this case, a small amount of blood, i.e. 100 ml/kg b.w., is sufficient for adequate replacement and in severe states even less is required (Poláček 1967).

When exchange has been completed, the infant is placed in an incubator and given oxygen as required. The bilirubin level must always be checked systematically at 12- or 24-hour intervals until it manifestly falls. If it rises above 20 mg% again, replacement must be repeated a second (and even a third) time. The indication graph is no guide for repeating exchange, the only criterion for which is a danger of the 20 mg% limit being exceeded. About 20% of cases of haemolytic disease in the Rh system do not need an exchange transfusion and can be treated conservatively — not forgetting to watch the bilirubin level.

Subsequently, up to the age of $8-10$ weeks, the red blood picture must be checked and if the Hb level drops below 8 g% a rh negative blood transfusion must be given. These check-ups are especially necessary in infants not given a replacement transfusion, as they often develop severe anaemia.

b) **Haemolytic disease in the ABO system.** As a rule, this disease can be anticipated only in infants born to mothers whose history shows a case of haemolytic disease due to incompatibility in the ABO system. This situation is rather exceptional, as in 50% of the cases even the fist infant is affected. If haemolytic disease in the ABO system is suspected, blood is sent for serological and biochemical tests, as for haemolytic disease in the Rh system. In positive serological tests, the mother's group is found to be O and the infant's A or (very seldom) B.

Since increased destruction of the blood cells does not start until the perinatal period, a prenatal anaemic form of the disease is virtually unknown and the newborn infant is liable only to an icteric form with a usually milder course. For the same reason, premature infants are rarely affected. The diagnosis is generally not established until after birth, on the basis of early (within 24 hours) and rapidly increasing jaundice. It is confirmed by a finding of blood incompatibility in the ABO system.

Therapy: Severe cases require blood replacement, which is almost always indicated by the observation technique, i.e. by studying the serum bilirubin level. Most cases can be treated conservatively and radiation therapy, using a suitable apparatus, produces good results. Blue or white "daylight" bulbs or lamps are employed and the infant is irradiated, in an incubator, with a dose of about 3,000 lux (at the level of its body). The best way is to irradiate the infant continuously until the bilirubin level falls. Light causes bilirubin in the organism to be converted to readily excreted non-toxic and diazonegative products (evidently dipyrroles). Its simplicity and manifest safety have made this the method of choice, especially for jaundice in premature infants and haemolytic disease in the ABO system. In mild cases, the administration of a $10-15\%$ glucose intravenous drip ($60-80$ ml/kg b.w.) until the bilirubin level falls has proved to be a satisfactory auxiliary method, although its mechanism is still obscure.

THE INFANT OF A DIABETIC MOTHER

The "diabetic foetopathy" syndrome is determined by the mother's metabolic disorder and relative immaturity of the foetus. The birthweight of these infants is higher than that of normal infants born at the same stage of gestation. Deposition of excess fat and glycogen during pregnancy makes the infant obese, but its obesity is also characterized by infiltration of the subcutaneous tissue reminiscent of Cushing's syndrome. If the syndrome is fully developed, the infant has a moon-face, with swollen lids and closed eyes, a double chin, powerful shoulder and a stocky body with a deep fat cushion. The skin is usually deep red and is often characterized by circumoral and acral cyanosis. Despite macrosomia, the infant appears immature and respiratory disturbances typical of the premature infant are generally the first pathological sign

206

of adaptation diffuculties. In the presence of a picture of asphyxial crises with inspiratory retraction, exspiratory grunting, tachypnoea and apnoeic pauses with cyanosis, atelectases occur and hyaline membranes disease develops. This state is usually accompanied by strikingly raised excitability.

The development of these signs depends on the time of birth and often on the form of delivery. The closer to term and the easier the birth, the smaller the incidence of respiratory disturbances.

In addition to immaturity, we find a tendency to vascular fragility and oedema. Severe metabolic disturbances in the mother lead to ketoacidosis and a difficult birth causes mechanical injury of the CNS. Intrauterine hyperglycaemia of the foetus is succeeded in the first hour of life by hypoglycaemia of the newborn infant which is due to the hyperplasia of the insular apparatus and to hyperinsulinism. In addition to postnatal functional disorders, the infant of the diabetic mother runs a raised risk of congenital deformities. At present, we do not know reliably how far the tendency of these infants to diabetes influnces their subsequent development.

To prevent the appearance and prolonged duration of hypoglycaemia, we introduced 10 % glucose nutrition from the 1st hour of life (orally or by tube, after first emptying the stomach). If, in the 1st hour, the blood sugar level does not fall below 20 mg %, early enteral nutrition is sufficent, but if hypoglycaemia recurs on the first day of life it is sometimes necessary to institute parenteral 10 % glucose nutrition (i.v. drip, total dose 65 ml/kg/day).

Both during and after delivery, the infant should be handled very sparingly, because of the sensitivity of its tissues and its tendency to eodema, haemorrhage and infection. Antibiotics are not administered preventively, but we look carefully for clinical signs of possible complications, which may develop even after the 14th day. All these infants are consequently kept in hospital for over 2 weeks. The infant is put to the breast after the 4th day, according to its own condition and the mother's milk supply. Measures for maintaining a normal body temparature and indications for the administration of oxygen, alkalizing, sedative drugs and antibiotics come under the same rules as for premature infants.

In recent years, increased administration of insulin during pregnancy has enabled obstetricians to postpone delivery of the infants of diabetic mothers to the limits of term. Most of these infants no longer have the typical appearance and their state immediately after birth requires nothing more than observation.

Premature infants born to diabetic mothers can be brought successfully through postnatal adaptation in intensive care units, but as perinatal mortality in this group diminishes, the risk of mild or severe neurological and psychological anomalies increases. Even in such cases, however, early determination of the disorder and systematic rehabilitation can achieve good results.

We can reckon with a growing proportion of fertile women with manifest and latent diabetes, and their children must receive special attention, both postnatally and later. The development of obstetrical prevention is constantly improving the early and late prognosis of these cases and the paediatrician's main task is becoming the prompt detection of psychomotor anomalies, with a view to early rehabilitation.

INFECTIONS OF THE NEWBORN INFANT

Infections have always been a very dangerous and important factor in the care of the newborn. At the outset of the present century, the high morbidity and mortality caused (mainly) by diarrhoeas, respiratory infection and classic bacterial infections (diphtheria, tetanus, staphylodermatitis) resulted in the adoption of strict isolation measures. Antibiotics have completely wiped out some infections, but they have also led to some neglect of basic hygiene and

Table 52. Infection routes and factors influencing invasion of infective agent into fetus and newborn infant

Infection routes	Infective agent		Additional unfavourable factors
Transplacentally	Viruses:	rubella herpes cytomegalovirus	Acute illness of the mother
	Spirochetes		
	Protozoa:	toxoplasmosis	
Infection from the birth canal	Ascending:	*E. coli* Staphylococci	Premature rupture of foetal membranes
	Gonococci		Protracted labour
	Candida		Obstet. manipulations
	Herpes		Asphyxia
	Listeria		
Infections after birth	Staphylococci		Bad hygiene
	E. coli		Contaminated: incubators
	Pseudomonas		respirators
	Proteus		Immaturity
	Viruses		Malformations
	Beta haemol. streptococci		Surgical problems

Congenital infections are manifested within 48 to 72 hours after birth (early or primary sepsis).

Late (secondary) sepsis is manifested after 48—72 hours.

to the appearance of antibiotic-resistant infections. In addition, we are finding more and more negative side effects of antibiotic therapy and our knowledge of the specific features of the immunulogical reactivity of the foetus and the newborn infant (which must be taken into account) is increasing. The routes of infection and the factors influencing the infiltration of infective agents into the organism are summed up in Table 52.

The foetus and the newborn infant are susceptible to most bacterial, viral, fungal and parasitic infections. In the newborn infant, infections can even be caused by organisms which, in later life, are regarded as non-pathogenic. Up to 1953, Gram-positive microorganisms (streptococci) were the commonest cause of infections, but today, Gram-negative microorganisms (*E. coli*, *Proteus*) are in the ascendancy. *Klebsiella* species are a frequent danger after surgical operations, while in damp environments, ventilators and in O_2 administration *Pseudomonas* is the greatest danger. In general, a foetus can be infected transplacentally or by direct introduction of a pathogen into its blood stream. An infant can swallow or inhale a pathogen, or the latter can infiltrate into its organism through injured skin or mucous membrane.

Specific features of immunological reactivity and defence of the newborn infant

The cellular response is limited by the low leucocyte count and functional immaturity of the leucocytes. The ability to select and localize cells at sites of inflammation is lacking. The polymorphonuclears have fewer amoeboid movements and reduced phagocytic capacity. The amount of the complement component C'5 is small. Limited phagocytosis together with low capacity for intracellular digestion and a delay in the appearance of inflammatory exudate allows the rapid invasion, spread and proliferation of an infective agent, especially in premature infants.

As regards the components of humoral immunity, the infant receives IgG transplacentally, in a concentration depending upon the amount possessed by the mother and upon the length of gestation. IgM and IgA containing specific antibodies to Gram-negative bacteria are not transmitted to the infant. The IgM value in the cord blood is less than 20 mg/100 ml and IgA is absent altogether. Raised IgM values in the cord blood are a sign of intrauterine infection, but even normal values do not exclude it. The determination of IgM in the cord blood is thus not a suitable screening test. After birth, IgA appears in a low titre. After antigenic stimulation the newborn infant forms IgM, but unlike adults, who then produce IgG, IgG does not appear until 20 – 30 days after IgM in the newborn infant.

The **signs** of incipient infection of the newborn infant are usually scanty and are similar for all infections. They include changes in tonus and colour, loss of appetite, vomiting, the appearance of icterus and hypothermia rather than pyrexia. The signs are not often typical for the aetiological agent and do not embrace the affected system (e.g. there may be convulsions without CNS involvement, gastrointestinal disturbances without an infection of the alimentary tract, etc).

The role of laboratory diagnosis

Although infection of a newborn infant calls for a quick decision on treatment and it is not always possible to wait for the results of laboratory tests, the latter are necessary and valuable. The first necessity is a full examination of the blood picture. Anaemia, fragmented erythrocytes, reticulocytosis and thrombopenia together with abnormal coagulation are indicative of a general infection. Cultivation tests are carried out with blood, cerebrospinal fluid, urine, an ear smear, gastric juice and, if required, skin lesion material. These are accompanied by a microscopic examination and by Gram staining. X-rays of the chest, the long bones and the skull are done. Serological tests comprise the determination of immunoglobulin and fluorescent antibody levels, biochemical determination of the pH, the blood sugar and calcium levels and, in the case of haemorrhage, clotting factors. The histology of the placenta, the umbilical cord and the foetal membranes is one of the most exacting examinations.

Therapeutic measures

In any treatment of a newborn infant we must bear in mind the specific features of its metabolism, such as slow clearance, low detoxication capacity, altered absorption, etc. Complex therapy is always essential, i.e. both against the infection and to counteract dehydration and shock. The preventive administration of antibiotics is not recommended.

The first condition for success is to transfer the infant to an intensive care unit. An incubator ensures both isolation and a supply of warmth, oxygen and moisture. Monitoring is today already a routine measure.

According to the results of the biochemical tests we ensure a supply of fluids and electrolytes and correct acidosis, hyponatraemia, hypoglycaemia and hypokalaemia. As well as improving anaemia, a blood transfusion stimulates phagocytosis and provides small amounts of antibodies. In severe

210

infections a replacement transfusion is sometimes necessarry. Gamma globulin is indicated only in cases of demonstrated agammaglobulinaemia.

Among the antibiotics, penicillin G remains the key one, but not procaine penicillin. In cases of primary sepsis we recommend its administration together with kanamycin, or kanamycin combined with ampicillin. Kanamycin in regarded as the most satisfactory for the treatment of Gram-negative infections. Ampicillin is not suitable for initial therapy, though only where there is demonstrated sensitivity. Kanamycin together with oxacillin are good for late sepses, which are most frequently caused by staphylococci. Gentamicin is not very efficacious for infections caused by Gram-negative organisms (*E. coli, Klebsiella, Pseudomonas, Proteus*), but there is little experience in its administration to newborn infants. Tetracycline should be excluded completely from the treatment of newborn infants and chloramphenicol should be used only with the greatest caution. Nystatin is satisfactory against *Candida* infections and has no side effects. Therapy is naturally supplemented by the usual hygiene and antiepidemic measures.

THE ANAEMIC AND PLETHORIC NEWBORN INFANT

Comparable values of red cell parameters at birth can be obtained from the cord blood. The mean haemoglobin value is 16 – 17 g/100 ml (range 13.5 to 20 g/100 ml) and the mean haematocrit value 53%. During the first few hours after birth, the red cell count, the haematocrit and the haemoglobin concentration in the venous blood increase as a result of placental transfusion, with subsequent adjustment of blood volume. The mean haemoglobin value on the first day is 18.4 g/100 ml and the mean haematocrit value 58%. On the following days these values slowly fall, reaching approximately the original cord blood values at the end of the first week. Capillary samples obtained by skin prick show higher values than simultaneously collected venous samples (mean haemoglobin value 20 g/100 ml, range 17 – 23 g/100 ml). The differences between capillary and venous samples are variable and venous samples should be obtained wherever possible.

Anaemia in the neonatal period is characterized by haemoglobin concentrations of less than 13 g/100 ml in venous blood, or less than 14.5 g/100 ml in capillary blood. It can be due to various causes, which can be divided into three aetiological categories:

I. *Haemorrhagic anaemia*, due to

(1) obsterical complications, e.g. placenta praevia, abruptio placentae, rupture of umbilical cord or vessels,

(2) occult haemorrhage from the foetus into the maternal circulation or from twin to twin,

(3) internal haemorrhage in the infant, usually caused by obstetric injury, e.g. intracranial or retroperitoneal haemorrhage, or rupture of the liver or spleen.

The rapid loss of blood is manifested in pallor or shock with irregular respiration, but the haemoglobin concentration may initially be normal. On the other hand, anaemia after chronic haemorrhage may be haemodynamically compensated and may be recognized only from laboratory findings in a pale infant.

The treatment of haemorrhagic anaemias depends on the degree and acuteness of the blood loss. Infants affected by severe anaemia after birth should receive an immediate infusion of the available fluid or a transfusion of 10 to 20 ml suitable whole blood/kg as soon as possible. Infants with chronic anaemia (the degree of which is usually milder) should be treated with iron or be given a whole blood transfusion.

II. *Haemolytic anaemias* are frequent in the neonatal period. They are commonly associated with hyperbilirubinaemia, which is usually the most prominent and first detected feature. Increased haemolysis is due either to maternal-foetal incompatibility in the Rh (rarely the ABO) blood group system, or to congenital or acquired defects of the red cells. These disorders are described in the chapter on the newborn infant with haemolytic disease.

III. *Impaired red cell production*, known as congenital hypoplastic anaemia, is a rare disease of unknown aetiology, which is sometimes detected after birth, but more commonly in later months. The diagnosis is confirmed by the finding of normocytic and normochromic anaemia with a low reticulocyte count and the absence of erythroid precursors in the bone marrow.

The age at which anaemia is found is of value in evaluation of the differential diagnosis. Marked anaemia at birth is usually the outcome of prenatal haemorrhage or severe isoimmunization in the Rh blood group system; the two disorders can be differentiated by the result of a direct Coombs test. Anaemia detected during the first two days is usually caused by internal or external bleeding, while if discovered later it is normally of haemolytic origin, particularly if associated with jaundice. The essential laboratory tests include haemoglobin determination, the reticulocyte count, a direct Coombs test of the infant's blood and examination of the maternal blood for the presence of foetal erythrocytes.

Polycythaemia in the neonatal period is a relatively rare feature, but it may be of clinical significance. It is best identified by the high haematocrit value, the normality limit of which is 60%. A venous haematocrit of over 65%, or a venous haemoglobin concentration of more than 22 g/100 ml, is evidence of polycythaemia. Capillary blood samples are less reliable, because they give falsely high haemoglobin and haematocrit values.

There are several causes of polycythaemia:

(1) Prenatal transfusion from twin to twin, or the maternal-foetal transfer of red cells.

(2) Intra-uterine hypoxia in small-for-dates infants, postmaturity or toxaemia of pregnancy.

(3) Various anomalies, such as Down's syndrome, D trisomia, diabetic foetopathies, adrenal hyperplasia, etc.

The aetiology of some cases is still obscure.

The signs of polycythaemia are mainly the result of increased blood viscosity, which may reduce the capillary blood flow in organs, including the lungs and the CNS and cause tissue hypoxia. The main signs are respiratory distress, cyanosis, heart failure, lethargy and convulsions. Dimished perfusion of the brain may well cause permanent damage to nervous and mental function. Many infants with polycythaemia, hovever, display no signs at all.

All polycythaemic infants should be carefully supervised and those with respiratory or CNS signs should be treated by reducing the haematocrit to about 60%. This is usually accomplished by removing about 10% of the blood and replacing it by the same amount of fresh plasma through a partial exchange transfusion.

THE GENETICALLY STIGMATIZED NEONATE

Despite all preventative efforts about 1.5 − 2% of all infants are born with congenital anomalies diagnosable **immediately** after birth. In absolute figures, this means that the number of infants born with congenital anomalies in 1972 must have been roughly as follows:

in France, Italy or England and Wales, about	12,000 − 17,000
Spain or Poland	9,000 − 12,000
Czechoslovakia	3,700 − 5,000
Belgium or Bulgaria	2,000 − 2,600
Austria or Sweden	1,500 − 2,200, etc...

The paediatrician thus encounters congenital anomalies relatively often and must be professionally prepared for them, i.e. he must be ready to answer the following questions:

(1) Is the anomaly lethal, conditionally lethal, or compatible with life?

(2) Can it be treated? If so, how? (e.g. if surgically, **which** specialist should operate and **when**?)

(3) Is it a gene-determined trait and thus likely to recur in siblings, or is it rather a random event in a single pregnancy, caused by the action of a teratogen (e.g. drugs, virus infenctions)?

The paediatrician can answer the first two questions relatively easily, whereas the others need special qualifications and comprehensive examination, which only **genetic counselling** can provide at the required level. Here knowledge and experience (both first-hand and acquired from the literature) are concentrated, links for any special tests (biochemical, cytological) are elaborated economically and schemes for evaluating the complete case analysis, i.e. for expressing a definite conclusion on the recurrence risk for further siblings, are drawn up (Tab. 53). The paediatrician does not analyse the familial genetic load in detail or calculate the risk figures nor does he determine the genotype of the members of the family and the proband. After organizing the appropriate care for the afflicted infant and informing the parents about it, he stresses the significance of genetic counselling and advises them on what will be required of them at the first visit, i.e. the pedigree of the mother's and father's side, the course of the pregnancy, the occupational and/or private life of both parents before conception and 3 months after it, etc. Table 54 shows a scheme of how the evaluation of the aetiology of some anomalies should be considered.

The scheme is simply a general guide. A more exact prognosis can be given only by a specialized laboratory, where all the peculiarities of the polygenic multifactorial system and the family's genealogy (e.g. the occurrence of spontaneous abortions in the family) are taken into consideration.

The paediatrician's normal duties comprise the reporting (registration) of selected structural congenital anomalies and the screening of some metabolic anomalies. These activities both belong to modern medicine, since they contribute to the working out of problems raised by genetic prognosis. Data banks in the field of population and/or clinical genetics will also benefit the recording of CA and the screening of metabolic congenital diseases. **All** newborn infants should be screened, but, in addition, maximum attention should be given to infants from families and/or parents identified as carriers of genes for certain metabolic diseases. Recessive mutant genes can be recognized in the carriers of some 20 such diseases; the children of these carriers are

Table 53. Recurrence risk of certain congenital anomalies

Type of congenital anomaly	Both parents healthy		One parent afflicted	
	1st child	2nd child	1st child	2nd child
Anencephaly	1:25 – 1:40	1:10 – 1:15	–	–
Spina bifida	1:40 – 1:50	1:10 – 1:25		
Microcephaly	1:50			
Cerebellar aplasia	1:50			
Cerebral palsy, all types	1:50			
Epilepsy, all types	1:30			
Mental defects	1:20 – 1:40			
Cataract	1:4			
Cleft palate	1:25		1:15	1:6 – 7
Hare lip	1:50		1:25	1:8
Hare lip + cleft palate	1:25		1:25	1:8
Megacolon	1:30 – 1:50*)			
Pyloric stenosis	1:10 – 1:30*)		1:15	1:5
Heart anomalies, all types	1:40 – 1:50	1:10 – 1:15		
Kidney agenesis	1:50	1:25		
Hypospadias	1:10			
Achondroplasia	1:40			
Arthrogryposis	1:20			
Osteogenesis imperfecta	1:20	1:2		
Down's syndrome caused by				
21/21 translocation	1:1			
D/G translocation	1:10			
21/22 translocation	1:20			
mosaic	1:20 – 1:40			
Juvenile diabetes	?	1:30	1:30	1:10

Explanation of columns (1st child, 2nd child): if the first child has, say, spina bifida, the risk for the next is 1 : 40 – 1 : 50, i.e. 2.5 – 2%. If the second child is affected, the risk for the next is 1 : 10 – 1 : 25, i.e. 10 – 4%.
*) With these traits, the recurrence risk depends on whether the first child to be affected is a boy or a girl.
By A. E. H. Emery: Elements of Medical Genetics, 2nd Ed., E. & S. Livingstone, Edinburgh and London, 1971.

high risk cases and require the appropriate examination after birth and special care during infancy.

The paediatrician (especially if he works in a nursery department) forms, together with the afflicted infant and its parents, a single unit, in which he is the first contact link. In the complicated and still relatively unexplored field of human teratology, it is essential for this link to be strong and operative.

Table 54. Types of examination of an afflicted infant and members of the family

Type of congenital anomaly	Type of examination	Subject(s) examined
Anomalies with known inheritance (autosomal and heterosomal, dominant and recessive)	genealogy	proband's family
Metabolic anomalies (known and suspected)	biochemical (for carriers) genealogy	proband, parents, siblings
Chromosomal defects (Down's, Klinefelter's, Turner's syndrome, etc.)	karyology dermatoglyphics genealogy	proband, parents
Multiple anomalies (syndromes) of known genesis (e.g. chromosomal, genic) or of unknown type	karyology genealogy occupational analysis	proband, parents
Repeated abortion, immature and stillborn foetuses	blood sugar (prediabetes) iodine level karyology	mother, possibly father
	genealogy immunoglobulins spermiogram occupational analysis	family parents father parents
Rubella embryopathy (cataract, deafness, mental retardation, heart defects)	dermatoglyphics immunoglobulins rubella antibodies	proband, mother
Heart defects	immunoglobulins virus serology (e.g. Coxsackie B_3, B_4)	mother
Pancreatic fibrosis Pyloric stenosis Exomphalos Diaphragmatic hernia	among others (see above), occupational analysis	father
Atresia of oesophagus and other parts of gastro-intestinal system (excluding anus and rectum), stenosis (atresia) of urinary system	immunoglobulins and other tests for infections (Coxsackie B_2, B_4)	mother
Gross skeletal defects	occupational analysis blood sugar attempted abortion? history of drug-taking	mother and her social and mental environment
Hydrocephalus	immunoglobulins toxoplasmosis (CFR)	

NEUROLOGICAL DIAGNOSTICS

IMPORTANCE OF NEUROLOGICAL EXAMINATION

It is a sad fact, but we have to admit that our knowledge of the morphological and functional development of the human nervous system is still largely fragmentary. Recent studies have refuted many older beliefs. We do not possess a completely verified, constant set of valid and adequate tests for detecting individual, clinically important functions of the nervous system in early infancy. Sometimes we fail to recognize exactly when a motor manifestation is already abnormal. Despite this, we are obliged to examine term, pre-term, small-for-dates, endangered and sick newborns and older infants, to submit a medical verdict on them, to treat them and to express an opinion on the prognosis. We are expected to be able to distinguish high risk from "normal" or non-risk infants. This is a very difficult task. It entails examining large groups of infants, detecting all the possible known and potential risks as accurately as possible, carefully choosing and/or suggesting the examination method and technique respectively and, after years of repeated examination and selection, describing the "normal" picture or the main features of the abnormal.

The problem does not concern only the children's neurologist. Child development must be studied from every aspect. We cannot confine our investigations solely to the development of gross and fine motor activity, which can be studied best in the first months. The development of all the other functions of the nervous system (e.g. visual, auditory function, etc.) is equally important, not to mention the need for studying the development of mental faculties. Study cannot be restricted to the neonatal period and infancy, but the children must be followed up until they start attending school and usually longer. Interdisciplinary team work is thus a prerequisite condition.

Pronounced lesions are usually evident at first glance, so to speak, but "mild" manifestations may go unrecognized for a long time. Quite frequently, the possibility of injury to the nervous system is suspected only from the case history. Repeated, careful examination will often confirm this suspicion or, conversely, negate it. It is known that even a fairly incontestable pathological finding in the neonatal period can sometimes soon "disappear", only to re-emerge later and often in a different form. If, in the interim, the infant is examined by routine methods only, the usually discrete finding will escape the examiner's notice.

The importance of neurological examination in the neonatal period has been summed up by various authors (Prechtl 1964, Joppich and Schulte 1968, Vlach 1969). Here we can only briefly enumerate the following aspects: a) its immediate diagnostic and therapeutic significance, b) its importance for determining the stage of development and/or the maturity of the CNS, c) its preventive-therapeutic significance (early rehabilitation), d) its prognostic significance, e) its importance for study of the development of reflexes and other phenomena and functions of the nervous system, f) its importance for assessing the infant's general condition.

Today it is generally acknowledged that careful, methodologically and technically correctly chosen neurological examination can readily reveal a small lesion or affection of the nervous system in the newborn infant. The examination method is thus an important factor. Its choice depends on our concept of the nervous system, on what we consider to be substantial and what not, on what we are looking for and studying, on our battery of tests, on whether our tests are valid, on their prognostic significance and on our own practical experiences, etc.

The "localization concepts" on which the neurological examination of adults is based are not capable of general clinical application in infants. They can be used, to some extent, for the spinal cord and brain stem areas. In modern pathophysiological analysis we no longer think in terms of centres, but of functional circuits, which can be evaluated clinically by a series of examination tests. We should not imagine that such an examination is by any means complete. Individual functional circuits can be examined by given tests of varying diagnostic value. For reasons of practical economy we are often obliged to choose only some of a series of reflexes or reactions. In this we follow a basic principle: according to our aim and general concept we choose the tests which we consider to be the most satisfactory. We may conceivably make gross mistakes through incomplete knowledge of the validity of the various possible tests. We may not utilize the right tests completely, or may not use them at all. Furthermore, we usually evaluate functions by different subjective and/or personal criteria and no doubt break up many functional units quite superfluously. In other cases we are unable to discriminate and/or select individual functions forming part of a large complex. For

218

practical reasons we mostly fall back upon the observation of fairly simple functions, e.g. the basic manifestations of spontaneous gross and fine motor activity, and examine changes in muscle tonus and "provoked" motility. Up to now, relatively little attention has been paid to different static and kinetic postural and movement patterns during infancy.

Another trouble is that the variable, and often still unknown, dynamics of development create behavioural manifestations in which the differentiation of a developmental and an incipient pathological change presents considerable difficulties. Many are of the opinion that two testing methods ought to be used — one for determining the level of development and the other for determining specific pathological changes. The two problems are not completely independent of each other. For instance, a pathological lesion often causes only developmental retardation at first, while, conversely, simple, uncomplicated psychomotor retardation may be accompanied by signs which we should regard as manifestly pathological in another stage of development. This means that our knowledge of all the components (fields) of development, together with their evolutional dynamics and variations, and our knowledge of pathological development of various functions and different sensorimotor manifestations ought to be as thorough as possible. At present, these questions are more or less in the research stage.

Our conduct of neurological examination

Our aim was to draw up an examination code covering the developmental and the neuropathological component. We chose tests which we considered to be essential for evaluating infants from high risk pregnancies. We are cognizant of all the pitfalls of our attempt. Our examination code is comparatively short, but its purpose is to detect the neurological development of individual infants relatively complexly. We do not claim that our system is definitive, or that it can be used unmodified for patients in the neurological departments of children's hospitals. When studying high risk infants, we want to detect, in a relatively short time, only the essential deviant features by a qualitatively and quantitatively standardized, **simple method,** to enable the results to be processed by mathematical machines. Our method must thus be subjected to criticism with these reservations.

In principle, we have used our own neonatal and infant examination technique, which was verified by years of experience and then published and filmed (Vlach, 1964, 1968). In the present monograph, however, from among whole series of tests we have included only those which we considered to be the **most satisfactory** and **essential.** For example, from among the tests used for evaluating muscular "tone" we have chosen only one of the five techniques advised by Thomas (1960), i.e. examination of extensibility, because it allows objective, quantitative assessment. We have chosen tests by which the infant's **development** and any **pathological signs** in the neonatal period and subsequent trimesters can be assessed. In further follow-up we have tried not to omit a single test from the series, to make sure of detecting the development of the observed phenomena. For later phases of development we were naturally obliged to add a number of tests.

Principles of examination technique

During the examination we try to proceed as **naturally** and **gently** as possible, so as not to affect the child's behavioural state. We are interested in:
(1) The child's condition and appearance (shape and proportionality of head, trunk and limbs; size of head, great fontanelle and sutures; auscultation of head, percussion sounds).
(2) Resting posture (position of head, trunk and limbs).
(3) Motility:
a) spontaneous: of head, trunk and limbs; facial expression, oculomotor innervation.
b) passive: the child remains passive and we actively move individual body segments. For example, we examine extensibility and determine whether it is normal, raised or lowered; at the same time we feel some resistance.
c) provoked: tonic myotatic (stretch) reflexes (e.g. the head-righting reflex); phasic reflexes (e.g. the Achilles tendon reflex);
exteroceptive reflexes (e.g. Galant's lumbar reflex).
To avoid upsetting the child unnecessarily at the outset of the examination, we begin with **observation.** We evaluate general condition and appearance, position and posture (with special reference to muscular tone) and spontaneous motility. We obviously record findings like strabismus, nystagmus and abnormal or pathological forms of movement, etc.
Inspection is followed by gentle **palpation.** We evaluate muscle consistence and test the extensibility of the individual body segments. We examine "passive" motility and also provoked motility (tonic stretch reflexes). We further palpate the head, fontanelles and sutures.
We then proceed to **auscultation** of the head and the large blood vessels.
We next carry out a **percussion** examination, using a percussion hammer or our own finger. We tap the head and compare the percussion sound over the right and left hemisphere and over the ventral and dorsal part of the skull. We observe any nociceptive reaction (as likewise in palpation by press-

ure on nerve origins and trunks). We further test phasic muscle (tendo-muscular, deep) reflexes – and hence provoked motility – by percussion. Idioneural excitability (e.g. Chvostek's sign, excitability of the radial nerve, etc.) and idiomuscular excitability can also be tested by percussion.

Lastly, we test exteroceptive reflexes, which are known to upset the child a little on occasion – surprisingly enough, far more than percussion-elicited proprioceptive phasic muscle reflexes. Cutaneous reflexes are elicited by **tactile stimulation of the skin** with a wooden stick or our fingers.

We examine the infant by the above method in the following sequence:

I.   First of all in the position in which the mother places it on the examining table, i.e. on its back – in the **supine position** (observation, then palpation, auscultation, percussion and cutaneous reflexes).

II.   We next take the infant by the hands and slowly raise it to a **sitting position.** When the trunk is at an angle of about 60 degrees to the table, we stop for a few seconds and carefully record the position of the head and trunk and of the upper and lower limbs. We then pull the infant into the full sitting position and, after a few seconds, further forwards, until its head tends to bend towards the table, or even touches it (e.g. in hypotonic infants). We also test a number of reflexes in the sitting position.

III.   We then carefully lower the infant from this position on to its back again and turn it over reflexly on to its abdomen, i.e. into the **prone position.** To do this we use two reflexes: (1) the neck-righting reflex on the trunk and, if this is not completely successful, (2) the rolling reflex. We next examine the infant in the prone position in the same sequence as before (observation, palpation, percussion and cutaneous stimulation). We thus again examine appearance, posture and passive and provoked motility. In addition, we carefully evaluate spontaneous motility by close observation.

When we have completed all the necessary examinations in this position, we proceed to the next (IV).

IV.   This position is known as **suspension.** With both hands, we lift the infant from position III (prone) above the level of the table into horizontal suspension. We examine a number of postural reflexes (e.g. Landau's reflex, the rolling reflex in suspension, Vojta's reflex and others). We next examine the infant in vertical suspension and then try to swing it, etc. Lastly, we carefully lower it until its feet are on the table.

V. In this, the **vertical** (upright) **position,** we examine the positive supporting (standing) reflex, the walking mechanism (stepping reflex), spontaneous standing, walking, etc.

At the very end we test a number of irritating and upsetting reflexes, such as Moro's reflex, with the infant again on its back.

In the course of time, we discovered, to our surprise, that infants found many completely painless tests and techniques disagreeable and upsetting and that the majority reacted to them by crying. These include the examination of certain extensibility phenomena and some tonic stretch reflexes, e.g. arms up testing, with the upper limbs pressed passively to the ears, tonic neck reflexes, etc. We therefore generally leave them until the end of the examination.

Although spontaneous motility, tremor, hyperkinesia and opisthotonus are mentioned on the first page of our code, we likewise do not evaluate them until the end of the examination, when we are better able to assess them.

Our examination technique is thus **standardized.** Its standardization is not rigid, however, but can be partly varied according to circumstances. In principle, it corresponds to the requirements and demands of Prechtl's school. We standardize the external environment, the infant's state and the intensity of stimuli and responses. We also standardize the **sequence** of the examination, not only as regards the **examination positions,** but also the **initial positions** of the body segments, i.e. of the trunk and limbs, and the **sequence of reflexes** and other phenomena in the various positions.

METHOD OF EXAMINING INFANTS FROM HIGH RISK PREGNANCIES

I. SUPINE POSITION

We draw a sketch like that in supplement.
Spontaneous motility:
- hypokinetic (infant absolutely calm, minimal motor activity)
- normokinetic (infant calm, but active)
- hyperkinetic (infant restless, cries frequently, motor hyperactivity)
Tremor:
- absent
- fine (amplitude not more than 2 cm, frequency about 6 – 7/s)
- gross (amplitude over 2 cm, frequency 3 – 4/s)
Hyperkinesia:
- absent
- choreoathetoid (more often choreiform or athetoid)
- tonic or clonic seizures

Pathological provoked motility:
- absent
- ankle clonus provoked when examining extensibility of ankle
- gross tremor of upper limbs (UL) in Moro's reflex
- exaggerated reflexogenic zone
- polykinetic responses in tendomuscular (tendon) reflexes
- other pathological responses

Opisthotonus (prolonged hyperextension of head when infant lies on side or abdomen or when reflex standing is tested):
- absent
- present

Strabismus (always evaluated to see whether or not it is paralytic):
- absent
- convergent, divergent

Nystagmus (always recorded):
- absent
- present

Anterior fontanelle: we determine size and measure length of sides

Arm-raising: we passively raise infant's UL, extended at elbows, so that inner surface of elbow touches ear lobe
- elbow joint touches ear lobe
- elbow joint cannot be brought into contact with ear lobe

Extensibility in shoulder joint (actually an attempt to test "scarf" phenomenon in both UL at once, i.e. we passively cross UL, wrapping them round neck as far as possible and evaluate distance between olecranons):
- olecranons in single vertical line
- do not reach vertical line
- cross over vertical line

Extensibility in elbow (we passively extend UL in elbow, evaluate angle between forearm and arm, holding limb with elbow supported, and record it):
- over 180°
- 180°
- 160° − 179°
- 90° − 159°
- under 90°

Extensibility in knee: with lower limb (LL) lying on table, we passively extend it in knee joint and evaluate leg-thick angle in presence of passive extension in hip joint. Angles recorded in same way as for extensibility in elbow joint.

Extensibility of ankle:
- dorsum of foot can be passively placed on anterior surface of leg
- cannot be placed on anterior surface of leg; in that case we evaluate and record angle between leg and foot axis

Abduction at hip joint (both LL are passively abducted at hip joint, with knees flexed at 90°; we evaluate the angle formed by the axes of the thighs):
- 180° (lateral condyles touch table)
- 150° – 179°
- 90° – 149°
- under 90°

Flexion at hip joint, with knees flexed:
- both LL folded protractor-wise on abdomen, i.e. knees and ventral surface of thighs rest on abdominal wall and flexed surfaces of LL likewise touch each other
- thighs cannot be made to touch abdominal wall

Flexion in hip joint with knees extended (heel-to-ear manoeuvre) (LL flexed passively in hip, without elevating buttocks; we measure angle between axis of trunk and LL):
- over 90°
- 90°
- 60 – 89°
- under 60°
- heel touches ear

Neck-righting reflex on head (we slowly rotate pelvis by 90°, turning infant on to side; rotation of head evaluated):
- head turned in same direction by up to 90°
- head turned by not more than 20°, or not at all

Reflexes: we test the following reflexes: nasopalpebral, masseter, palmar grasp, Babinski's sign, Juster's sign, digital, biceps, abdominal, patellar, plantar, medioplantar, Achilles tendon, Rossolimo's, plantar grasp. Evaluation:
- response positive (even small response, if clinically evident)
- response negative

II. SITTING POSITION (traction test)

The infant is slowly pulled up by its hands to a sitting position and when the trunk forms an angle of 60° with the table, head, trunk, UL and LL posture are examined.

Head position (control):
- head drops into retroflexion
- head in line with trunk
- head anteflexed

UL posture (angle of elbow joint measured):
- 180°
- 90° – 179°
- 60° – 89°
- under 60°

LL posture: angle of knee joint measured; evaluation as for UL.

Bending sideways in sitting position: reflex response of supporting limb to passive deflection of trunk to side studied. Evaluation:
- infant does not support itself
- supports itself on elbow, with UL abducted
- supports itself on clenched hand, with UL extended and abducted
- supports itself on palm

Rocking on buttocks: sitting infant is rocked passively backwards and forwards. Posture of UL and LL evaluated.

Posture of UL during rocking on buttocks (angle of elbow joint evaluated):
- 180°
- 160° – 179°
- 90° – 159°
- under 90°

Posture of LL during rocking on buttocks; angle of knee joint evaluated in same way as for UL.

Anteflexion of trunk from sitting position (we passively bend the head and trunk slowly forwards between the extended and slightly abducted LL):
- head and trunk can be anteflexed down to table
- not as far as to table

III. PRONE POSITION

We change the infant from the supine to the prone position by means of two reflexes: the neck-righting reflex on the trunk (NRRT) and the rolling reflex.

NRRT: passive rotation of head by 90° induces successive rotation of trunk. Posture of shoulder, pelvis, UL and LL studied.

Shoulder:
- no elevation, shoulder remains on table
- shoulder raised from table by up to 60°
- shoulder raised from table by over 60°

Pelvis:
- relevant hip not elevated
- hip lifted from table

Bracing on bottom UL:
- infant braces itself on elbow
- bracing does not occur

Top UL (angle of elbow joint and stroke performed by UL evaluated):
- flexed (90°), no stroke
- extended (160° – 180°), no stroke
- swung (limb actively swung from backward to forward position)
- any other response

Top LL:
- flexed (in knee and hip joint, about 90°)
- extended (in knee and hip joint, 160° – 180°)
- stepping forward (active movement, semi-extended LL describes curve into kneeling position, i.e. flexion)
- any other reponse

Bottom LL:
- flexed (knee and hip joint about 90°)
- extended (knee and hip joint about 160° – 180°)
- any other reponse

Rolling reflex (Vlach): infant passively rolled over from back on to side and reflex response of head, UL and LL studied.

Head:
- turned together with trunk
- turned after trunk

Head-raising:
- infant does not raise head
- infant lifts head from table

Bracing on bottom UL:
- infant does not brace itself
- braces itself on elbow
- arm abducted, flexed in elbow
- arm extended upwards
- arm adducted

Top UL: evaluated as in NRRT
Top LL: evaluated as in NRRT

226

Bottom LL: evaluated as in NRRT
Passive abduction of top LL with infant lying on side:
 — passive abduction easily possible
 — bottom LL raised when abduction attempted
 — any other response
Spontaneous turning over from supine to prone position:
 — yes
 — no
Spontaneous turning over from prone to supine position:
 — yes
 — no
Prone position: we draw a sketch
Elevation of head:
 — for over 30 s
 — for less than 30 s
Bracing on UL:
 — infant does not brace itself
 — braces itself on elbows
 — braces itself on clenched hands, with both UL extended in elbow
 — braces itself on palms, with both UL extended in elbow
Spontaneous crawling, neonatal type (UL, LL):
 — alternating crawling movements, mainly of LL, later also of UL, not necessarily with locomotor effect
 — no crawling movements of UL or LL
Symmetrical tonic neck reflex: we passively bend the head gently back into maximum possible retroflexion, at the same time slightly raising the trunk. We evaluate:
 — flexion at elbow joints
 — extension at elbow joints
Elevation of buttocks: we grip the infant just above the pelvis and raise the buttocks above the table. We evaluate the angle of the hip joints (between trunk and thighs):
 — less than 90°
 — 90° – 120°
 — 120° – 180°
 — over 180°
Interscapular reflex (Vlach): using tactile stimulation of the paravertebral skin in the thoracic area, we evaluate:
 — absence of motor response
 — trunk response (isolated incurvation of upper trunk)

— complete response (incurvation of trunk, with flexion of limbs on stimulated side and semi-extension on controlateral side; the head tends to rotate towards the flexed limbs)

IV. SUSPENSION

Suspension in prone position: we draw a diagram
Axial suspension: in this study we examine the LL only (the angle of the hip joints)
  — flexion (90° and less)
  — semi-flexion (90° – 180°)
  — extension (180° and over)
Lateral suspension (modified after Vojta): 5 s after lateral suspension we examine the infant's LL. We evaluate:
  — flexion of top LL
  — extension of top LL
  — both LL directed forwards
  — extension of LL with abduction
Symmetry in lateral suspension:
  — on changing from one to other position, reciprocal posture of LL remains unaltered
  — asymmetry on changing position (change in reciprocal posture)
Placing reflex: in axial suspension we stimulate the dorsum of the foot against the edge of the table. We evaluate:
  — infant flexes LL, then braces plantae against table and extends LL
  — no reaction

V. UPRIGHT (VERTICAL) POSITION

From suspension, we stand the infant on the table.
Supporting reflex: we stand the infant on the table and evaluate:
  — no response
  — extension of LL
  — extension of LL and trunk
  — extension of LL, trunk and head
Standing on tiptoe: when examining the supporting reflex we evaluate foot posture:
  — infant stands on toes, with tendency to opisthotonic posture of trunk
  — stands on plantae

Walking reflex (stepping reflex):
- take at least one step with each LL
- no step

VI. LAST REFLEXES

Examined sometimes in the supine, sometimes in the sitting position.
Optical blink (dazzle) reflex: a bright light, shone on the infant's face, provokes:
- closing of eyelids
- no reaction
Following light:
- the infant follows a moving light above the examination table (distance about 60 cm)
- does not follow the light
Opticofacial reflex:
- the infant reacts by blinking when a hand is suddenly brought close to its eyes (from 40 cm to 5 cm in 1 s)
- does not react
Following of objects:
- the infant follows a horizontaly moving object 60 cm above its head over a distance of 1 m
- does not follow the object
Acousticofacial reflex:
- the infant reacts to a clap of the hands 20 cm from its ear by blinking
- does not react
Reaction to soft sound:
- the infant turns its head towards to source of the sound
- does not react
Symmetrical tonic neck reflex:
- passive anteflexion of head in supine position produces change in limb posture
- no change in limb posture
Asymmetrical tonic neck reflex:
- passive rotation of head by 90° with fixed shoulders and 5 s maintenance of this position produces change in posture of one or more limbs
Withdrawal reflex:
- tickling (pricking) soles elicits triple flexion of LL
- reflex not elicited

Moro's reflex: elicited by jerking infant suddenly in caudal direction; response of UL and LL evaluated
  - phase I: extension of UL less than (more than) 90°
  - phase II: flexion of UL less than (more than) 90°
  - LL in phase I: flexion (extension)

At the age of 8 months we further examine:

I. SUPINE POSITION

Locomotion:
  - infant lies still or moves limbs spontaneously without locomotor effect
  - pushes off from surface of table with LL

II. SITTING POSITION

If sat up, infant remains sitting without support:
  - for at least 1 min
  - less than 1 min or not at all
Unaided sitting up:
  - does not sit up
  - draws itself up from supine position by holding side of cot
  - turns over from back on to side or abdomen using one UL as support
  - turns over from back using UL as support

III. PRONE POSITION

Unaided, spontaneous rolling:
   turns over on to abdomen and again on to back at least 3 times in succession in same direction
  - not able to roll
Active locomotion:
  - crawls at least 25 cm, mainly by means of LL
  - crawls mainly by means of UL
  - crawls on all fours, supported on kness and on palms of extended UL
  - any other form of locomotion
  - no locomotion

Bending in "all fours" position: using gentle pressure, we deflect the trunk left and right or backwards and forwards and study the reaction of the supporting limbs:
- infant loses balance, falls in direction of pressure, examiner feels no resistance
- maintains balance, offers resistance, reaction of supporting limbs recorded

IV. SUSPENSION

Parachute reflex:
- no change in UL posture
- UL extended to table for support
- UL extended in elbows and abducted

Reaction of hands in parachute reflex:
- no reaction
- infant supports itself on clenched hands
- supports itself on palms

"Wheelbarrow" test:
- in the final position of the parachute reflex the infant takes 2 "steps" on its hands; angle between trunk and table about 25°.

V. UPRIGHT (VERTICAL) POSITION

Standing reaction: from vertical suspension we stand infant on table
- infant stands actively, LL extended in knees
- LL not extended

Maintenance of balance:
- if held under axillae, infant stands at least 30 s without "giving" at knees
- cannot support weight, "gives" at knees

Supported standing:
- infant stands in play-pen about 30 s, holding on with one or both hands
- does not stand

Bending in upright position: holding infant in vertical position under axillae, we bend it from side to side or backwards and forwards and observe LL movements
- takes step with supporting limb
- does not take step

Supported walking:
- takes 6 steps if held by one or both hands
- does not walk

Independent walking:
- not yet able to walk unaided
- takes about 6 steps without support

VI. LAST REFLEXES

Startle reaction: the infant responds to a sudden supra-threshold stimulus by a holokinetic (Moro-like) body movement; if often bursts into tears
- reacts
- does not react

Test of mental development during neurological examination:

In supine position puts great toes into mouth: yes − no
Voluntary hand grasp: yes − no
Puts toys into mouth: yes − no
Laughs out loud: yes − no
Vocalization: yes − no
Reaction to own name: yes (orientative motor reaction) − no (no motor reaction)
Reaction to change of voice: yes (change in infant's facial expression) − no
Cube-grasping: yes (in palm, with 1st and 2nd finger) − no
Bead-grasping: yes − no
Cube transfer from one hand to other: yes − no
Bites solid food: yes − no
If fed, takes food from spoon: yes − no
Drinks from held cup: yes − no
Performs trained elements (e.g. "bye-bye"): yes − no

At the age of 18 months we further examine:

V. UPRIGHT (VERTICAL) POSITION

Independent (unaided) standing: we evaluate the width of the base, i.e. the position of the LL in relation to the width of the pelvis, the position of the feet and dexterity when standing

Base:
- wider than pelvis
- same width as pelvis
- narrower than pelvis

Position of feet:
- tips turned inwards
- feet held parallel
- tips turned outwards

Dexterity when standing:
- picks up ball from ground
- catches rolling ball

Independent (unaided) walking: We make a note of when the child started to walk unaided, watch it walk a distance of 20 m and record:

Stability of walking:
- falls down while walking
- does not fall

Speed:
- walks slowly, still falls down
- runs without falling
- runs quickly without falling

Position of UL during walking (we draw a sketch):
- UL abducted in shoulder and flexed in elbow
- UL abducted in shoulder and extended in elbow
- UL held loosely beside body
- UL perform accompanying movements during walking

Length of steps: we measure heel-to-heel distance in cm

Rhythm of walking:
- steps regular and of equal length
- long steps alternated with short
- any other response

Angle of knee on loading supporting limb:
- LL remains extended in knee joint
- knee is semiflexed

Hip drops when supporting limb is loaded:
- yes
- no

Hip rotated when stepping forward:
- yes
- no

Treads:
- on toes
- on whole of sole
- on heel
- in some other manner

Dexterity in walking:

180° turn:
- does not turn
- takes two steps to turn
- takes three steps
- needs more than three steps to turn

Walking up and down stairs:
- with support
- without support
- changes feet
- puts same foot first
- unable to negotiate stairs

Tests of mental development during neurological examination:

Keeps self clean:
- yes
- no
- partly

Dribbles:
- yes
- no

Builds tower with bricks:
- no, does not play, scatters bricks
- yes, we record the number of bricks used to build the tower

Eats unaided with spoon:
- yes
- no

Drinks unaided from mug:
- yes
- no

Investigates contents of hollow object:
- yes
- no

Imitates observed actions:
- yes
- no

At the age of three years we further examine:

II. SITTING POSITION

Synergy of LL in spontaneous sitting up: if the child rises from the supine to the sitting position without using its UL (or with only slight assistance from the examiner), the LL are raised from the table. We evaluate the angle formed by the LL and the table and the symmetry of elevation of the LL:
  - synergy ($\leq 30°$)
  - asynergy ($> 30°$)
  - assymmetry of LL

Push test: we give the sitting child a rapid push backwards, thereby putting it off its balance, and observe
  the reaction of the UL:
  - UL extended and abducted
  - any other response
  the reaction of the LL:
  - extension together with abduction
  - any other response

Reflexes: We additionally test the triceps r., the finger flexors r., the Achilles tendon r. and Vítek's summation phenomenon and evaluate them in the same way as in the younger age groups.

Taxis of UL: with closed eyes, the child touches the tip of its nose with its index finger:
  - yes
  - no

Diadochokinesia of UL: the child holds its arms in the front stretch position and alternately turns its palms from supination to pronation:
  - yes, turns both UL in unison
  - no, movements asymmetrical

IV. SUSPENSION

Diagonal suspension: We suspend the child diagonally at an angle of 45° and 5 s later we evaluate the position of the LL:
  - LL dangle
  - LL extended
  - any other response

V. UPRIGHT (VERTICAL) POSITION

Stands unsupported on narrow base with eyes closed:
- — yes
- — no

Dexterity in standing:

UL: throws ball with both hands
- — yes
- — no

throws ball with one hand
- — yes
- — no

LL: stands 3 s on heels
- — yes
- — no

stands 3 s on tiptoe
- — yes
- — no

stands 3 s on the one leg
- — yes
- — no

Jumping and hopping: hops with feet together
- — yes
- — no

jumps down 1 step with feet together
- — yes
- — no

hops on one foot
- — yes
- — no

Walks 4 m unaided with eyes closed
- — yes
- — no

Dexterity in walking:

Can walk on heels
- — yes
- — no

Can walk on tiptoe
- — yes
- — no

Can walk along line for distance of 4 m
- yes
- no

AUXILIARY EXAMINATION METHODS

When an infant is born after a high risk pregnancy, with its CNS jeopardized by one or more high risk factors, a period of longitudinal study of its psycho-motor and neurological development begins for the team of doctors. The differential diagnostic aspects which have to be resolved during this study may be simple, or very complex. This is due to the variability of the picture from the first moments after birth, to age-related variation of the signs and to differences in the degree of involvement. Intact and damaged structures reciprocally influence each other, thereby producing different pictures, from simple disharmony, to given, more or less typical syndromes. We repeatedly ask ourselves whether the findings are merely the outcome of the presumed risk, or whether they are due to some other, coincident CNS disease of meta-bolic or genetic origin, etc.

The answer cannot be a purely medical one. The problem of the jeopardized or manifestly traumatized infant has an impact on family life and serious social consequences. The answer to the parents, who are often very young, must be as concrete as possible, since they will want to know whether, and with what safety, they can have another child. This makes auxiliary, and often very complicated, examination methods necessary. We must perform these examinations at the appropriate time and consider the information they can give and what contribution they can make to our conclusions.

When an infant is born we know the prenatal risk factors, the details of the course of the birth and the neonatal and neurological findings for the first 24 hours. These determine the infant's risk score, its prospects of survival and the degree of possible CNS damage. Present-day knowledge of the pathology of the neonatal period leads to more frequent cooperation between the children's neurologist and the paediatrician, and hence to a more active approach in examination, the indication of auxiliary methods and the choice of treatment.

When selecting our examination tactics, we proceed, on principle, from less to more exacting methods.

In the neonatal period, biochemical tests are the basic method. They include evaluation of the milieu intérieur and of any anomalies (alkalosis and acidosis, alone or combined). We must know reliably the values of mineral metabolism and osmolarity. We follow bilirubin levels vary carefully; the causes of hyper-bilirubinaemia must be determined and the differential diagnosis weighed. Blood sugar levels are determined as a matter of course. Liver tests should also be performed and the development of clotting factors should be studied in relation to all types of bleeding.

The neurologist attempts to correlate changes in these basic biochemical values in both the clinical and the electroencephalographic picture.

Examination of the cerebrospinal fluid gives information on the actual state of the CNS. It excludes the possibility of an inflammatory condition or confirms possible haemorrhage. In classic examination we evaluate the number of elements and the age of the RBC, total protein, sugars and chlorides (in this order, according to the amount of fluid available). Astrup's method of examining the cerebrospinal fluid tells us a great deal, particularly regarding respiratory centre control. This requires further clinical experiences and correlates, however. The fluid is obtained chiefly by lumbar puncture.

The range of indications for other forms of puncture (suboccipital, ventricular) is very small. As intensive care in specialized units increases, there will no doubt be an increase in the indications for ventricular puncture for suspected haemocephalus, with the possibility of drainage, in the same way as for fontanelle puncture in subdural hematomas, on the basis of lateralization findings in the neurological and encephalographic examination.

Intraparenchymal bleeding (haematoma) is an extremely serious, and diagnostically very complex, question. The first, orientative information is provided by echoencephalography (a shift of the middle echo), while arteriography gives more reliable findings. Where the findings are confirmed, neurosurgical puncture can be undertaken.

In the neonatal period, echoencephalography can be used, with some elaboration, to measure the width of the ventricles and their expansion in hydrocephalus and to look for a haematoma echo.

Pneumographic examination is indicated in the neonatal period primarily where intracranial and (still more frequently) spinal malformations are suspected. It is undoubtedly indicated more often in large, specialized intensive care units. X-rays of the skull and spine and examination of the optic fundus are further basic methods in the neonatal period. A craniometric study is also included. Screening tests of the urine for congenital metabolic defects are carried out automatically.

Electroencephalography is already an important method in the neonatal period and, together with specialized neurological examination of the newborn infant, i.e. with auxiliary examination methods in the broad meaning of the term, it forms the foundation for further study of the development and electrogenesis of the CNS, or the development of abnormal signs. The importance of electroencephalography in early postnatal ontogenesis is increasing. It is used for actual, acute diagnostics. Here we look primarily for signs indicative of lateralization, for focal signs compatible with possible involvement of the hemispheres and for signs indicative of brain stem involvement or cerebral oedema. Correlation of the EEG, which in this phase takes about 30 min, together with the heart and respiration rate, with the paediatric and neurological clinical picture usually forms the basis for the initiation of further therapeutic and examination methods.

When an acute state has been brought under control, a classic polygraphic examination, including EEG, is indicated. A standard examination lasts at least 90 minutes and includes electromyography of the mental muscle and the recording of eye movements, as well as heart and respiration rate and EEG. The elaboration of this graph, particularly in relation to the development of the REM and non-REM stages of sleep, is the starting point in the determination of electrogenesis and prognostic considerations.

In a longitudinal study from infancy to toddler age, we determine whether the presumed risks influenced the child's psychomotor development or not. We also confirm or refute whether any abnormality of development (retardation, mental change, the appearance of pathological phenomena) is the outcome of previously determined risks, or whether it is due to a coincident, developing, serious neurological disease of a degenerative, metabolic or expansive character. The attempt to reduce everything to a single denominator, to a reliably known and sometimes multifactorial risk, is the greatest diagnostic pitfall, since it may cause us to miss the correct therapeutic indications (e.g. in an infant with an indisputably pathological birth accompanied by a fractured humerus and retarded psychomotor development, phenylketonuria was overlooked and was not diagnosed until two years later).

Detailed neurological examination forms the basis of study of the development of endangered children. It evaluates the child from the aspect of motor and mental development, detects muscular tone and the development of pathological movements in the initial stages and signals the onset of known syndromes, from simple psychomotor retardation to minimal cerebral dysfunction and the typical picture of infantile cerebral palsy (ICP).

The majority of auxiliary examinations are indicated by the children's neurologist in conjunction with the responsible paediatrician. In this period we also proceed from less to more exacting examination methods.

Here again, biochemical tests form the basis, in particular mineral values (chiefly calcium and phosphatase values with reference to rickets, an often forgotten possible cause of psychomotor retardation). We examine the optic fundus and look for retinal haemorrhage, pigmentation and atrophy of the papillae of the optic nerve.

239

Straight X-ray examination is important. In X-rays of the skull we study the state of the sutures, growth of the skull in given planes, the shape of the fossae and the thickness of the skull, or changes in its character, and look for intracranial calcifications. In the straight spinal X-ray we exclude the possibility of malformations. A detailed craniometric examination is an inseparable part of examination of a skull with an abnormal shape or abnormal growth.

Further diagnostic techniques which cause the patient no stress are echoencephalography and translumination. Translumination is very useful in the case of a suspected subdural haematoma and for diagnosing hydrocephaly and other abnormalities of the contents of the cranium (e.g. large cysts, etc). Echoencephalography detects a shift of the middle echo and the growth dynamics of hydrocephaly (measurement of the width of the ventricles) and often helps in the diagnosis of a subdural haematoma by means of the haematoma echo.

EEG examination holds an important place in the spectrum of auxiliary examination methods, its applicability increasing with age. A longitudinal study detects progress or retardation of electrogenesis, which has fixed criteria, within a given range, for individual ages. A frequency analysis can be used when determining the theta-alpha quotient. In the course of the study, different types of abnormalities become more distinct or, conversely, vanish and specific epileptic graphoelements appear. The character (type) of the epileptic sign, e.g. hypsarrhythmia, indicates the degree of severity and prognosis of the disease.

Fontanelle puncture is a fairly frequent diagnostic operation in infancy. Where psychomotor development is retarded, the clinical picture shows signs of lateralization and there is a finding in the EEG or some other auxilliary examination, it should be done as a matter of choice. In our experience, there has been an increase in the incidence of subdural haematomas and hygromas in recent years − not, apparently, merely from improved diagnosis.

Both pneumoencephalography and ventriculography are used in this period chiefly for the diagnosis of hydrocephaly (to determine its aetiology and types). Scintigraphy, with intrathecal administration of the tracer, will show whether it is communicating or non-communicating. As the child grows older, we use pneumoencephalography to investigate residua of CNS damage, e.g. various malformations, agenesis, symmetrical periventricular atrophy or atrophy of only given parts of the ventricular system. We exclude the possibility of an expansive process. The cerebrospinal fluid is naturally examined as well.

Arteriography (visualization of the CNS vascular bed) is employed less often. We mostly make it with the methods mentioned above, partly because of the technical difficulties of examining little children. With advancing age its indication range and practical uses widen, particularly for suspected vascular malformations and tumours in the posterior fossa. Electromyography is also being used with increasing frequency in infants and toddlers, in the differential diagnosis of muscular diseases, e.g. to decide whether a paretic sign is of neurogenic or myogenic, peripheral or central origin and whether it contains a metabolic or some other component. Biopsy is also often needed to decide the nature of muscular diseases. It is likewise required, for histological tests, in certain serious CNS diseases of degenerative or metabolic origin. In serious cases we therefore indicate sternal puncture and removal of a liver, rectum or appendix sample. Brain biopsy is very rarely indicated.

We have given a brief survey of auxiliary examination methods used in child neurology. Some of them today require superspecialization in this post-graduate field. The treatment of a child with serious problems is thus a matter for a whole team, which should include a psychologist, a geneticist and, if need be, other specialists, as well as a paediatrician and a children's neurologist.

PSYCHOLOGICAL DIAGNOSTICS

SPECIFIC FEATURES OF THE PSYCHOLOGICAL EXAMINATION OF VERY YOUNG CHILDREN

The latest studies of the development of organisms underline the significance of the first phases of life for later development. The quality and quantity of the first stimuli (early stimulation) strongly influences the further development of physical and mental capacities.

The aim of diagnosis of an infant's mental and motor development is to determine the course of development of the infant's behaviour, i.e. whether it deviates from normal and, if so, to determine the quality and quantity of the defect. It helps in determining the causes of defects and in the choice of suitable therapeutic measures.

The principle of developmental diagnostics is comparison of the child's behaviour in a given situation with the behaviour of a representative sample of children of the same age, under the same conditions. For this purpose, suitable, objectively determinable and comparable criteria of behaviour are required. We require that developmental criteria should not only enable us to determine the level of different components of mental development, but also help us to distinguish the extent to which that level is determined by heredity and the extent to which it is dependent on learning i.e. on exogenous conditions. Behavioural criteria, which depend more on endogenous maturation and less on learning, are diagnostically suitable, although we know that all behaviour is in some measure influenced by learning. The authors of diagnostic methods attempt to quantify the level of behaviour development and their quantitative measure is usually the age at which a given criterion appears in the child population. They assume that the sooner the criterion appears (or disappears), the better the quality of the child's development. Before a criterion can be used in diagnostic practice, it must be standardized, i.e. it must be defined and determined in a representative sample of the child population.

There are other features of child development, however, in which the important criterion is not age, but the form and intensity in which they are present in the child. For instance, the ability to concentrate, or relationships to people, are features of behaviour which develop slowly and the authors of diagnostic methods look for different ways of determining their quality and measure their quantity.

The level of culture and civilization varies in different countries and in different periods and influences the child's development in a different way. Developmental diagnostic techniques standardized under given cultural conditions cannot therefore be applied to social conditions other than those for which they were originally determined.

In development tests for the youngest children, different forms of behaviour in known situations, e.g. play are assessed. Another feature of development tests for infants is their nonverbal character; the extent to which speech can be used for communication is very limited in these children. When choosing tests for infants, precedence should be given to tasks requiring the least possible interference on the part of the examiner, as this could strongly influence the child's behaviour and hence the results of the examination. Series of tests for determinating the level of an infant's mental and motor development must enable the quickest possible examination, since these children are not capable of cooperating well for more than 20 – 40 minutes.

When examining infants, we proceed differently than for older children. The main principle is to examine them only if they have slept well, are fed, relaxed, healthy and in a good mood. Unless these conditions are fulfilled, the reactions of the infants will not show the true level of their mental and motor development. The success of psychological examination also depends on the examiner's skill to contact the infant. It is easier for the child to adapt to the new situation when familiar elements in the text situation are included, e.g. by allowing the child to sit on its mother's lap, by letting it hold its favourite toy, etc. Very often, we can admit a reasonable compromise between the need to maintain standard conditions for all children and the need for adjusting them to the child's state. In infancy, subjective conditions are more important than the exogenous, objective conditions. It often happens that the child does not respond in the test situation, although its mother claims that, at home, it usually responds to the given stimulus. The mother's information is usually correct and should therefore be included in the records. In many cases we could not manage without the mother's information at all and without her assistance we should hardly be able to find out whether the child already asks to be put on the pot, etc.

Behaviour and its assessment

At an early age, it is very difficult to distinguish different functions or factors of later mental development. It is relatively easy to distinguish motor behaviour, but its relationship to mental functions in adults is very slight. There is, however, a correlation between tests of motor abilities and mental tests at an early age. There are various reasons for this. Tests of motor development allow us to evaluate the degree of neuromuscular coordination, which is also the basis of fine sensorimotor adaptation (regarded by many authors as the origin of later intellectual functions). Motor skills allow the child to enlarge the environment by which it is influenced. This means that the child is stimulated to more and more interactions with the environment and that its mental development is thereby positively affected. That is why the mental development of infants whose movements are restricted for a considerable length of time, for orthopaedic reasons, for instance, is usually temporarily retarded. The evaluation of motor development, as a part of psychological examination, is also very important, because disturbances of motor coordination are often the first sign of deviation from normal mental and motor development.

Apart from the motor development scale, development tests attempt to evaluate other components of child behaviour. Gesell (1947) differentiates adaptive behaviour, language and social behaviour. For him, adaptivity is the biological equivalent of intelligence and he evaluates it according to the degree of fine sensorimotor adaptation to objects and situations. For example, in the 4th week the child follows a toy in the midline and diminishes activity in response to a sound stimulus. In the 16th week the hands approaches an offered toy, the infant regards a toy in its hand and looks at a small object (a pellet). At 28 weeks, the hands move towards a bell and grasp it and hold two cubes more than momentarily. At 40 weeks the infant plays with two cubes, touches cube in cup, approaches to a pellet with its index finger and grasps a bell by handle. At 52 weeks it tries tower of two cubes, releases a cube into a cup and tries to insert a pellet into a bottle. Gesell defines languge as all visible and audible forms of communication – vocalization, gestures, words, understanding. As social behaviour child's reactions to the social culture in which it lives are defined. For example, at 4 weeks the infant's activity diminishes when spoken to by an adult, at 16 weeks it smiles when it looks at an adult and "recognizes" its own bottle, at 28 weeks it takes solid food and at 52 weeks it begins to cooperate in dressing. Gesell evaluates all components of behaviour separately and thus avoids too great generalization of behaviour.

In another development test for the smallest children, Bühler (1932) evaluates a) sensory perception (reactions to optic, acoustic and tactile stimuli), b) social behaviour, in which capacity for social contact, ability to respond

244

verbally and non-verbally to instructions and language are differentiated, and c) learning, which she interprets as an experience-induced change in behaviour. Under this she evaluates a) practical memory (e.g. looking for a lost object), b) verbal memory (after the age of 1 year), c) imitation (e.g. imitative banging on a drum with a stick), d) activity with objects in which, in addition to proper activity (e.g. opening a box at 11 – 12 months), persistence is also evaluated, and e) mental production, i.e. the use of tools (at 11 – 12 months the infant pulls a toy by means of a string) and the understanding of relations (e.g. at 11 – 12 months dragging a toy from under a screen).

Today, N. Bayley's development test (1969) is frequently used. In addition to a motor development scale, this test includes a separate mental development scale and a scale for evaluating the child's behaviour during examination. The mental scale evaluates the development of perception, the beginnings of learning and solving problems, the development of vocalization and verbal communication and the first signs of ability to form generalizations and classifications, as the basis of abstract thinking. For evaluating development during the first year of life, 21 different situations are defined, in which the child's reactions are assessed, e.g. its reactions to optic and acoustic stimuli, complicated manipulation with cubes, a spoon, two toys, pellet, etc.

In order to be able to evaluate an infant's development, it is necessary to use one of the developmental tests. For the psychological examination of a one- -year old we should allow about 45 minutes. In paediatric routine this is usually not possible. We therefore need screening methods which will shorten the psychological examination procedure. By means of these methods we can determine whether the course of development is normal or abnormal. If we find an aberration, it is necessary to send the child for a more detailed psychological examination.

Table 55 shows reactions characteristic for the given months of the first year of life. We have supplemented it by another table (Table 56), which gives the borderline criteria of neuropsychic development in the 3rd, 6th, 9th and 12th month. When drawing up this table, we paid attention chiefly to reactions whose absence at the given age may be taken as a serious sign of deviation from normal development. The given reactions occur in the great majority (over 90 %) of normal children. For example, if, in the third month, an infant does not lift its head when lying in the prone position, does not vocalise or smile in response to the examiner's talk, or does not follow objects with its eyes — reactions present in the majority of normal infants — we do not wait, but immediately send the child for special examination.

The sixth month is characterized by the beginning of locomotion (the infant rolls on to its side and often to a prone position), by the beginning of sitting up (the head and arms cooperate when the child is pulled up into a sitting position)

Table 55. Table for determining an infant's mental and motor development

Month	Development of gross motor activity	Development of perception, hand movements and playing	Development of language and social behaviour
1	In prone position, lifts head momentarily, usually rotates the head to one side. Occasionally lifts the pelvis and performs crawling movements with his legs	Hand clenches on contact with a toy. Regards a toy held in its line of vision and pursues its movements in through an arc of 90°	Occasionally vocalizes small throat noises and single vowel sounds such as "ah", "eh". Regards momentarily the face of person who comes into its line of vision
2	In prone position, holds the head lifted about 10 cm at least 5 s. If held vertically, supported around the chest under the axillae, keeps head erect	Retains toy briefly (over 10 s). Pursues moving toy with eyes through an arc of 180°	Smiles in reply. Follows moving persons in near distance
3	In prone position, keeps head lifted more than momentarily, curves back in lumbar region, props himself on arms	Holds toy more than momentarily and waves it. Regards hands. Looks for source of sounds	Begins to vocalize in reply. Smiles and shows excitement to voice
4	In prone position, arms extended, sometimes rolls passively to supine. If pulled up into sitting position, head erect, steady. If held under arms, sustains a small fraction of weight	Regards toys in hand. Approaches hand tentatively towards proffered toy	Vocalizes spontaneously, begins to laugh out loud when teased
5	Rolls unaided from supine to prone position. When prone, his weight is on his abdomen and hands. If pulled into sitting position, retracts head, stretches legs forward. If held under arms, sustains a great part of weight	Approaches hand to toy with assurance. Transfers it from one hand to other and puts it into mouth. Turns head in direction of sounds	Vocalizes and calls out. Distinguishes gentle and severe shades of speech and facial expression
6	When prone, lifts one hand. Rolls actively from abdomen to back. Grasps offered fingers and pulls itself up. If held under arms, supports whole of weight for a short time on feet and "bounces" (does knee-bends)	Can hold one toy in either hand	Vocalizes and utters vowels and consonants, begins to join them in syllables. Behaves differently to familiar persons and strangers. Establishes contact by vocalizing
7	When prone, rotates right and left on umbilical axis (pivots). Holding a second person's fingers pulls itself up into sitting and also standing position	Takes cube in each hand itself, inspects toys, using wrist movements. Bangs table with toys	Babbles syllables (ba, ma, da, va). Looks at one named object. — Understands game of "peep-bo"

246

Table55 (cont.)

Month	Development of gross motor activity	Development of perception, hand movements and playing	Development of language and social behaviour
8	Creeps on abdomen and bounces on knees. Sits unaided, but unsurely. Stands firmly holding a railing	Begins to grasp small objects with thumb and index finger. Pushes cube with cube	Repeats syllables ba-ba-ba etc. and begins to duplicate (ba-ba). Looks at more (about 5) named objects. Understands game of "bumps-a-daisy"
9	Crawls. Sits with good control and sits up without holding. Stands up holding play-pen	Touches details on toy. Bangs toy with toy	Patacakes
10	Begins to walk sideways round furniture	Removes cubes from bowl, opens and empties drawers and boxes	Understands: "Give it to me!", "Wave bye-bye!"
11	Walks forwards holding furniture and walks when held by both hands	Inserts objects into boxes and holes. Pulls toy towards itself by means of string	Can point to its arm, foot and to other specified persons and things. Understands praise and repeats activity to be praised
12	Walks when held by one hand. One step without holding when moving e.g. from chair to couch	Grasps 2 cubes in hand. Inserts small object (e.g. a pellet) into bottle	Says 1—2 words. Responds correctly to simple commands, e.g. "Fetch your spoon!" Understands and responds to "Mustn't!" Imitates, e.g. dusting

and by a good postural compensation in the prone position (the child lifts its chest high and props itself on its forearms or palms and holds its head firmly erect). The child distinguishes between known persons and strangers, vocalises while playing, and turns itself in the direction of sounds. It plays with toys, grasps an offered rattle and transfers it from one hand to the other. As a rule, it is also capable of grasping a toy in both hands and of holding it for a short time.

At nine months the infant sits steady and begins to sit up. If it does not sit with good control at this age, we do not draw any conclusions from the fact as long as the other indicators are present. At this age the infant must, however, be capable of standing supporting its full weight on its feet (not only the toes) when held under the arms. Most children also stand if held by only one hand, and pull themselves up on to their feet, holding rail. Fine sensorimotor adaptation to objects makes further progress (the child handles two toys simultaneously and can grasp small objects with its thumb and index finger). In

Table 56. Borderline criteria of infant's mental and motor development

Month	Development of gross motor activity	Development of perception, hand movements and playing	Development of language and social behaviour
3	Holds head in the midline when supine. In prone position lifts head	Follows moving object with eyes and head	Observes adult, smiles and vocalizes in reply
6	In prone position holds head, props himself on its forearms and raises chest. Rolls to side. When pulled to sitting position, head is in good alignment with the trunk	Turns towards sounds, grasps rattle. Transfers rattle from one hand to other	Vocalizes while playing
9	Rolls on to stomach. Sits with good control. If held under arms, places full weight on feet	Grasps cube in each hand	Vocalizes syllables
12	Stands if held by one hand. Stands up by furniture makes stepping movements holding it	Bangs cube with cube	Duplication of syllables (da-da). Patacakes

language, we often find duplication of syllables (ma-ma, da-da, etc.). The child is capable of carrying out a number of verbal instructions, but it is amazing how few children of this age are stimulated in this way. If an infant of this age does not babble, it should be examined in greater detail.

A one-year-old sits with good control, stands up by means of the cot-side, etc., stands if held by one hand and takes steps round the sides of the play-pen. It can often walk if held by one or both hands and (less frequently) may walk alone. Most children also crawl, but there are some who only make attempts to crawl, and only for a short time. The way the child grasps is of great diagnostic value; the thumb should be opposed to the fingers and small objects should be grasped only with the thumb and the index finger. The children often throw toys out of the cot, but will occupy themselves quietly for several minutes with toys or objects. The beginnings of mediated behaviour start to appear at this age, e.g. the child pulls a toy towards itself by a string. Imitation of various activities also progressively develops, understanding of speech increases and the child begins to utter words. The extent of understanding and the number of words the child utters both depend largely on stimulation, so that when we evaluate the development of speech we must know the child's environment. If, at one year, we do not find beginnings of understanding, and if the child's vocalisation does not contain at least duplication of syllables, it is necessary to send the child for a more detailed examination.

DELAYED EFFECTS
IN HIGH-RISK-PREGNANCY CHILDREN

SOCIO-ECONOMIC FACTORS

Statistical analyses in western countries have demonstrated that various, completely non-medical influences, grouped under the definition "socio-economic factors" also participate in perinatal mortality and morbidity. Among the most important of these non-medical high risk factors are low level socio--economic conditions and unmarried mothers and their negative effect is manifested chiefly in a raised incidence of premature births.

In western studies, pregnant women are divided into 5 family income groups. The incidence of premature births in the first three groups (professional workers, office workers, shopkeepers) is low (4.6 %). In the fourth (qualified manual workers) it is 7.9 % and in the fifth group (labourers) it is as high as 10.3 %. If the economic situation were the decisive factor, this high risk factor ought not to be felt at all in Czechoslovakia, owing to the small differences in the incomes of the above groups and the higher basic income limit. No such studies exist there, however, and there is therefore no objective evidence in support of this hypothesis.

The raised incidence of premature birth among unmarried mothers in western analyses is probably the outcome of several factors. The possible influence of inadequate antenatal care was excluded when it was found that the incidence of premature births in a group of unmarried women who received good antenatal care was still double that for married women (Butler 1969). The data of intensive care units show that these departments admit three times as many infants of unmarried mothers as of married mothers (Pierog et al. 1970). Since the majority of unwanted pregnancies in unmarried women are terminated in Czechoslovakia by legal abortion, this high risk factor is no longer of quantitative significance there. Even there, however, it remains a high risk factor, chiefly as regards the risk of more frequent prematurity (Štembera et al. 1974).

Employment, as a high risk factor for pregnant women, is too complex a question for us to be able to give clear cut answer. In Czechoslovakia, where the percentage of women who continue working during pregnancy is high, it is a very important question. An extensive sociological analysis carried out in England among married women of the same age, and belonging to the same social group, showed that premature labour occurred in 11.1 % of those who worked longer than 28 weeks during pregnancy, in 8.4% who worked for a shorter period and in only 4.7% of those remaining at home (Stewart, 1955). Other, later authors (Trampuz 1963, Ahvenainen et al. 1963) arrived at similar conclusion. If we do not take special high risk environments, e.g. work with toxic substances in chemical laboratories (Sapák et al. 1964), into account, we can find no greater predisposition to premature labour in any given form of employment, in either Czechoslovak (Pontuch et al. 1964) or other, extensive analyses (Watteville 1963). It seems rather to be the extra strain (the second "job", i.e. housework after returning home, insufficient rest and sleep) and the greater probability of contact with other negative factors (bad transport conditions, various situations at work) which constitutes the high risk premature labour factor. It is for our sociologists to produce some sound studies on this problem and the prospects future. Their results could furnish new points of view and provide objective material, e.g. on which to base a change in the time for taking maternity leave prior to the infant's birth, etc.

Poor antenatal care on an average, a relatively high percentage of extra-institutional births and consequent high perinatal mortality are problems which involve the gipsy question directly in perinatal problems. We know nothing at all about perinatal morbidity among gipsies, or of the part it plays in certain indexes which point to deficiencies in improvement of the quality of this section of the Czechoslovak population (a low mean IQ, low cultural standards, etc.). From the standpoint of the number of Romanies in Czechoslovakia (270,000, i.e. 1.6% of the total population, in the Czech Socialist Republic only 62,000 i.e. 0.6%), the inclusion of the gipsy question in this chapter might, at first glance, seem to be superfluous. Regarding the Romany population explosion in Czechoslovakia, however, this question appears in a very different light. In the Czech Socialist Republic there is only 1 Romany to 161 other members of the population, but in birth statistics the proportion is 1 to 14, so that, today, half the Romanies are children under the age of 15 and 22 % of the children in children's homes are of gipsy origin. This question, as a whole, obviously exceeds the scope of the present book. Instructions for its resolution were issued to all national committees in a government decree (No. 279/1970).

In most of the advanced countries, perinatal mortality was found to be higher in large towns than in the country. Although, on the surface, this may appear paradoxical, since good perinatal care is easier to concentrate in densely populated areas, where it should produce better results, the above finding applies also to Czechoslovakia. On the other hand, it should be borne in mind that some non-medical, and even certain medical, risks are concentrated precisely in large towns. Similar regional differences also exist. For instance, North Bohemia is characterized by a concentration of large industrial towns, while other regions have a largely rural population. The sociological studies recommended above might help to provide an answer to the question of whether the higher perinatal mortality in such regions is the price we have to pay for "progress".

The developing child interacts continously with the family environment. We must therefore pay attention to the various ways in which the family, as a community, influences his development. A good knowledge of the environment is an important factor in an analysis of late effects, especially in a long-term study, in which changes during development can be detected.

The significance of an inquiry into the social and economic conditions of high-risk-pregnancy children consists in:

a) the need to characterize the children from the social aspect, and

b) the possibility of discovering factors specific for a given population which might play a role in the development of given conditions.

It is not easy to investigate the social environment and we do not yet possess any uniform criteria for its evaluation. In Czechoslovakia, these problems come under the Department of Family Care of the Ministry of Labour and Social Affairs, which carries out extensive cross section and long--term studies. Important results have been obtained in a long-term study of the influence of family factors on child development and growth (Bouchalová 1964, Kapalín 1969).

Working under the auspieces of the International Children's Centre in Paris there are 8 groups, from different European, African and American countries, which study child development in small series (of up to 200 children) by the same methods and meet regularly to evaluate and compare their results. The methods by which all these teams evaluate the socio-economic situation were elaborated by Graffar (1956). They are based on a system of simple, reliable and objective data and on the principle that classification by occupation provides a true picture of a family's degree of education and of its economic situation and culture. Graffar chose five criteria for evaluation: employment, education, source of income, type of dwelling and place of residence. For each of these factors he fixed a five-grade scale. He recommended that the socio-economic environment should be classified by adding the individual evaluated factors, combining the results in five qualification classes according to the final number of points. The purpose of Graffar's system is to allow reciprocal comparison of the social, hygienic and cultural environment of the children whose development is being studied. It has the advantage of being comprehensive, but combination of the results tends to obliterate differences in the importance of the individual criteria and it cannot be adopted under our conditions without modification.

The questionnaire used by the Institute for Care of Mother and Child, Prague-Podolí, for evaluating the influence of the environment on child development in long-term prospective studies for the quantification of risk factors comprises the fundamental socio-economic characteristics, i.e. the age, education, occupational status and income of the child's parents, data on family structure and living conditions. We also determine the course of the mother's pregnancy, her mental and physical working stress (high risk workplaces) and the health of the nearest blood relatives:

(1) **Family structure:**
    siblings: none
    (sex, age)   (1)   (4)
                          (2)
                          (3)
    family lives alone
    family lives with grandparents
    family lives with other relatives
    other data:
    data of marriage:
    whether previously married: father..., mother.... (widowed, divorced)
    stepchildren of father...., mother.... (sex, age):
    living, not living with family

(2) **Child's father:**
    age: education:
    employment:
    working hours: shifts
                      daytime
                      other times
    income (net):   compulsory payments for other children:
    other family incomes (except mother's):
    father's birthplace:
    length of residence at present address (type of community):

(3) **Child's mother:**
    age: education:
    employment:
    income (net):

change of employment during pregnancy:
unfitness for work during pregnancy:
date of commencement of maternity leave:
how long mother intends to remain at home after child's birth:
working hours: shifts
        daytime
        other times
journey to work: on foot, transport (from):   minutes:
workplace: office, factory, others:
working environment: dusty, noisy, cold, smoky, others: (high risk)
mother smoked: prior to pregnancy, how many cigarettes daily – during
        pregnancy, how many daily
physical (mental) strain imposed by employment: constant
        occasional
        none

finds housework: exhausting
        sometimes tiring
        not tiring
help given by family: regularly
        occasionally
        not at all
time spent away from town during pregnancy:
Saturdays and Sundays: mostly in country
        mostly in town
mother's mental state during pregnancy:

(1) influence of workplace:
(2) family relationships:
(3) financial and dwelling situation:
(4) important events which affected mother strongly:
accidents, injuries during pregnancy:
parenthood planned, not planned:
whether mother wants further children: yes
        uncertain
        no (reason)
mother's birthplace:
length of residence at present address (type of community):
employment of mother's father at time of her brith:

(4) Dwelling conditions:
cooperative flat, own house, state-owned flat, others:
house new, moderately old, old

dwelling inhabited by: immediate family
extended family
others
number of rooms: number of persons:
kitchen: own, shared, kitchenette, adapted corner, other arrangements:
conveniences: lavatory,   bathroom,   water supply
own, shared, inside dwelling, outside dwelling
heating: central, stoves, other forms
dweling: dry, damp, light, dark
remarks:

(5) **Health of family:**
child's father:
child's mother:
child's siblings:
father's parents:
father's siblings:
mother's parents:
mother's siblings:
remarks: date of investigation:

The above data are obtained straight from the mother, either in the maternity hospital (home) at the time of the child's birth, or on the occasion of a visit
to the family by a regular health visitor. Further control inquiries are made
when the child is 18 months and 3 years old. Their purpose is to determine
changes in basic socio-economic factors – in occupational status, in the
morther's employment, in the parents' income, in living conditions and in
family structure, the births of another infant and the type of care of the child
(i.e. whether he is looked after by the mother or some other person, or whether
he attends a nursery school).

FIRST SIGNS OF DEFECTS IN THE DEVELOPMENT
OF MOTILITY

In an infant with a prenatally or perinatally acquired CNS disturbance we
observe in the neonatal period defects in autonomic function (disturbances of
respiration, circulation and thermoregulation) and absence of oral reflexes,
which, if they persist for any length of time, markedly influence the infant's
viability. Not until they have subsided can we evaluate other signs which

enable us to assess the gravity of CNS injury. These include absence of Moro's reflex or the grasp and sucking reflex, for example, but in that case the CNS is usually seriously damaged.

CNS disturbances which do not endanger the infant's life in the neonatal period are not manifested until later. The development of a CNS defect can be evaluated by comparing the motor development and postural attitude of the afflicted infant with development in a healthy infant. The development of the healthy infant and its motor and postural development form an objective criterion for assessing pathological motor development in the infant with CNS damage. We must also bear in mind that progress or retardation of motor development is closely associated with progress or retardation of mental development.

Compared with a normal infant, the infant with CNS injury may display poor spontaneous motor activity. This is observed mainly in infants with a hypotonia syndrome. Conversely, in infants with a hypertonia syndrome we sometimes see increased spontaneous motility. In the early postnatal phase, muscular tone is a very valuable guide in distinguishing pathological states.

Changes in provoked motor responses observed on changing the infant's postural attitude are another very valuable indication of a pathological state. They include, for example, opisthotonic head-holding, which appears when the infant's position is altered, e.g. if it is rolled (or rolls) on to its side, or is rocked on its buttocks. If the infant lies in the prone position, the doctor may sometimes erroneously evaluate opisthotonic head-holding as a sign of incipient head-righting. In our experience, however, in opisthotonic head-holding the neck is extended asymmetrically and not symmetrically. This can often be demonstrated by placing the infant in the prone position. It extends its neck assymmetrically, thereby causing retraction of one shoulder and a swinging movement of the arm. As a result, the infant rolls over spontaneously from prone to supine position, even in the first trimester, i.e. at an age when the normal infant is not yet able to do so.

Pathological motor responses are also found in postural reflexes in infants with CNS damage. In the rolling reflex, when the infant is turned passively on to its side, in a healthy infant of less than 3 months we find flexion of the lower limb which is on top when it is rolled over (the top lower limb). In an infant with CNS injury, this limb may be pathologically extended.

Differences are also found in Vojta's postural reflex, for which the infant is grasped under the arms and is turned horizontally on to its side, so that it is laterally suspended. This manoeuvre provokes reflex motor responses in the upper and lower limbs. In a heatlhy infant of less than 3 months, the arms are spread as in Moro's reflex, while the bottom lower limb is held extended, with the toes flexed, and the top lower limb is held in triple flexion, with the toes extended. In a pathologically developing infant of the same age, these responses of the top lower limb are absent, i.e. the limb remains extended, or responds incompletely or more slowly.

Another sign of motor involvement in infants with CNS injury is delayed development of righting mechanisms. At about 6 weeks, the normal infant is capable of symmetrical extension of the neck; at 3 months neck extension is better, the infant carries its weight on its forearms, clenching of the fists relaxes and adduction of the thumbs begin to disappear. Extension of the neck and the placing of weight on the forearms are the first basic components of righting mechanisms in ontogenetic development. If one or both are absent, it means that the infant is not developing normally.

The elicitation of tonic neck reflexes disappears during the first 3 months. Persistence of these reflexes in the second trimester and later is always a pathological sign. The same applies to reflex crawling. Moro's reflex likewise disappears at the end of the third month. If, during the first 3 months, Moro's reflex can be elicited very easily by any environmental stimulus, e.g. simple contact, a slow change in position, a weak acoustic stimulus, etc., we regard this as a sign of hyperexcitability of the CNS.

In the traction test, we evaluate the way in which the infant holds its head and limbs. In the first 3 months its head drops back, or is in line with its trunk, its upper limbs are held semi-extended and its lower limbs are flexed. At the end of the second trimester, the infant already pulls itself up into a sitting position, with its head anteflexed and its upper and lower limbs synergically flexed. In hypertonia syndromes, at the end of the first trimester, instead of flexion of the lower limbs we find extension and adduction; the trunk and neck are sometimes also extended and when passively raised to a sitting position the infant braces itself opisthotonically on its heels and lifts itself "en bloc". In the first and second trimester, we evaluate extension of the lower limbs, with adduction of the thighs, as a sign of pathological development of motility.

At the end of the first trimester we pay attention to symmetrical holding of the head. In the second trimester, we regard persistent preferential holding of the head to one side as a sign of retarded motor development. The same applies to fist-clenching, with the thumb adducted in the palm. Towards the end of the second trimester, the upper limb grasp reflex starts to disappear and is gradually replaced by voluntary grasping.

At the end of the second trimester, the infant, if placed in the prone position, must be able to support itself on its extended elbows and open hands. Absence of these motor abilities is a sign of impaired development of motility.

When studying an infant's motor development, we must also look for a hemi-syndrome. This means that we determine delayed development or pathological responses in provoked motility in only one limb, or in both limbs on the same side. Examples of this are a weaker response by one upper limb in Moro's reflex, unilateral persistence of fist-clenching, or stereotypic use of one side when rolling over on to the side or into the prone position (the affected limbs are those which remain underneath during rolling). The spontaneous motility of the affected limbs is poorer. In afflicted infants, in the second trimester we still find asymmetrical extension of the neck in the prone position. Parents often draw our attention to premature dominance of one upper limb, i.e. the healthy one, although infants are generally held to be "ambidextrous" up to the end of their first year.

Careful observation of spontaneous motor activity, evaluation of posture, examination of extensibility and the evaluation of reflex responses to a change in the postural situation will help us to determine certain anomalies even during the first and second trimester in infants with suspected CNS damage. They do not allow us to express a definite opinion on the size and extent of the injury, or on its further development and prognosis, but they do enable us to detect an infant with impaired motility and to institute early and timely specific rehabilitation therapy.

DEVELOPMENT OF MOTILITY AND ITS STIMULATION IN INFANTS WITH PERINATAL CNS INJURY

Movement is a fundamental property of matter. The movement of living matter is controlled. In the lowest organisms, movement is a reaction to chemical and other changes in the external and internal environment. In more highly organized animals, including man, it is controlled by the nervous system. As the nervous system continuously improves and matures, both phylogenetically and ontogenetically, the motility of living organisms likewise develops and becomes more intricate. This also applies to man.

In man, motility is completely based on, and develops from, fundamental movement patterns formed progressively throughout prenatal ontogenesis and during subsequent postnatal development. The development of human motility starts in the foetus. The first signs of foetal motility are of reflex origin, i.e. they are responses of the foetus to stimulation from both the external and the internal environment. These reflex responses are important for development of the infant's and adult's whole further voluntary movements. Even in the foetal period, movement is not the movement of single muscles, but already has the character of generally coordinated movement (movement pattern). According to research by Minkowski (1967), Hooker (1967) and Humphrey (1967), foetal motility begins in the $7^1/_2$ week of menstrual age, is of a purely reflex nature and develops as an expression of the functional capacity of "matured" neuromuscular structures. According to Hooker, foetal reflex movement patterns develop in a craniocaudal direction, i.e. motility of the cervical spine appears first and is followed by the thoracic and then the lumbar spine; motility of the upper extremities appears before motility of the lower extremities. Foetal motor reflex movement patterns become the basis for the development of postnatal motor activity.

If we are to be able to determine retardation of motor development in the infant and to recognize signs of pathological motility in infants with pre- and perinatal CNS injury in time, we must know and carefully follow the sequence and manner of the development of motility in the normal, healthy individual. It is extremely important to know the time sequence and way in which the healthy infant learns and performs its first movements, so that we can tell whether and when, in a high risk infant, there is any delay in the onset of individual motor manifestations. A delay in the appearance of righting mechanisms in the infant with CNS injury means that the infant lacks the basic prerequisite postural conditions for the performance of voluntary movements of the trunk and limbs and pathological motor signs start to appear, e.g. in limb movements. Certain elements in the development of the normal infant allow us to assess pathological motor development in an afflicted infant. This gives us an objective criterion for evaluating and determining the level of motor development.

According to Bobath and Bobath (1962), pathological muscular tone is caused by poor control of the postural situation in the individual with CNS injury. The degree to which the individual fails to control the postural development scale determines the development of pathological movement patterns and, at the same time, the development of pathological muscular tone.

If we succeed in assuring correct development of postural functions by rehabilitation, pathological movements need not develop very far in the infant with CNS injury. Consequently, it is very important to diagnose retardation of righting mechanisms in the infant in good time, so as to be able to initiate specific rehabilitation as soon as possible. Following patterns of normal motor development, we try to conduct rehabilitation of the afflicted infant so as to avoid the development of pathological motor stereotypes, which are very resistant to correction once they are fixed.

The modern rehabilitation of motor disturbances caused by perinatal CNS injury is based on findings on normal motor development of the healthy infant. We try to maintain and regulate the sequence of the development of motility in accordance with physiological conditions. We utilize reflex mechanisms present in early infancy as an aid to induce correct movement patterns. In infants with perinatal CNS injury, the gradually maturation of higher CNS structures inhibiting reflex mechanisms is to some extent retarded. We can therefore still utilize these reflex mechanisms in the rehabilitation of infants with CNS injury at a time when they are already inhibited in the healthy infant by interconnection of higher levels of the CNS, which cause them to disappear when these higher controlling structures begin to function.

If we are to be able to diagnose a motor disturbance in infants from high risk pregnancies and to grasp the basic principles of the rehabilitation of infants with a central disturbance of motility, we must take into account the manner in which motility develops in the healthy individual.

The motor activity of the newborn infant is reflex in character. Some neonatal reflexes are simple spinal reflexes, while others are more complicated mechanisms controlled at brain stem level. The newborn infant lies mostly in the supine or side position, with its upper and lower limbs flexed and its fists mainly clenched. It can move its head to one side or the other and often turns its head preferentially to one side. If we pull it up passively to a sitting position, its head drops back, because control of head posture is absent. If placed in the prone position it turns its head to one side, but is incapable of symmetrical extension of its neck, which is the first basic righting mechanism. When rotating its head to the side, the child extends its neck asymmetrically. The spontaneous movements of the newborn infant can be characterized as apparently aimless and uncoordinated movements of the upper and lower limbs. As a rule, the newborn infant does not perform isolated movements with one limb, but its whole body is usually in motion. This stage, which is known as the stage of holokinetic motility, lasts up to the end of the 2nd month of life.

Other manifestations of the newborn infant's motility are of a purely reflex nature, e.g. the sucking, rooting and Moro's reflex and the withdrawal reflex, which is actually brisk triple flexion of the lower limb in response to nociceptive stimulation of the sole. If the infant is held vertically, the walking (stepping) reflex can be elicited by contact of its soles with the examination table. This is reflex complex movement controlled at spinal cord level. Reflex crawling, seen in the prone position, is regarded as a phylogenetically old form of locomotion. It is a very intricate movement pattern involving the newborn infant's whole locomotor system. In most newborn infants we can elicit the tonic neck reflexes described by Magnus and de Klejn, which can be either asymmetrical or symmetrical. Asymmetrical tonic neck reflexes are elicited by passive rotation of the head to one side. This causes increased extensor tone of the limbs on the side to which the face is turned and increased flexor tone on the other side ("fencer" position). Symmetrical tonic neck reflexes are elicited by anteflexion and dorsiflexion of the infant's head. Anteflexion produces increased flexor tone of the upper extremities and increased extensor tone of the lower limbs, while in dorsiflexion the reverse occurs.

Another reflex which can be elicited in the newborn infant is the neck-righting reflex on the trunk. This can be elicited by passive rotation of the head to one side, which causes reflex rotation of the whole trunk to the same side, thereby keeping the body oriented in relation to the head. Similarly, passive rotation of the pelvis causes the trunk and head to rotate to the same side; this is known as the neck-righting reflex on the head. These two reflexes both participate in the further development of motility and induce the infant to turn first on to its side and later to the prone position and back again. In time, these movements lose their reflex character and become voluntary. In voluntary movement the trunk no longer rotates "en masse", however, but the shoulders, trunk and hips rotate successively, accompanied by movements of the upper and lower limbs.

At six weeks, symmetrical extension of the neck begins to appear when the infant is in the prone position, i.e. the infant starts to raise its head. This is the first stage in the motor mechanism of erect posture. It is also an essential stage. If the first link of the postural mechanism is not formed, the infant's whole motility develops in a pathological manner. By the end of the first three months the infant can hold its head symmetrically erect better and longer. Simultaneously, hand-mouth coordination occurs for the first time and the infant begins to put its hand to its mouth. At the end of the first three months, reflex crawling and preferential turning of the head to one side decline and Moro's reflex, the walking reflex and tonic neck reflexes disappear. As predominance of flexor tone diminishes, the infant no longer holds its upper and lower limbs flexed when lying in the supine position. If the head-righting mechanism does not appear by the end of the third month, and if the above reflexes persist, we must take the possibility of motor retardation and of central disturbance of motility into account.

At the beginning of the second trimester the infant is able to rotate its head to both sides and begins to turn over on to its side. If we pull it up into a sitting position, its head no longer drops back, but remains in line with the trunk (better control of head posture). The hands are no longer held so tightly clenched and hand-mouth coordination develops and improves, concurrently with the development of vision. In the prone position, the infant can extend its neck symmetrically and bears its weight on its forearms. Righting mechanisms advance from the neck to the interscapular area. In the upper limbs they shift towards the tip. Flexion of the lower limbs, characteristic for the newborn infant, relaxes and in the prone position the buttocks are at the level with the head, whereas in the newborn infant they are higher than the head, owing to pronounced flexion of the lower limbs.

The ability to turn over from the supine to the prone position develops gradually during the second trimester. This is no longer a reflex mechanism evoked by a neck-righting reflex, but in time it becomes voluntary, i.e. it is already controlled by higher levels of the CNS. The infant at first rotates its head voluntarily to one side and raises it, the shoulder on top is rotated forwards, the free upper limb is swung out and the body is proped on the elbow of the bottom upper limb; simultaneously, rotation of the trunk continues and the top lower limb is crossed over and propped on the knee. We can thus see how complicated it is for even a normally developing infant to turn over to the prone position. It needs complex motor coordination, which is formed during the infant's development. This requires the formation of postural tone, which helps to keep the body erect against the force of gravity. Its first link is extension of the neck.

By the end of the second trimester, righting mechanisms have reached the lumbar spine. In the prone position, the infant supports itself on its extended elbows, with open hands, its head and trunk are held erect and its lower limbs are mildly abducted and propped on the knees. In the upper limbs, the appearance of active grasping is accompanied by disappearance of the grasp reflex. The infant actively pulls itself up into a sitting position, with its head slightly anteflexed and its upper and lower limbs flexed.

In about the 7th month, hand-mouth coordination is replaced by foot-mouth coordination. The infant begins to take an interest in its feet, inspects them and, with the help of its hands, pulls them up to its mouth. If placed in the sitting position, it remains there for a while, at first still with lumbar kyphosis. Balance reactions in the sitting position develop, first of all forwards and at 8 months sideways. The righting mechanism now advances to the lower limbs, to the area of the knees, and the infant gets up on all fours. It begins to crawl, first of all backwards, as a rule, probably because the motor activity of its upper limbs is more advanced at this stage and initiates the movement, so that the infant, bracing itself on its upper limbs, pushes off and its lower limbs take a step backwards. A few days later it also starts to crawl forwards. At 9 months, righting mechanisms reach the tips of the lower limbs and the infant begins to stand up in its cot, holding on to the side. At about 10 months it begins to take steps (with support). One hand is moved sideways along the side of the cot and the lower limbs successively follow. The grasp reflex of the lower limbs also disappears at this stage. In the second half of the fourth trimester, balance reactions in standing are formed and when these are fully developed, at about the end of the 12th month, the infant takes its first independent step.

The development of fine motor activity, i.e. of manipulation, begins in the

6th month with the appearance of voluntary grasping. The infant seizes objects in the ulnar part of its whole palm, with pronation of the forearm. Between the 7th and 8th month it is able, in the prone position, to transfer its weight to one extended upper limb and free the other for manipulation. It is interesting to note that voluntary movements of the individual fingers also appear at this stage, still with the forearm held prone. As ability for supination of the forearm develops, the thumb and index finger acquire the ability to grasp in a more mature manner, with finger-thumb apposition (pincer grasp, "forceps" grasping). At about 10 months the development of grasping is completed by the appearance of mature grasping, with opposition of the thumb and with partial supination of the forearm.

When studying infants born after a high risk pregnancy, every paediatrician ought to evaluate the development of the infant's motor activity through regular examinations. He should instruct the mother to lay the infant, during the first three months, in the prone position regularly, several times a day, gradually prolonging the time. At this stage the infant cannot turn over to the prone position by itself and if it is not placed there the basic head-righting mechanism cannot appear, since motor skills are formed as a result of stimulation from the external environment. Similarly, an infant which does not turn its head to both sides by itself must be trained to do so by tempting it with brightly coloured toys, sounds, light, etc. If the neonatal type of preferential head-holding still persists in the third month, we must try to correct it, as it may cause deformation of the head and sometimes facial asymmetry. Strabismus is often seen in these infants. Furthermore, if the head is rotated to one side for the greater part of the day, asymmetrical tonic neck reflexes result in continued predominance of extensor muscle groups in the limbs on the side to which the face is turned and of flexor muscle groups in the limbs on the occipital side of the head. This leads to asymmetrical distribution of muscular tone in the right and left limbs and to unequal development of motility and may even cause a hemi-syndrome. When studying infants from high risk pregnancies, we found that continued preferential holding of the head to one side at 3 months was very often associated with motor retardation, that development of the head-righting mechanism was delayed, that the infant did not prop itself on its forearms and that the upper and lower limbs were held asymmetrically in both the supine and the prone position. We explained to the mother that rotation of the head to the side opposite to the preferential side must be actively stimulated by means of toys, sounds and light (e.g. by turning the infant, in the cot, towards a light shining from the side opposite to the preferential side). Control examination at 8 months showed that most of these infants had caught up on their motor development and that the posture and motility of the limbs were no longer asymmetrical.

262

Asymmetrical distribution of muscular tone in the limbs likewise leads to asymmetry in further development of motor activity, i.e. in turning over on to the side and to the prone position. The infant begins to turn over mainly on to one particular side. It also grasps objects with only one hand. If we explain to the mother that she can stimulate the infant to turn over on to the other side by placing it on its back, grasping its leg and rotating the pelvis to the unused side by means of the lower limb, she can induce rotation of the trunk and shoulder by means of a head-righting neck reflex. If this is repeated for a few days, the swinging movement of the top upper limb and righting on the elbow of the bottom upper limb will be induced.

If we see poor head control when the infant is pulled into a sitting position, we encourage the mother to perform this exercise. In many infants, its frequent repetition improves the situation. By pulling the infant, in the sitting position, forwards, sideways and obliquely, we train head balance reactions.

The above instructions can be given to mothers in whose infants we find only motor retardation. If retardation persists beyond the second trimester, we usually also find some elements of pathological motor activity. An infant whose righting mechanisms are not properly developed and which thus does not have the postural conditions for normal development of motility, still feels the need for motor expression — first of all with its upper limbs (reaching for objects) and later with its lower limbs. It reacts in this way to the demands of the external and the internal environment, using its imperfect postural abilities to do so. This forms the starting point for the development of pathological motor activity. If we train such individuals in the use of the basic righting mechanisms, we may succeed, after the basic postural situation has been brought under control, in achieving normal development of voluntary movements and in correcting pathological muscular tone in the limbs.

In pathological individuals in whom retarded or defective development of righting and postural mechanisms occurs during ontogenesis, we often find a neonatal type of muscular tone situation. Voluntary movements are effected on a background of coordination mechanisms belonging to tonic neck reflexes and labyrinthine tonic reflexes. Pathological motility develops. In the most severely afflicted infants, the tips of the limbs are completely incapable of movement. The fist remains clenched, the thumb is adducted in the palm and the development of fine motor activity — voluntary grasping — is inhibited.

Infants from high risk pregnancies in whom pathological distribution of muscular tone appears, children with incipient signs of spasticity, markedly hypotonic infants in whom motor stimulation does not succeed in achieving the development of righting mechanisms, even at the beginning of the third trimester, and infants in whom the paediatrician finds manifestations of pathological motility must, of course, be seen by a children's neurologist and sent by him to a qualified physio-therapist specialized in the rehabilitation of motility in children with CNS defects.

The rehabilitation of such children must take the developmental aspect of motility into account. It begins with training in individual elements of motility at the level for which the given individual has the necessary postural conditions. Its aim is to induce and train the whole sequence of righting mechanisms and, when a given postural level has been attained, to start the training of balance mechanisms at this level. When these basic requirements have been fulfilled, but not before, the child is taught the basic elements of voluntary movement at the respective postural level. Today, in Czechoslovakia, we make use of different combinations and modifications of the experiences of Temple Fey (1964) and Bobath and Bobath (1962) in the treatment of central motility disturbances.

The utilization of modern neurophysiological findings and adherence to the basic schemes of normal development of human motility seem to yield the best results in ensuring optimal motor development of a child with CNS injury, which is more frequent in infants from high risk pregnancies. The paediatrician's task is to look among endangered infants for those in whom motor development is retarded or follows a pathological course and to see that they are given early, specific and rational rehabilitation care. If they are detected between the second and third trimester of life, there is real hope that specific rehabilitation will be able to improve their development. The prospects for successful rehabilitation depend on the development of the child's intellect, however. For instance, if the child is seriously mentally defective, the results of even regular physical therapy will be influenced by the degree of the mental disorder.

MINIMAL CEREBRAL DYSFUNCTION
(MINIMAL BRAIN DAMAGE)

Unlike infantile cerebral palsy, which we should be able to diagnose very early because the clinical (especially the motor) signs are already evident in the first year of life, minimal cerebral dysfunction (minimal brain damage), in the opinion of most specialists, cannot be diagnosed until after the 3rd year. Infantile cerebral palsy is often clinically evident from the abnormal motor signs and psychomotor retardation already in the first weeks, and in particularly severe cases from the first days of life, whereas in minimal cerebral dysfunction gross motor development displays practically no striking anomalies and it is therefore much harder to recognize it in the first years.

The term "minimal cerebral dysfunction" (MCD) is mostly employed for impaired or abnormal behaviour and learning difficulties at school. A routine neurological examination shows no marked neurological signs, but a very careful, detailed and specific examination sometimes reveals "minimal" signs.

The adjective "minimal" might lead one to imagine that the trouble is negligible and unimportant, but in fact, the problem is a very serious one. Many authors put the incidence of MCD at 20% of the whole child population. The condition is usually recognized when the child starts attending kindergarten, but often not until he begins attending school. Superficially, these children do not appear to be abnormal and the same demands are made on them as on other schoolchildren. They are unable to cope with all the requirements, however, and further, secondary signs (psychological, emotional, of character, etc.) consequently develop. If the root of the matter is not discovered in time, the sequelae may well become permanent. A late or wrong diagnosis may result in such children developing into anomalous individuals with no inhibitions, with flaws of character, into law-breakers, alcoholics and other "degenerates".

The term MCD can be applied to children of almost average, average or slightly over-average intelligence who display mild to severe learning disabilities and behavioural disturbances associated with functional anomalies of the CNS. The manifestations of these anomalies, which can be combined in varying ways, include disturbances of perception, conceptualization, speech, memory, attention, affectivity and sometimes motor activity. They are thus signs which we also encounter in infantile cerebral palsy, epilepsy, mental backwardness, blindness, deafness, etc. Some authors regard the signs of MCD as being largely genetically determined, others as a manifestation of biochemical disorders or perinatal CNS lesions, or as the outcome of bad education, while often they have to admit that they simply do not know the cause. Sensory deprivation can likewise produce a picture of MCD. In many respects, therefore, it presents aetiological analogies with infantile cerebral palsy. Our authors, who often use the term "mild children's encephalopathy", believe the disease to be organic by nature and to consist in small, scattered, permanent lesions of the brain tissue.

The clinical signs are usually very varied. Most authours give the frequency of the individual characteristics in the following sequence: (1) hyperactivity, (2) perceptual-motor impairment, (3) emotional lability, (4) general coordination defects, (5) attention disorders (short attention span, distractibility, perseveration), (6) impulsiveness, (7) disorders of memory and thinking, (8) specific learning disabilities, with special reference to reading, counting,

265

writing and spelling, (9) disorders of speech and hearing and (10) equivocal neurological signs and EEG irregularity.

Glós (1969) regards the following signs as the commonest:

(1) **Hyperactivity.** This is probably the main sign. The children are unable to sit still and continuously pursue some activity; they play with their fingers, hands or some other part of their body and keep touching objects. Many of them are strikingly talkative, disturb lessons, keep getting up from their seat, etc. This is "situation hyperactivity", i.e. inadequate in the given situation. In addition to hyperactive children we also find hypoactive and bradykinetic children, however.

(2) **Perceptual-motor impairment.** This is caused by disturbances of the visual, auditory and tactile systems. Impairment of visual perception is manifested not only in reduced ability to reproduce drawn images, but also in inability to differentiate the image from the background. Impaired auditory perception is manifested in wrong reactions to sound, in inability to synthesize the acoustic manifestations of speech into meaningful semantic units and consequently in difficulties in speech functions. It is presumed that tactile perception is also impaired, but so far no exact studies are available. Perception disturbances are regarded as one of the main causes of poor progress at school.

(3) **Emotional lability.** The children's mood is unstable (as far as it is possible to speak of stable mood in connection with children at all). They burst into tears too often, e.g. for minor frustrations or conflicts. At other times they are over-excitable and even aggressive. Another group displays extreme passivity. These children are unwontedly "good", obedient, timorous and anxious.

(4) **Impulsivity.** The children react impetuously, without considering and analysing the situation, i.e. unsuitably, incorrectly and disproportionately. Such impulsivity is often a source of conflict situations, so that the children are unpopular and create animosity and hostility round themselves. Antisocial tendencies are an extreme example of this development.

(5) **Disorders of attention and concentration.** The children have a short attention span, are inattentive, unconcentrated and distractable and their interest wanders from one thing to another. Any side stimulus, however weak, readily attracts their attention. They lack perseverance and their performance is consequently below standard. Impaired concentration is further manifested in imperfect capacity for abstract thinking, because concrete stimuli predominate. Disorders of attention also include over-concentration, i.e. "concentrative perseveration", when the children find it hard to turn their attention from a given object in the proper direction rquired by the instantaneous situation.

(6) **Disturbances of thinking and speech.** The children are incapable of thinking in the proper direction and sequence. Their thoughts jump about, precipi-

tately and often illogically. They do not properly comprehend abstract concepts like space and time and in practice they therefore often confuse yesterday with tomorrow, above with below, etc. Their speech is accompanied by agrammatisms and their verbal symbols are inaccurate, often artificial and wrongly constructed. Their articulation is imperfect and arrhythmical. They often stammer.

(7) **Neurological signs.** In some children considered to be afflicted with MCD, a detailed, specific examination will show small, soft or mild "organic" neurological signs. We cannot conclude from their presence whether there is necessarily an anatomical lesion of the CNS, however. For instance, it is well known that a number of "pyramidal" phenomena (especially "irritative") can be provoked in normal, healthy infants and that, during later development, they disappear, in different sequences, at different rates and in an individually different manner. Some of them are still regarded as physiological at about 5 years.

According to Rutter et al. (1970) we should look for "soft" neurological symptoms and signs, e.g. if there are difficulties in distinguishing the right side from the left, for retarded development of speech, perception and coordination and for auxiliary and associated movements, such as mirror movements, etc. Wolfik (1973) divides the signs of MCD into 3 groups.

(1) **Motor disturbances.** Under these he groups physical hyperactivity, clumsiness, impaired coordination of gross motor activity, e.g. in hopping, jumping and ball-throwing, or of fine motor activity, e.g. in writing, tying up shoelaces or putting food to the mouth, disturbances of equilibrium and balancing and, lastly, "minimal" signs of cerebral palsy, such as faint indications of spasticity, ataxia or athetosis.

(2) **Perception difficulties.** Here he includes impaired attention and imperfect perceptional cognitive function, especially visual and auditory (e.g. in figure--background discrimination), which, if not adequately developed, can lead to disturbances of learning how to spell, read, write and count.

(3) **Behavioural disturbances.** He divides these into a) primary, including reduced control of affectivity and impulse, poor tolerance of frustration, disorganization and untidiness, altered reactivity and emotional lability, and b) secondary, which include the psychological overlay produced by constant setbacks in learning tasks at school and inability to keep pace or compete with fellow pupils. The psychological signs are the outward manifestation of an inner feeling of helplessness.

Precise neurological examination requires attentive cooperation on the part of the patient. Since we cannot expect this from the small, inattentive, distrait and unconcentrated children with whom we have to deal in MCD, the examination methods are different from those used for adults.

The most frequent **neurological** signs in MCD are considered to be strabismus or other disturbances of oculomotor innervation, disturbances of associated movements, dysdiadochokinesia, general faulty coordination, clumsiness, lefthandedness or mixed laterality, certain pyramidal signs, choreiform or other types of hyperkinesia, however small their degree, speech disorders, dyslalia and stammering, mild abnormalities in the elicitation of tendon (deep) reflexes and disturbances of symbolic functions.

Some years ago (Vlach et al. 1971) we carried out a neurological examination of a group of 10-year-old children followed up by the Institute for Care of Mother and Child because they were diagnosed at birth as premature and small-for-dates.

Fifty of the children were premature, 30 were small-for-dates at birth and 50 were the controls. We carried out the examination without knowing to which group the respective child belonged. We questioned each on his (her) symptoms and found that only one child suffered from headaches of a vasomotor character and that one was under treatment for epileptic seizures.

The objective neurological examination was standardized. We evaluated the cranial nerve findings, including Chvostek's sign, upper and lower limb reflexes, irritative "pyramidal" phenomena, abdominal reflexes, taxis, idiomuscular excitability, dermographia, spinal (trunk) posture, standing on one leg with closed eyes, hopping on one foot, small combined flexion, diadochokinesia and "muscular tone", i.e. the consistence and extensibility of the muscles and passivity of the limb segments. We also recorded eyelid and finger tremor in Mingazzini's test and "restless static innervation" (Tab. 57).

In 5 groups of phenomena we found a marked difference between the percentual incidence of abnormal responses in the premature and control children, to the detriment of the former. A difference of 100% or only slightly lower was regarded as marked. In this case, a marked difference was found in the group of irritative "pyramidal" phenomena, faulty trunk posture, standing on one leg, hopping on one foot and finger tremor. When we compared the small-for-dates with the control children, we found a markedly higher percentage of abnormal responses in 2 groups of phenomena, to the detriment of the small-for-dates children. In a similar comparison of the premature and small-for-dates children, we found marked differences in 6 groups of phenomena — in 4 to the detriment of the premature children (irritative pyramidal phenomena, spinal posture, standing on one leg and hopping on one foot) and in 2 to the detriment of the small-for-dates children (abdominal reflexes and diadochokinesia) (Tab. 58).

We then divided the children in all 3 groups into 6 subgroups, according to the gravity of the neurological findings: children in whom the neurological findings were **normal,** children with **minor organic findings** (small, scattered

268

Table 57. Phenomena tested

Phenomena groups No.	Phenomena tested	Resultant responses considered to be abnormal
1	Cranial nerves	Labial reflex, fixation nystagmus (5″), 1st degree nystagmus, mild strabismus, weakness of convergence, increased axial reflexes, deafness
2	Chvostek's sign	
3	Upper and lower limb reflexes	Raised (with extended elicitation zone), diminished
4	Irritative "pyramidal" signs	Thumb-chin r., palm-chin r., Hoffmann's r., Juster's sign, Foix-Marie sign, Babinski's sign, Vítek's sign, Rossolimo's reflex, ankle pseudoclonus
5	Taxis (finger-nose, heel-knee)	Inaccurate, not smooth, with small intention tremor before reaching target
6	Abdominal reflexes	Very brisk, depressed, areflexia
7	Idiomuscular excitability	Very pronounced
8	Defective spinal (trunk) posture	Mild scoliosis, flattened spine, excessive lordosis--kyphosis, "angel's wings"
9	Standing on one leg with eyes closed	Less than 5 seconds
10	Hopping on one foot	Less than 4 metres
11	Small combined flexion	Marked elevation of lower limbs
12	Eyelid tremor	
13	Finger tremor	
14	Restless static innervation	Postural restlessness, especially in acral parts of extremities, choreiform of athetoid restlessness, grimacing, choreiform movements of tongue, twitching of muscles or groups of muscles
15	Adiodochokinesia	Limbs and tongue
16	Signs of hypotonia	Lowered muscle consistency, higher extensibility, reduced resistance
17	Vegetative signs	Cutis marmorata, acral parts of extremities cold and sweaty, Marañon's spots, slight cyanosis of acral parts of extremities

signs of "pyramidal", extrapyramidal and taxis involvement), children with **minor organic findings associated with clumsiness** (evaluated from standing and hopping on one leg), children **merely clumsy** in the same respect, i.e.

269

Table 58. Abnormal responses in groups of children examined

Pheno-menon No.	Phenomena tested	Controls		Premature		Small-for-dates	
		number of abnormal responses	%	number of abnormal responses	%	number of abnormal responses	%
1	Cranial nerves	11	22	15	30	3	10
2	Chvostek's sign	25	50	25	50	12	40
3	Reflexes on UL and LL	31	62	26	52	16	53.3
4	Irritative "pyramidal" signs	3	6	15	30	4	13.3
5	Taxis	10	20	13	26	5	16.7
6	Abdominal reflexes	16	32	12	24	13	43.3
7	Idiomuscular excitability	7	14	1	2	–	–
8	Defective spinal posture	6	12	12	24	4	13.3
9	Standing on one leg	5	10	11	22	3	10
10	Hopping on one foot	5	10	12	24	2	6.6
11	Small combined flexion	–	–	1	2	–	–
12	Eyelid tremor	8	16	6	12	1	3.3
13	Finger tremor	6	12	12	24	5	16.7
14	Restless static innervation	17	34	14	28	8	26.7
15	Adiadochokinesia	4	8	4	8	6	20
16	"Hypotonia"	1	2	1	2	–	–
17	Vegetative signs	9	18	8	16	4	13.3

without any other minor organic neurological signs, and children qualifying as cases of manifest **mild children's encephalopathy.** In one child the diagnosis came under the heading **"congenital developmental defects".**

In comparison of the various groups (Tab. 59), it is remarkable that the proportion of children with "soft" organic findings (No. 2+3+4) was approximately the same (about one third – 30%, 30%, 36.6%) in all 3 groups, i.e. premature, small-for-dates and control. Mild children's encephalopathy appeared in the premature group only. It consisted in a very "fruste" hemiparetic, paraparetic and extrapyramidal syndrome and occurred in 4 children. We considered it very interesting that **clumsiness** sometimes accompanied a small organic defect (No. 3) but was otherwise a completely isolated finding (No. 4), independent of other "organic" neurological signs. It occurred in all 3 groups.

We were therefore particularly interested in clumsiness. We found it together with other, minor neurological signs (No. 3), though not in every case (No. 2), so that it cannot automatically be qualified as the outcome of a small organic neurological lesion. In a few clumsy children, we failed to detect any other, even small abnormalities in the objective findings (No. 4), e.g. of the type of minimal cerebellar or vestibular signs. Of the 4 children described as having mild children's encephalopathy, 3 were clumsy.

Clumsiness thus occurred both in children with minor pyramidal and extrapyramidal findings (though not in all) and in children with small cerebellar-

Table 59. Neurological findings in compared groups of children

No.	Neurological findings	Number of children		
		C (control group)	P (premature)	SFD (small-for-dates)
1	Findings normal	35	30	19
2	Minor organic findings	6 ⎤	5 ⎤	6 ⎤
3	Minor organic findings plus clumsiness	6 ⎬ 15 (30%)	9 ⎬ 15 (30%)	4 ⎬ 11 (36.6%)
4	Isolated clumsiness	3 ⎦	1 ⎦	1 ⎦
5	Mild perinatal children's encephalopathy	–	4	–
6	Congenital developmental defects	–	1	–
		50	50	30

-vestibular signs (though again not in all), but also in children without any neurological findings. Clumsiness cannot be diagnosed only by the classic neurological examination technique. Suitable new tests for it will have to be found and it will probably need to be reclassified. It may prove necessary to regard clumsiness unaccompanied by any other neurological findings as a kind of "special" syndrome, since it also occurred in the control group.

The pathophysiology of this isolated clumsiness is unknown. We know from daily practice that there are extremely skilled, dextrous children and children who are the exact opposite, without our being able to discover anything pathological in their history or in the usual objective findings. Considerable individual differences no doubt exist within the limits of what can be regarded as "normal". We have so far virtually no valid standardized norms for different phenomena at different ages. They change with age and from child to child. For instance, anomalous deep muscular reflexes were strikingly frequent in the control group also.

The results showed that the premature children were prognostically the most at risk.

It is extremely important to diagnose MCD in time, by both medical and psychological methods. Proper attention is now being paid to it all over the world and simple screening tests and questionnaires have been elaborated and are already available. Everything is still in the initial stages, of course. The enormous differences in the symptomatology also require differentiation of therapeutic and educational methods and the whole approach must be strictly specialized.

INFANTILE CEREBRAL PALSY

Infantile cerebral palsy (ICP) is a set of clinical syndromes comprising disturbances of motor activity, sensitivity, sensory perception, affectivity, intelligence and character and epileptic seizure manifestations. It is not a nosological unit in the classic meaning of the term. Its aetiology is not uniform, but is very varied, often multifactorial and complex. It is mostly caused by lesions formed in the early phase of ontogenesis and thus belongs to the diseases in whose aetiology high risk pregnancy holds first place, although reliable and definitive determination of which pregnancy risks constitute the main danger for the origination and evolution of ICP and which phase of pregnancy is particularly dangerous is at present impossible. It will no doubt be a long time before the last word is spoken, because clinical diversity and heterogeneity, and hence anatomical differences, will not allow complete detection and explicit definition of all the aetiological factors.

The disturbances are chronic. The course of ICP is usually stationary, because the anatomical lesions do not change essentially, and yet the clinical picture changes during the first years after birth. The time when the disease is diagnosed and the subsequent treatment are naturally very important. If therapy is undertaken early, many secondary defects can be avoided and some disturbances rectified, as the undamaged parts of the young brain are believed to be capable of taking over the function of the injured parts. The development of the brain *per se* plays an important role in the course of the disease, because many areas of the brain do not begin to function properly for some time after birth and a defect in these areas is not necessarily clinically determinable before that. This means that many disturbances may not be clearly evident immediately and/or soon after birth, or even for some months. The clinical manifestations of minor defects may actually take years to appear.

ICP undoubtedly has many aetiological factors. As regards time, **prenatal** factors can be said to include those which influence the germ cell and thus lead to gametopathies, factors acting during the embryonal period and leading to embryopathies and factors causing foetopathies. In addition to harmful factors existing before fusion of the gametes and those acting during pregnancy, there are also **perinatal** and early **postnatal** factors (many authors actually extend the danger period to the first two years). Understandably, prematurity plays an important role. Cerebral anoxia and haemorrhage seem to be of considerable aetiopathogenic significance in ICP. It is thus evident that there is no typical pathomorphological substrate for ICP. Alongside haemorrhage and encephalomalacia, prenatal and postnatal encephalities, meningitis, dysrhaphic states, various congenital malformations such as microgyria, pachygyria, cerebellar malformations, porencephalia, ulegyria, cystic degeneration, circumscribed and diffuse atrophic sclerosis, status mormoratus and different rare morphological pictures are described.

Clinically, the motor defect is usually the most striking in the first months. Sensitivity, sensory and psychological disturbances are not particularly evident in the earliest phase of development. The afflicted infants develop slowly and psychomotor retardation is diagnosed. In forms of ICP characterized mainly by a motor defect, **impaired muscular tone and postural and coordination disturbances** are usually an early feature. They are expressed in abnormal posture and in anomalous verticalization, equilibrium and locomotor abilities. Muscular dystonia, dyskinesia, incoordination and paresis are frequent manifestations.

Muscular tone is maintained reflexly, i.e. it depends both on the relevant afferentation and the function of brain stem and higher tonoregulative centres and on efferentation. During the evolution and maturation of these components (especially the regulative centres), muscular tone changes and the physiological posture and position of the individual segments of the child's body consequently change as well. In pathological developmental situations, the whole scale of tone evolution alters. Muscular tone is differently distributed and the posture and position of the trunk and limbs are consequently also different. As well as these static patterns, postural reflexes and spontaneous movement patterns are affected. Static and dynamic patterns are closely associated, since movement is actually a change of position and, conversely, position represents arrested movement. In addition to retardation or arrest of normal motor development, ICP is therefore generally characterized mainly by the persistence of primitive motor synergies and pathological postural reflexes leading to unusual, incoordinate and even bizarre motor manifestations inhibiting the development of normal forms of movement.

Motor evolution thus does not follow the normal course, in which several stages can be differentiated. Bobath (1966), for instance, distinguishes: (1) a phase in which the infant learns to control head movements, (2) a gradual increase in extensor tone towards an antigravity posture, (3) perfection of balance reflexes of the head, trunk and lower limbs for maintaining equilibrium when sitting, standing and walking, (4) release of the hands for fine, purposive movements, (5) acquisition of the ability to turn on one's own axis and to move the lower and upper limbs alternately when walking. Hines (1940) divides early motor development into two phases: (1) holokinetic and (2) ideokinetic. Lesný (1959) subdivides the ideokinetic phase into 3 periods: monokinetic, dromokinetic and kratikinetic. Some authors divide infant motility simply into reflex and voluntary. In the development of motility, Ingram (1959) distinguishes a 1st flexion stage, a 1st extension stage, a 2nd flexion stage and a 2nd extension stage. Vojta describes (1) a "phylogenetic" stage, or stage of reflex locomotion, (2) a stage of transition from the phylogenetic to the ontogenetic, or of conscious contact with the environment, (3) a stage of preparation for human locomotion and (4) a stage of verticalization and bipedal locomotion.

Each of these classifications is artificial and in many respects forced and incomplete, emphasizing only one part of the facts and omiting many others. Each is subjective and is made to fit the author's aims. The period between the neonatal phase and the stage of erect bipedal locomotion could undoubtedly be divided in some other way. For instance, we could speak of (1) **a phase of primitive reflexes,** (2) **a stage of verticalization and locomotion on all fours** (including turning over from the supine to the prone position and balance reflexes) and (3) **a phase of erect, balanced bipedal standing and walking.**

In ICP, inadequate inhibition by damaged higher centres causes the release or persistence of lower postural reflex mechanisms which, according to Bobath (1966) coexist with muscular hypertonia in spastics and with intermittent dystonia in athetotics. The main released tonic reflex mechanisms are the tonic labyrinthine reflex, tonic neck reflexes (asymmetrical and symmetrical), the supporting reflex, and associated reactions. These **impair the onset and development of righting and equilibrium reflexes.**

Vojta vindicates his locomotor principle in the development of motility. He claims that every locomotor manifestation has 3 basic motor components: postural, righting and phasic, which are coordinated in ontogenesis and develop according to fixed laws. In developmental motor disturbances, all 3 are affected. Their disturbance can be diagnosed soon after birth, in particular from impairment or abnormality of postural reflexes indicative of a **disturbance of central coordination.** Lower brain stem coordination patterns then come to the fore. Spontaneous movements are performed in primitive and stereotype patterns.

In addition to this central motor coordination disturbance, in clinical evaluation and assessment we can use a seemingly simpler sign, such as **muscular tone.** This was studied in detail by André-Thomas (1960) and, from a different aspect, by Ingram (1959). In our examination procedure, after finding motor or psychomotor retardation in an infant we first of all look for its simple, "semeiological" cause and in the first phase of our pathophysiological analysis we emphasize the role of muscular tone in the origination of motor retardation. To put it very simply, we realize that motor retardation is accompanied by abnormal muscular tone and determine and diagnose either muscular hypertonia or hypotonia.

There are various clinical tests by which **hypotonia,** and hence a "floppy" infant can be diagnosed. In the case of **hypertonia,** in clinical practice we differentiate spastic and plastic hypertonia.

We speak of **spastic** hypertonia when a muscle, if stretched, offers springy, elastic resistance, which, in a given phase of stretch, suddenly relaxes. This is known as the clasp-knife sign (phenomenon). In **plastic** hypertonia, flexor tonus usually predominates on both the lower and the upper limbs (as distinct from spasticity, in which, in man, extensor tonus predominates on the lower limbs). In passive stretching, but also in shortening, the muscles offer unchanged, wax-like resistance, which, in general, does not alter throughout the whole range of the movement. If very marked (in the flexors and extensors), this resistance is called muscular rigidity. Sometimes the examiner, during passive stretching, feels staccato resistance (the cogwheel sign).

As already mentioned, there are situations and/or conditions in which the infant is now hypertonic, now hypotonic. Here, alongside hypertonia, we find "central" muscular hypotonia, which can also occur separately, of course. When the abnormal tonus situation has been diagnosed, the diagnosis of ICP is then confirmed by a number of **developmental postural reflexes.**

In Czechoslovakia, many doctors still distinguish 4 **forms** of motor involvement in ICP: a) diparetic, b) hemiparetic, c) hypotonic and d) extrapyramidal. Very often we find mixed forms. The diparetic and hemiparetic form are spastic forms. The former mainly affects the lower limbs, the latter, as a rule, mainly one side, the upper limb being held flexed and the lower limb usually extended. In the hypotonic form, the muscles feel flabby (floppy), the elicitation of reflexes is good, spastic signs are often present and the children are generally of low intelligence. There are several types of extrapyramidal form: choreatic, athetotic, choreoathetotic and rigid. The athetotic form is characterized by muscular hypotonia or dystonia in the first 2 trimesters, by variability of muscular tone and by persistence of primitive and bizzare Moro-like postures and movements. Apart from this simple clinical classification, there are two others which are very well known and internationally recognized. In 1956, the American Academy for Cerebral Palsy named the following types: spastic, athetotic, rigid, atactic, with tremor, atonic, mixed and unclassifiable. In 1958, British authors published the following classification: (1) spastic infantile cerebral palsy, (2) dystonic ICP, (3) choreoathetotic ICP, (4) mixed forms, with signs of all the first three, (5) atactic ICP and (6) atonic diplegia.

For routine clinical practice, the Swedish classification originally elaborated by Hagberg (1972) seems to be more satisfactory. It distinguishes: (1) spastic syndromes (hemiplegia, diplegia and tetraplegia), (2) dyskinetic syndromes (mainly athetotic and mainly dystonic) and (3) ataxic syndromes (congenital ataxia and ataxic diplegia). In 1972, Hagberg added another syndrome, which he called the dysequilibrium syndrome, to the third group. As distinct from ataxia, in which, according to Hagberg, the coordination of voluntary movements is impaired as a result of muscular dyssynergy, in the dysequilibrium syndrome the child is incapable of, or finds difficulty in, maintaining its position and balance owing to impairment of postural reflexes. The Swedish concept of the classification of ICP refuses to recognize the hypotonic form as such and points out that hypotonia is merely a transitional or dominant sign in a given period of earliest postnatal development. It likewise does not recognize a purely cerebellar form. In the dysequilibrium syndrome, Hagberg found cerebellar atrophy and/or hypogenesis in the pneumoencephalogram. Lesný (1972) divides ICP into spastic and nonspastic forms, including the hypotonic, dyskinetic and rigid form among the latter. In addition, in his monograph, he describes symmetrical cerebellar hypogenesis as a separate nosological unit. In our opinion, "symmetrical neocerebellar syndrome" would be a more appropriate term.

For children's neurologists, the classification of ICP could be supplemented by a pathophysiological consideration on the responsible motor **coordination circuits** and by the assumption that the clinical picture and/or syndrome, *en gros*, is chiefly a manifestation of the coordination circuit which still functions relatively sufficiently, or which has been released from higher control. It would be then possible to speak of predominance of manifestations of the spinal coordination circuit, the inferior brain stem circuit, the superior brain stem circuit or the subcortical circuit.

In the past few years, starting in 1970, we have followed up more than 1,000 infants at risk from birth up to the present day. The oldest are now over 3 years old. All were born in the Institute for the Care of Mother and Child. Neurological examinations were carried out in the neonatal period (in the first week after birth) and at the age of exactly 3, 8, 18 and 36 months, in the standardized manner described above. At present, we are able to publish only the results obtained from the processed data from over 700 infants and toddlers followed up from birth to the age of 18 months (Vlach et al. 1974). Significant corrections will be made at the age of 3 years (Tab. 60).

The preliminary results permit a certain degree of optimism. They demonstrate that, among the infants born to our groups of mothers (who were well looked after and treated very thoroughly in the Institute during pregnancy), the majority of those diagnosed as being at risk or endangered very early and given early treatment progressed satisfactorily: the percentage of serious findings (= ICP) is relatively very small, i.e. 1.6% of the whole series at 18 months. The percentage of normal infants rose from the 3rd to the 18th month. The sharp decline in the proportion of slight neurological deviations in the course of time is very impressive. The retardation percentage differs according to aetiology, e.g. in premature infants it decreases, while in others

276

Table 60. Neurological assessment of children at risk (including prematures)

Age Neurol.findings	Newborn (%)	3 months (%)	8 months (%)	18 months (%)
Normal	58.2	42.5	49.9	51.9
Retardation	4.1 (prem.)	25.4	37.2	43.8
Neurol. deviat.	35.3	30.9	11.2	2.7
Serious	2.4	0.7	1.7	1.6
+		0.5		
	100	100	100	100

it increases. At 18 months, retarded infants are recruited mainly from the group with neurological deviations, the percentage of which is by then diminishing. As far as we can tell at present, the percentage of retarded children among the 3-year-old is decreasing and the percentage of normal children is increasing.

As mentioned above, in addition to motor involvement, disturbances of sensitivity, including both superficial and deep and discriminative sensitivity, disturbances of sensory functions, gnosis, praxis, speech, intellect, affectivity, body scheme, finger agnosia, etc. are virtually inseparable parts of the signs of ICP. Small patients can be of low intellingence and hard to educate and can display behavioural disturbances. Epileptic seizures are frequent. Therapy must be instituted very early indeed. Since the treatment is highly specialized and differentiated, it can be entrusted only to qualified specialists.

SUPPLEMENT: SCREENING OF AN INFANT'S PSYCHOMOTOR DEVELOPMENT

The paediatrician encounters delayed motor or psychomotor development relatively often. The sooner such a diagnosis is made, the better the chances for early and successful treatment. Retardation of motor development is a sign of involvement not only of the locomotor system, but also of sensory functions, intellect, the endocrine system, enzymatic regulation, etc. It is a wide problem extending into the spheres of psychology, sociology and economics as well as medicine.

In routine practice, when the paediatrician examines dozens of little children every day, he ought to have at his disposal a small set of examination tests enabling him to diagnose motor or psychomotor retardation in a short time. The same applies to doctors working in clinics for infants from high risk pregnancies.

As a rule, only one test is regarded as a diagnostic screening test, e.g. screening determination of phenylketonuria. On the other hand, there are internationally recognized screening methods covering over 100 data, e.g. the DDST (Denver Developmental Screening Test, 1967), which is an excellent diagnostic instrument precisely for determining psychomotor development. It is relatively laborious and time-consuming, however, and is thus generally unsuitable for daily, routine paediatric practice.

We therefore attempted to give the paediatrician a simpler and shorter battery of tests for determining an infant's psychomotor age. We chose tests which would roughly detect the main features of all the clinically important aspects of development. They are fairly simple and can be learnt without special training, merely by reading the instructions. The examination method is standardized and allows an infant's psychomotor development to be assessed with a fair degree of accuracy in 3 – 5 minutes.

The method stresses the need for natural and unforced examination. Like our neurological examination method, it starts with the infant in the supine position, after which the infant is gently pulled up by the hands into a sitting

278

position; it is then carefully replaced on its back, turned over reflexly into the prone position, raised above the table (horizontal and vertical suspension) and finally placed on its feet (vertical position). Moro's reflex is tested last, because it usually upsets the infant.

The infant can be examined in all the above positions at any age (month) and the findings can be compared. As it develops, its position and its spontaneous, passive and provoked motility alter. It acquires more and more new skills and its mental faculties develop. The method covers the basic aspects of development and includes motor, sensory, speech and adaptive-social tests; it takes development into account.

In the columns for the various months we find simple sketches showing the developmental positions of the head, trunk and limbs. If the head is rotated mainly to one side, the position of the nose is indicated by a tiny line. Black circles for the hands denote a fist, white circles relaxation of the fingers. Completely extended fingers are not drawn in a special manner. The presence of individual components of the test is indicated by ticking off or ringing a plus sign, absence a minus sign. The responses are thus evaluated only as positive or negative, so as to facilitate processing of the results.

EXAMINATION PROCEDURES

Family history

Neurological or other diseases in near and distant relatives.
Disturbances of psychomotor development in members of family.

Personal history

Illnesses of mother prior to pregnancy.
Condition of the mother.
Number of pregnancy.
Course of pregnancy (any infections or contact with infections, toxaemia).
Course and mechanism of labour (delivery).
Birthweight and birth length.
Resuscitation.
Sucking on first days after birth.
Respiratory disturbances or convulsions during neonatal period.

	1 month	2 months	3 months	4 months	5 months	6 months
I. Supine position	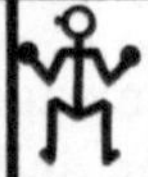 Strab. + – Facial symmetry + – Sym. spont. motility + – Hyperabduc. of LL + – Grasp reflexes + –	Follows with eyes + – Smiles + –	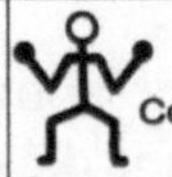 Coos + – Reacts to sound + – (Orientation reflex, or, on contrary, becomes still)	Turns towards sounds + – Plays with hands + –	Reaches for toys + – Puts toy into mouth + –	Finds source of soft sound with eyes + –
II. Sitting position (traction response)	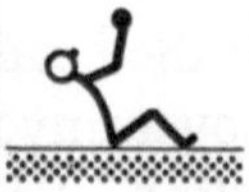		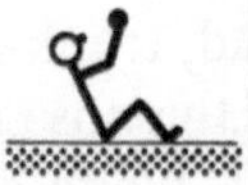			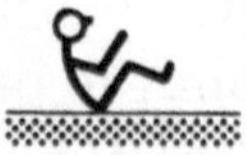
III. Prone position	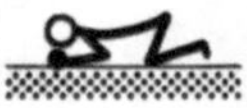	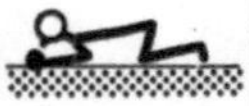	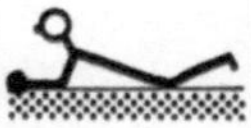			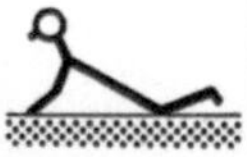 Rolls over on to abdomen + –
IV Horizontal suspension Vertical suspension	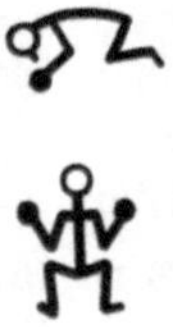		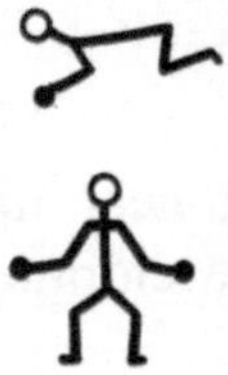			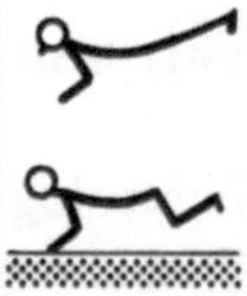 "Parachute" reflex + –
V. Vertical (upright) position	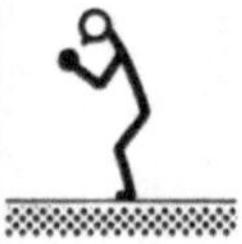 Reflex standing + –		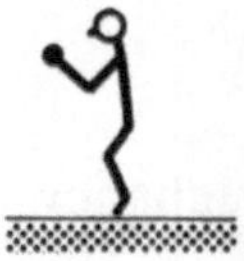	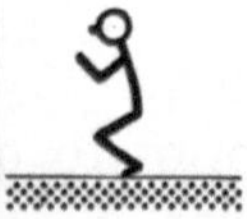 Cannot support body weight + –		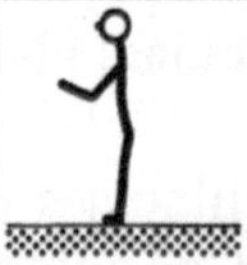 Supports body weight if held under axillae + –
VI. Startle reactions	Moro I, II + – asymetry + –	Moro + –	Moro + –	Moro ∅		

Fig. 26. Screening of psychomotor development (after Vlach, Čiperová and Dolanský).

280

7 months	8 months	9 months	10 months	11 months	12 months
Plays with feet + – Utters syllables + –	Repeats syllables + –	Doubles syllabes + –		Utters one meaningful word + –	Uses at least 2 meaningful words + –
	Sits up unaided + – Eats roll + – Bangs bricks together + – Turns round when name called + –	Pick up button + –	Performs movement when asked (pat - a - cake, bye - bye, etc) + –	Can put cup properly on table + – Throws toys down + – Hands or points to about 3 known objects + –	Picks up bead with finger and thumb (oposition) + –
"Pivoting" position and/or movements + –	Maitains "wheelbarrow" position + – Crawls + –	Crawls on all fours + – "Gliding"		Crawls up on to step or other surface 20 cm high + –	"Landing"
Supports body if held by hands + –	Stands holding side of play - pen + –	Stands up unaided beside furniture + –	Walks round furniture holding on with both hands + –	Walks round furniture holding on with one hand + –	Stands without support + –

Icterus neonatorum.

Any infections, especially if accompanied by pyrexia.

Fits, cramps, seizures, unconsciousness.

Injuries.

Post-vaccination reactions.

Signs of pathological motor development

Pronounced hypotonia:
- "scarf" sign (UL), hyperabduction of LL,
- "armadillo" (anteflexion of trunk) sign (trunk and LL),
- absence of flexion posture of UL and LL in neonatal period.

Pronounced hypertonia:
- persistence of fist-clenching beyond first trimester,
- impaired abduction in hip joints,
- impairment of dorsal flexion in ankle joint (up to at least 90°).

Persistence of preferential turning of head to one side beyond first trimester.

Persistence of neonatal type motility beyond first trimester.

Persistence of tonic neck reflexes after the 4th month ("fencer" posture).

Explanatory notes to Fig. 26

I. SUPINE POSITION

The sketch (1st month) is clear. Strabismus: + = present, − = absent. Facial symmetry: + = face symmetrical, − = any form of asymmetry, including facial nerve paralysis. Spontaneous motility: symmetrical +, otherwise −.

Hyperabduction of lower limbs (LL): + = LL flexed at right angles in hip and knee joint, can be freely (pathologically) abducted until outer surface of knees touches table; ringed − = extent of abduction smaller.

Grasp reflex of upper and lower limbs (UL, LL): + = present, − = absent. All the signs enumerated must be examined in all subsequent months. They are omitted from the table to save space, but it is essential to test them. There is sufficient space in the individual columns to enter them if they are pathological. Only the grasp reflex merits extra remarks. It disappears from the hands during the second trimester and from the feet in the fourth.

The text for the 2nd month needs no explanation.

In the 3rd month we again have a sketch. The head is physiologically already in the median position and the hands are unclenched. The infant reacts to a not very strong acoustic stimulus by heightened attentiveness ("stiffening"), i.e. it responds (orientation reflex), but does not turn in the direction of the source.

The tests for the other months are perfectly clear and require no further comments. The supine position alters, flexion posture of the limbs is progressively relaxed and the hands are unclenched. The infant produces spontaneous movements, so that its posture and position are no longer so constant as in the first three months.

II. SITTING POSITION (traction response)

See sketches. In the 1st month, we slowly pull the infant up by its hands, stopping for a while when its trunk forms an angle of about 60° with the table. We record head, trunk and limbs position. The head drops back, the UL and LL are flexed (the LL more) and the hands are held clenched or grip our fingers. Changes in the 2nd month are small and we have therefore left this space blank, so that the examiner can draw in his own observations. In the 3rd month the head is in line with the trunk, the UL are held semi-extended, the fingers are more relaxed and flexion of the LL is relatively smaller than in the 1st month.

A gradual change occurs, so that at 6 months, when the infant is seated, the head is anteflexed, the infant pulls itself up by its UL (which are thus again flexed) and it grasps our hands voluntarily. The LL are flexed, high above the table. At 9 months, the infant anteflexes its head when sitting up and draws itself up powerfully by its hands, with its LL semi-extended above the table. At 12 months the head and UL behave similarly, but the LL are extended and only slightly above the table. The text does not need any explanation.

III. PRONE POSITION

See sketches. At 1 month the head lies on the table and is rotated to the preferential side, the buttocks are higher than the head and shoulders, the limbs are flexed beneath the trunk and the hands are clenched.

At 2 months the head is occasionally raised (for the time being a trifle asymmetrically) and the limbs, which still remain beneath the trunk, are less flexed.

At 3 months the infant holds its head erect in the median position and braces itself on its forearms; the hands are unclenched and the pelvis rests on the table.

At 6 months the infant supports itself on its open palms, with the UL extended in the elbows. The LL are semi-extended on the table. The head is raised in the median position, at an angle of 90° to the table.

At 7 months the infant, from time to time, raises its body in a concave arch, lifting all its limbs from the table, and sometimes, by means of one of them, turns on the axis passing through the umbilicus, i.e. it pivots.

At 8 months, if we raise the infant's hind quarters as shown in the sketch, it supports itself on its extended UL. When crawling, it moves forwards or backwards, with its abdomen on the table, using all its limbs.

The rest of the sketches and text require no comments.

At 12 months the infant crawls very quickly and nimbly and keeps its balance if deflected.

IV. SUSPENSION

In suspension, the prone infant is raised above the table on our hands, held under the abdomen in the horizontal plane or under its arms (vertically), i.e. it is not hung by its hands. Posture in the 1st month can be seen from the sketch.

At 3 months, when suspended horizontally, the infant already holds its head above trunk level (the first sign of Landau's reflex), the hands are unclenched and flexion of the limbs diminishes. In axillary suspension it holds its head erect.

At 6 months, Landau's reflex is positive – the head and LL are held higher than the trunk, the UL are semi-extended and the hands are unclenched. If the infant is suddenly lowered obliquely from this position, head first, towards the table, it extends its UL and supports itself on its open palms (the "parachute" reflex). In subsequent months Landau's reflex slowly disappears; the head remains higher than the trunk, but the limbs are abducted as if the infant were gliding.

At 12 months, the head remains extended in horizontal suspension; the limbs are likewise extended in the elbows and knees, but they point towards the table as if in readiness for landing.

V. VERTICAL (UPRIGHT) POSITION

At 1 month, reflex standing (positive supporting reflex) can be elicited. If placed on the table so that the whole of its plantae touch the surface, the infant straightens first of all its LL, then its trunk and lastly its head. Its UL are flexed and its hands clenched.

At 3 months we find only traces of this reflex mechanism; the infant stands on its toes and the outer margin of its feet and its hands are unclenched. It can barely carry its weight.

At 4 months reflex standing disappears, the head and trunk are held erect through the influence of a vestibular reflex, the LL are weak – slightly flexed below the trunk – and the feet do not rest on the whole of the sole.

At 6 months, if held under the arms to prevent it from falling, the infant actively stands on its LL, which can now carry the weight of the body. The trunk and head are held erect.

The rest of the sketches do not need explaining.

VI. STARTLE REACTIONS

The last to be tested is Moro's reflex, which disappears at the beginning of the second trimester. We found that we obtained the most satisfactory response if we gripped the infant gently by the thighs or pelvis and suddenly pulled it towards us.

In evaluation we tick off or ring a plus or minus sign, according to whether the respective phenomenon is positive or not. For instance, if the infant, at 6 months, cannot find a sound source in position I, we mark it off as minus and then examine all the phenomena, in the same position, for the 5th or even the 4th month. We may, for example, find that, in the supine position, the infant corresponds developmentally to an infant of 4 months. If its position differs from the one in the sketch, we modify the latter with a red pencil to show how the infant really lies. In subsequent examinations we draw or modify the figures in some other colour.

In this way we can determine, in a relatively short time, whether an infant's psychomotor development is retarded, and to what degree. Premature infants are evaluated not according to their calendar age, but according to their corrected age, i.e. we subtract the number of weeks by which they were born too soon. If, in infants born at term, repeated examination still shows retardation, we call in the relevant specialist (children's neurologist, psychologist, orthopaedist, ophthalmologist, otorhinolaryngologist or phoniatrician). We thus ensure early identification of developmental anomalies ar abnormalities and make it possible to begin therapy and rehabilitation at an age when the undamaged parts of the infant's brain are still capable of taking over the functions of destroyed or injured areas.

REFERENCES

Ahvenainen, E. K., and *Kunnas, M.:* Mortality of premature infants by distance of transportation, place of delivery and urban versus rural origin. Ann. Paediat. Fenn. *9*, 97, 1963.

Acharya, P. T., and *Payne, W. W.:* Blood chemistry of normal fullterm infants in the first 40 hours of life. Arch. Dis. Child. *40*, 430, 1965.

Althabe, O. Jr., Schwarz, R. L., Pose, S. V., Escarcena, L., and *Caldeyro-Barcia, R.:* Effects on fetal heart rate and fetal pO_2 oxygen administration to the mother, Amer. J. Obstet. Gynec. *98*, 858, 1967.

Althabe, O. et al.: Influence of rupture of membranes on compression of the fetal head during labour. In: Perinatal Factors Affecting Human Development, PAHO Scientific Publ. No 185, Washington DC., 143, 1969.

Andreas, H.: Geburtshilfliche Operationen und das retrospektive Schicksal der so geborenen Kinder. Zbl. Gynäk. *81*, 145, 1959.

Asherman, J. G.: Traumatic intra-uterine adhaesions. J. Obstet. Gynaec. Brit. Emp. *57*, 892, 1950.

Avery, M. E.: The lung and its disorders in the newborn infant. Saunders, Philadelphia, 1968.

Babson, S. G., Kangas, J., Joung, N., and *Bramhall, J. L.:* Growth and development of twins of dissimilar size at birth. Pediatrics, *33*, 327, 1964.

Babson, S. G., and *Benson, R. C.:* Primer on prematurity and high-risk pregnancy. Mosby, St. Louis, 1966.

Backmann, A., and *Unnérus, C. E.:* Some factors influencing the rate of prematurity. Acta obstet. gynec. scand. *42*, 211, 1963.

Baillie, E. P., Meehan, A. J., and *Tyack, A. J.:* Treatment of premature labour with orciprenaline. Brit. med. J. *IV*, 154, 1970.

Barnes, A.: Discusion to: *Cannel, D. E.*, and *Vernon, C. P.:* Congenital heart disease and pregnancy. Amer. J. Obstet. Gynec. *85*, 749, 1963.

Baršić, E., Kurjak, A., Latin, V., Telišman, S., and *Polak, J.:* Cigarette smoking in pregnancy: its influence on short and log-term prognosis of perinatal complications. In: Perinatal Medicine, edit. Z. Štembera, Avicenum, Prague/G. Thieme, Stuttgart, 267, 1975.

Baumgarten, K.: Die Wehenhemmung. Praxis (Bern) *58*, 519, 1969.

Baumgarten, K.: Über die Hemmung der Wehentätigkeit bei drohender Frühgeburt. Congr. Danubiensis Primus. Collection of Abstracts, Bratislava, 12, 1970.

Bayley, N.: Manual for the Bayley scales of infant development. Psych. Corp., New York, 1969.

Bärtschi, R., Hüter, J., and *Römer, V. M.:* Der Einfluss von intravenösem Oxytocin, Methyloxytocin und Desaminooxytocin auf die Wehentätigkeit, die fetale Herzfrequenz und das fetale actuelle pH. Geburtsh. u. Frauenheilk. *32*, 826, 1972.

Beard, R. W.: Maternal-fetal acid-base relationships. In: Diagnosis and Treatment of Fetal Disorders. Edit. K. Adamsons, Springer New York, 1968.

Benirschke, K.: Chromosomal studies on abortuses. Trans. New Engl. obstet. gynec. Soc. *17*, 171, 1963.

Berg, D., Kronenberger, G., and *Kubli, F.:* Statistische Untersuchungen zur subpartalen Azidose des Feten. Arch. Gynäk. *209*, 34, 1970.

Berg, D.: Schwangerschaftsberatung und Perinatologie. G. Thieme Verlag, Stuttgart, 1972.

287

Bernard, A., Vaništa, J., and *Prošek, V.:* Infection and noninfection jaundice in the gestation period (in Czech) Čs. Gynek. *32,* 502, 1967.

Bhagwanani, S. G., Fahmy, D., and *Turnbull, A. C.:* Quick determination of amniotic fluid lecithin concentration for prediction of respiratory neonatal distress. Lancet *II,* 66, 1972.

Bienkiewicz, L., and *Kieszkiewicz, T.:* Relation of complicated pregnancy and labor to developmental disorders in children. Int. J. Gynaec. Obstet. *8,* 181, 1970.

Bishop, E. H.: Maternal heart volume and prematurity. J. Amer. med. Ass. *187,* 7, 500, 1964.

Bobath, K., and *Bobath, B.:* An analysis of the development of standing and walking patterns in patients with cerebral palsy. Physiotherapy *48,* 144, 1962.

Bobath, K.: The motor deficit in patients with cerebral palsy. Clinics in Develop. Med. No 23, Spastics Society & Heinemann Med., London, 1966.

Boden, W., and *v. d. Crabben:* Wehenhemmung mit einer neuen beta-adrenergen Substanz. Med. Welt. N. F. *21,* 1342, 1970.

Boensen, I., and *Gudbjerg, C. E.:* Incidence of premature deliveries among women with small heart volumes. Dan. med. Bul., *517,* 234, 1958.

Bolte, A., Bachmann, K. D., and *Kühn, G.:* Die fetalen Herzaktionpotentiale und ihre diagnostische Bedeutung. Arch. Gynäk. *203,* 133, 1966.

Bolte, A. et al.: Kindliche Hirnschäden nach operativen Geburten. Arch. Gynäk. *205,* 110, 1968.

Bolte, A.: Die pränatale fetale Elektrokardiographie. Gynäkologe *2,* 63, 1969.

Bouchalová, M.: Research in dwelling and health conditions in families in Brno (in Czech). Reports of State Population Commission *3,* 51, 1964.

Bozděch, V., Jíra, J., and *Martínek, V.:* Complement fixation reaction in toxoplasmosis (in Czech). Čas. Lék. čes. *100,* 872, 1961.

Bretscher, J.: The micro-analysis of fetal blood samples. In: Perinatal Medicine, edit. P. J. Huntingford, G. Thieme, Stuttgart 122, 1969.

Brosens, I., and *Gordon, H.:* The estimation of maturity by cytological examination of the liquor amnii. J. Obstet. Gynaec. Brit. Cwlth *73,* 88, 1966.

Brown, J. B., and *Beischer, N. A.:* Urinary oestriol excretion as a measure of foetal welfare. Fifth World Congress of Gynaecology and Obstetrics, Edit. C. Wood, Butterworths, Australia, 75, 1967.

Browne, A. D. H.: Optical Amnioscopy. In: Perinatal Medicine. Ist Europ. Congr. Berlin. Stuttgart /New York/ London, G. Thieme Acad. Press. 11, 1969.

Brugger, A. A., Esplugues Requena, J., and *Bedate Alvarez, H.:* Accion espasmolitica uterina de algunos simpaticomimeticos. Acta ginec. (Madr.) *17,* 185, 1966.

Bruns, P. D., and *Taylor, E. S.:* Comparative study of uterine contractility, urinary estrogen-pregnandiol levels and myometrils disappearance time of radioactive sodium in full-term pregnancy and premature delivery. Ann N. Y. Acad. Sci. *75,* 785, 1959.

Brutar, V.: Intraveneous infusion of oxytocin (in Czech). Čs. Gynek. *35,* 102, 1970.

Butler, N. R.: In: Perinatal Mortality. Edit. N. R. Butler and D. G. Bonham. Livingstone, Edinburgh and London, 1963.

Butler, N. R., and *Alberman, E. D.:* In: Perinatal Problems. The Second Report of the 1958 British Perinatal Mortality Survey. Livingstone, Edinburgh and London, 1969.

Butler, L. J., and *Reiss, H. E.:* Antenatal detection of chromosome abnormalities. J. Obstet. Gynaec. Brit. Cwlth, 77, 902, 1970.

Bühler, Ch., and *Hetzer, H.:* Kleinkindertests. J. A. Barth, Leipzig, 1932.

Caldeyro-Barcia, R. et al.: In: Effects of Labor on the Fetus and the Newborn. Pergamon Press, Oxford, 1964.

Caldeyro-Barcia, R., Mendez-Bauer, C., Poseiro, J. J., Escacena, L. A., Pose, S. V., Bienarz, J., Arnt, J., Gulin, L., and *Althabe, O.:* Control of human fetal heart rate during labor. In: The Heart and Circulation in the Newborn and Infant. Edit. D.E. Casseles. Grune & Stratton, New York, 7, 1966.

288

Caldeyro-Barcia, R. et al.: Correlation of intrapartum changes in fetal heart rate with fetal oxygen and acid-base state. In: Diagnosis and Treatment of Fetal Disorders (ed. Adamsons K.) Springer, New York, 1968.

Caldeyro-Barcia, R., Magana, J. M., Castillo, J. B., Poseiro, J. J., Mendez-Bauer, C., Pose, S. V., Escarcena, L., Casacuberta, C., Bustos, J. R., and *Giussi, G.:* A new approach to the treatment of acute intrapartum fetal distress. In: Perinatal Factors Affecting Human Development. PAHO Scientific Publication, Washington DC. No 185, 248, 1969.

Campbell, S., and *Newmann, G. B.:* Growth of the fetal biparietal diameter during normal pregnancy. J. Obstet. Gynaec. Brit. Cwlth *78*, 513, 1971.

Cannel, D. E., and *Vernon, C. P.:* Congenital heart disease and pregnancy. Amer J. Obstet. Gynec. *85*, 744, 1963.

Carr, D. H.: Chromosome studies in spontaneous abortions. Obstet. and Gynec. *26*, 308, 1965.

Carr, D. H.: Chromosome anomalies as cause of spontaneous abortion. Amer. J. Obstet. Gynec. *97*, 283, 1967.

Chard, T.: Human placental lactogen levels as a guide to foetal well-being during pregnancy. The Radio-chemical Centre Ltd. Amersham, Buck, England, Medical Monograph No. 8, 1973.

Cherry, S. H., Kochwa, S., and *Rosenfield, R. E.:* Characteristics of the amniotic fluid proteins in erythroblastosis foetalis. Obstet. and Gynec. *27*, 590, 1966.

Chiladze, Z. A., and *Bujiashvili, C. N.:* The uterine fetus state registration. Int. J. Gynaec. Obstet. 8, 238, 1970.

Churchill, J. A.: The relationship of epilepsy to breech delivery. Electroencephal. Clin. Neurophysiol. *11*, 1, 1959.

Clements, J. A., Platzker, A. C. G., Tierney, D. F., Hobel, C. J., Creasy, R. K., Margolis, A. J., Thibeault, D. W., Tooley, W. H., and *Oh, W.:* Assessment of the risk of the respiratory distress syndrome by a rapid test for surfactant in amniotic fluid. New Engl. J. Med. *286*, 1077, 1973.

Clifford, S. H.: Postmaturity with placental dysfunction. J. Pediat. *44*, 1, 1954.

Cobo, E., and *Kafury, S.:* Inhibición de la contractilidad del utero en la amenaza de parto prematuro, mediante et uso de orciprenalina (Alupent^R^). Informe preliminar. Rev. colomb. Obstet. Ginec. *21*, 111, 1970.

Constane, R., Rust, Th., and *Willi, H.:* Diabetes and pregnancy. Acta diabetol. lat. VIII, 26, 1971.

Cooper, L. Z., Green, R. H., Krugman, S., Giles, J. P., and *Mirick, G. S.:* Neonatal thrombocytopenic purpura and other manifestations of rubella contracted in utero. Amer. J. Dis. Child. *110*, 416, 1965.

Coyle, M. G., and *Walker, J.:* The physical and mental development patterns of school age children whose mothers had oestriol assays performed in pregnancy. Int. J. Gynaec, *8*, 174, 1970.

Crabben, V. D. et al.: The early diagnosis of the placental insufficience by the new dehydroepiandrosteron--sulfate load test to the cardiotocography, placental histology and other methods relating thereto. Acta endocr. (Kbh.) Suppl. *138*, 244, 1969.

Csapo, A. I.: The molecular basis of myometrial function and its disorders. Proc. Int. Congr. Gynec. Obstet. Geneva. 693, 1954.

Csapo, A. I.: The mechanism of myometrial function and its disorders. Modern Trends in Obstetrics and Gynaecology, London, Butterworth & Co. 20, 1955.

Curzen, P., and *Morris, J.:* Heat-stable alkaline phosphatase in maternal serum. J. Obstet. Gynaec. Brit. Cwlth *75*, 151, 1968.

Dawes, G. S.: Foetal and neonatal physiology. Year Book Med. Publ., Chicago, 1968.

Düssler, C. G.: The effect of ACTH on the maternal oestriol excretion pattern in normal pregnancy an in cases of intrauterine foetal death. In: Intrauterine Dangers to the Foetus. Excerpta Medica Monograph, Amsterdam, 280, 1967.

Delaney, J. J., and *Makowski, E. L.:* Management of the pregnant diabetic. Acta diabetol. lat. VIII, 1, 1971.

Diczfalusy, E., and *Lauritzen, Ch.:* Östrogen beim Menschen. Springer, Berlin, 1961.

Dittrich, J. et al.: General developmental neurology (in Czech). Avicenum, Prague, 1971.

Dlhoš, E., and *Raffaj, J.:* Our therapeutical proceeding in prolonged pregnancy (in Czech). Čs. Gynek. *34,* 69, 1969.

Donald, I., and *Brown, T. G.:* Demonstration of tissue interfaces within the body by ultrasonic echo sounding. Brit. J. Radiol. *34,* 539, 1961.

Douglas, C. P. et al.: Investigation into the sugar content of endometrial secretion. J. Obstet. Gynaec. Brit. Cwlth 77, 891, 1970.

Döring, G. K.: Die Übergangsstörungen des Neugeborenen und die Bekämpfung der perinatalen Mortalität. Ed. Ewerbeck. G. Thieme, Stuttgart 1965.

Dráč, P., and *Nekvasilová, Z.:* Premature termination of pregnancy after previous interruption of pregnancy (in Czech). Čs. Gynek. *35,* 332, 1970.

Dudenhausen, J. W., Kynast, G., and *Saling, E.:* The absorption of amino acids via the umbilical cord. In: Perinatal Medicine. Third Europ. Congr. Perinat. Med. Lausanne, Ed. H. Bossart, L. S. Prod'hom. H. Huber, Bern-Stuttgart-Viena, 320, 1972.

Dumermuth, G.: Elektroencephalographie im Kindesalter. Thieme, Stuttgart, 1968.

Duniewicz, M., and *Potužník, V.:* Importance of standardization of agglutination reaction in brucellosis (in Czech). Prakt. Lék. *44,* 466, 1964.

Effer, S. B.: Management of high risk pregnancy. Canad. med. Ass. J. *101,* 55, 1969.

Eggimann, U.: Uterussedation mit dem Vasodilatator Dilydrin. Gynaecologia (Basel), *168,* 476, 1969.

Ehrenfeld, E., Brzezinski, A., Braun, K., Sadowsky, E., and *Sadowsky, A.:* Heart disease in pregnancy. Obstet. and Gynec. *23,* 363, 1964.

Eskes, T. K. A. B.: Abortion and catecholamines. Ned. T. Verlosk. *70,* 465, 1970.

Ezes, H.: Elimination urinaires hormonales et cytologie vaginale au cours des grossesses. Bull. Ass. Gynéc. Obstét. franç. *6,* 137, 1954.

Fay, T.: Some correlation between the appearance of human fetal reflexes and the development of the nervous system. Growth and maturation of the brain. Elsevier, Amsterdam, 93-135, 1964.

Feldstein, M. S., and *Butler, N. R.:* Analysis of factors affecting perinatal mortality, a multivariate statistical approach. Brit. J. prev. soc. Med. *19,* 128, 1965.

Finberg, L.: Dangers to infants caused by changes in osmolal concentration. Pediatrics, *40,* 1031, 1967.

Finnilä, I. J., Tervilä, L., Vartianen, E., Kivalo, J., and *Väyrynen, M.:* The influence of oxygen and vasodilator therapy on uterine blood flow and fetal blood gases. In: Proceedings of XIII Intern. Congress of Pediatrics. Vol. I. Perinatology. Wiener Med. Akad., 51, 1971.

Fischer, W. M.: Untersuchungen zum Säure-Basen-Gleichgewicht im fetalen Blut vor der Geburt. Arch. Gynäk. *200,* 534, 1965.

Fischer, W. M., Halberstadt, E., Rüttgers, H., Berg, D.: Kardiotokografie. G. Thieme Verlag, Stuttgart 1973.

Fischer, W. M.: Fetale Herzfrequenzmuster vor intra- und postpartalem Fruchttod. Arch. Gynäk. *214,* 202, 1973.

Frankenburg, W. K., and *Dodds, J. B.:* The Denver developmental screening test. J. Pediat. *71,* 181, 1967.

Frazier, T. M.: Cigarette smoking and prematurity: a prospective study. Amer. J. Obstet. Gynec. *81,* 988, 1961.

Frazier, T. H.: Research Metodology and Needs in Perinatal Studies. Ch. C. Thomas, Springfield, 1966.

Fuchs, F., Fuchs, A. R., Poblete, V. F., and *Risk, A.:* Effect of alcohol on threatened premature labor. Amer. J. Obstet. Gynec. *99,* 627, 1967.

Gaál, J., Komáromy, B., Mihály, G., Mocsáry, P., Pohanka, Ö., and *Surányi, S.:* The continuous and synchronous recording of foetal acid-base balance and foetal heart rate during delivery. In: Intra-uterine Dangers to the Foetus. Edit. J. Horský and Z. K. Štembera, Excerpta Medica Foundation, Amsterdam, 361, 1967.

Gamissans, O., Esteban-Altirriba, J., and *Gómez, S.:* Estudio de la accion uteroinhibidora de un nuevo β--adrenergico derivado de la orciprenalina en clinica obstetrica. Acta ginec. (Madr.) *19,* 445, 1968.

Garrow, J. S.: Radioactive selenomethionine uptake test as a measure of intrauterine growth rate. Int. J. Gynaec. Obstet. *8,* 140, 1970.

Gazárek, F., Skácel, K., Podivínský, R., Lhoták, J., Sklenářová, L., Lubušský, D., and *Křikal, Z.:* Influencing the acid-base equilibrium of mother and foetus (in Czech). Čs. Gynek. *34,* 543, 1969.

Gazárek, F., Skácel, K., and *Křikal, Z.:* Use of intravenous infusion of oxytocine for induction and in course of labour (in Czech). Čs. Gynek. *35,* 97, 1970.

Gesell, A., and *Amatruda, C. S.:* Developmental diagnosis. P. B. Hoeber Inc., New York, 1947.

Glós, J.: Minimal cerebral dysfunction in children (in Slovak). Psychol. Patopsychol. Dieťaťa *4/4,* 335, 1969.

Gluck, L., Kulowich, M. V., Borer, R. C. Jr., Brenner, P. H., Anderson, G. G., and *Spellacy, W. N.:* The diagnosis of the respiratory distress syndrome (RDS) by amniocentesis. Amer. J. Obstet. Gynec. *109,* 440, 1971.

Gold, É. M.: Identification of the high-risk fetus. Clin. Obstet. Gynec. *11,* 1069, 1968.

Goodwin, J. W., Dunne, J. T., and *Thomas, B. W.:* Antepartum identification of the fetus at risk. Canad. med. Ass. J. *101,* 458, 1969.

Graffar, M.: Une méthode de classification sociale des échantillons de population. Courrier CIE *6,* 455, 1956.

Greene, J. W. Jr., Duhring, J., Smith, K.: Placental function tests. Amer. J. Obstet. Gynec. *92,* 1030, 1965.

Gutwirth, J., and *Machová, J.:* Investigation of prematurely born children in school age (in Czech). Čs. Gynek. *37,* 225, 1972.

Hagberg, B., Sanner, G., and *Steen, M.:* The dysequilibrium syndrome in cerebral palsy. Acta paed. scand., suppl. No 226, 1972.

Hammacher, K.: Neue Methode zur selektiven Registrierung der fetalen Herzschlagfrequenz. Geburtsh. u. Frauenheilk. *22,* 1542, 1962.

Hammacher, K.: Früherkennung intrauteriner Gefahrenzustände durch Elektrokardiographie und Tokographie. In: Die Prophylaxe frühkindlicher Hirnschäden. Ed. R. Elert und K. A. Hüter, Thieme, Stuttgart, 1966.

Hardy, J. B.: Viral infection in pregnancy: A review. Amer. J. Obstet. Gynec. *93,* 1052, 1965.

Havránek, F., Dyková, H., and *Tichý, M.:* The fate of pregnant women treated for sterility (in Czech). Čs. Gynek. *32,* 269, 1967.

Heinrich, J.: Zur Problematik der elektronischen Geburtsüberwachung auf grundlage der direkten fetalen Elektrokardiographie. International Symposium in Medical Electronics. ČVTS Ostrava 1970.

Hellman, L. M. and *Filistr, L. P.:* Analysis of atropine test for placental transfer in gravidas with toxemia and diabetes. Amer. J. Obstet. Gynec. *91,* 797, 1965.

Henderson, M., Entwisle, G., and *Tayback, M.:* Bacteriuria and pregnancy outcome. Amer. J. publ. Hlth *52,* 1887, 1962.

Hendricks, C. H., Cibils, L. A., Pose, S. V., and *Eskes, T. K.:* The pharmacologic control of excessive uterine activity with isoxsuprine. Amer. J. Obstet. Gynec. *82,* 1064, 1961.

Herre, D. H., Horký, Z., and *Jutzi, E.:* Stoffwechselführung und Geburtsleitung bei 300 Entbindungen diabetischer Schwangeren. IV. Int. Symp. über Diabetesfragen, Karlsburg 1965. Karlsburg, Institut für Diabetes, 53, 1966.

Hines, M., and *Boynton, E. P.:* The maturation of excitability in the precentual agens of the young monkey (Macaca mulatta), Pub. Carnegio Inst. *518,* 309, 1940.

Hodari, A. A.: Chronic uterine ischaemia and reversible experimental "toxemia of pregnancy". Amer. J. Obstet. Gynec. *97,* 597, 1967.

Hodr, J., and *Brotánek, V.:* Changes of actography and fetal heart rates in premature deliveries. In: Intrauterine Dangers to the Foetus. Exc. med. Found., Amsterdam, 343, 1967.

Hodr, J.: Uterine activity and metabolism (in Czech). Thesis, Prague 1970.

Hodr, J., Brotánek, V., Štembera, Z. K., and *Jouja, V.:* Changes of biochemical indices after oxytocine and methyloxytocine infusion (in Czech). Čs. Gynek. *35,* 70, 1970.

291

Hodr, J., and *Židovský, J.,* Relation between vaginal cytotypes, monitored foetal-heart sounds and changes of uterine circulation in diagnostics and treatment of placental insufficiency (in Czech). Čs. Gynek. *39,* 360, 1974.

Hofbauer, H.: Die Bedeutung von Fruchtwasseruntersuchungen für die Diagnose und Therapie des Morbus haemolyticus neonatorum. Zbl. Gynäk. *78,* 1707, 1956.

Holley, W. L., and *Churchill, J. A.:* Physical and mental deficits of twinning. In: Perinatal Factors Affecting Human Development. PAHO Scientific Publ. No 185, Washington DC, 24, 1969.

Honn, E. H., and *Wohlgemuth, R.:* The electronic evaluation of fetal heart rate IV. The effect of maternal exercise. Amer. J. Obstet. Gynec. *81,* 361, 1961.

Honn, E. H.: Instrumentation of fetal heart rate and fetal electrocardiography III. Fetal ECG electrodes. Obstet. and Gynec. *30,* 281, 1967.

Honn, E. H.: An atlas of fetal heart rate pattern. Harty Press, New Haven, Conn. 1968.

Hooker, D.: The Prenatal Origin of Behavior. Lawrence, Kansas Press, 1952. cit. Development of normal motor behavior. M. J. Jacobs, Amer. J. Phys. Med. *46,* 41, 1967.

Horák, C., Pačín, J., and *Dovala, F.:* Our therapeutical proceeding in prolonged pregnancy (in Czech). Čs. Gynek. *34,* 69, 1969.

Horská, S., Štembera, Z. K., and *Vondráček, J.:* The effect of ATP on the fetus in danger during labour. J. Obstet. Gynaec. Brit. Cwlth 77, 998, 1970.

Horská, S., and *Štembera, Z. K.:* Treatment of hypoxic foetuses by a combination of ATP and O_2 (in Czech). Čs. Gynek. *37,* 322, 1972.

Horský, J., and *Zwinger, A.:* Effect of new gestagens on the fuctional ability of the endometrium in habitual abortion. Com. I. Congr. Obst. Ginec. Bucuresti, 96, 1969.

Horský, J., and *Šabata, V.:* Principles for the induction of labour in prolonged gestation (in Czech). Čs. Gynek. *34,* 75, 1969.

Hradecký, L., Šach, J., and *Špringer, V.:* Fetal electrocardiography (in Czech). Čs. Gynek. *29,* 493, 1964.

Huch, R., Huch, A., and *Lübbers, D. W.:* Transcutaneous measurement of blood P_{O_2} — method and application in perinatal medicine. J. perinat. Med. *1,* 183, 1973.

Hudcovič, A., et al.: Induction of labour in cases of prolonged gestation (in Czech) Čs. Gynek. *34,* 73, 1969.

Hughes, E. C.: The nutritional value of the endometrium for implantation and in habitual abortion. Amer. J. Obstet. Gynec. *59,* 1292, 1950.

Hughes, E. C.: Nutritional physiology of the endometrium. Advances in Obstetrics and Gynecology, Vol. I., Edit. by S. L. and C. C. Marcus, Williams and Wilkins Co., Baltimore, 3, 1967.

Humphrey, T.: Embryology of central nervous system with some correlations with functional development. Ala. J. med. Sci. *1,* 60, 1964, cit. sec Development of normal motor behavior, M. J. Jacobs. Amer. J. phys. Med. *46,* 41, 1967.

Hunscher, H. A., and *Tompkins, W. T.:* The influence of maternal nutrition on the immediate and long-term outcome of pregnancy. Clin. Obstet. Gynec. *13,* 130, 1970.

Hüter, J., Rippert, Ch., and *Meyer, C.:* Wehenhemmung mit welchem Beta Mimetikum (Berotec[R], Ritodrine[R], Dilatol[R]). Geburtsh. u. Frauenheilk. *32,* 97, 1972.

Chamberlain, G.: Brit. J. Hospit. Med. *3,* 556, 1970.

Chan, W. H., Willis, J., and *Woods, J.:* The value of the nile blue sulphate stain in the cytology of the liquor amnii. J. Obstet. Gynaec. Brit. Cwlth *76,* 193, 1969.

Ingram, T. T. S.: Muscle tonus and posture in infancy. Cerebr. Palsy Bull. *5,* 1959.

Ittrich, G.: Eine Methode für die klinische Routinebestimmung der Harnöstrogene. Zbl. Gynäk. *82,* 429, 1960.

Jacobson, L., and *Rooth, G.:* Sodium bicarbonate administration during labour. The effect on the electrolytes and acid-base balance of mother and foetus. In: Intra-uterine Dangers to the Foetus. Edit. J. Horský and Z. K. Štembera. Excerpta Medica Foundation, Amsterdam 471, 1967.

Jacobson, L.: Studies on acid-base and electrolyte components of human foetal and maternal blood during labour. Student litterature, Lund 1970.

Janovský, M. et al.: Die Reaktion der Frühgeborenen und der Säuglinge auf die Natrium- und Volumendepletion. Mschr. Kinderheilk. *118*, 293, 1970.

Joppich, G., and *Schulte, F. J.:* Neurologie des Neugeborenen, Springer, Berlin, 1968.

Josimovich, J. B., and *MacLaren, J. A.:* Presence in the human placenta and term serum of a highly lactogenic substance imunologically related to pituitary growth hormone. Endocrinology *71*, 209, 1962.

Jung, H., and *Niebel, B.:* Der Wehenschmerz unter dem Einfluss von Valium-Roche und die Objektivierbarkeit durch das Algo-Tokogramm. Geburtsh. u. Frauenheilk, *26*, 937, 1966.

Jungmanová, Č.: Reactivity of placental vessels upon methyloxytocin *in vitro* (in Czech). Research report IV/2b, 45, 1974.

Kaiser, E., Werner, P. H., van der Crabben, H., and *Werner, Ch.:* Neuer Hormon-Belastungstest bei Plazenta-Insuffizienz. 7th int. Congr. clin. Chem., Geneva/Evian 1969; Vol 3: Hormones, Lipids and Miscellaneous, Karger, Basel, 6, 1970.

Kapalín, V.: Physical and psychical development of the contemporary generation of Czech children (in Czech). Academia, Prague, 1969.

Kass, E. H.: Bacilluria in pregnancy. Lancet I, 46, 196

Kittrich, M., and *Pospíšil, J.:* Cytological contribution to the diagnosis of loss of amniotic fluid (in Czech). Čs. Gynek. *31*, 325, 1956.

Kittrich, M.: Sectio caesarea in the case of pelvis delivery (in Czech). Čs. Gynek. *35*, 543, 1970.

Kittrich, M.: Estimation of the fetal weight by ultrasound (in Czech). Čs. Gynek. *36*, 588, 1971.

Kittrich, M.: On the determination of fetal maturity from the analysis of the amniotic fluid. Clinician, *36*, 444, 1972.

Knapp, R. C., Shapiro, A., and *Reading, P. E. Jr.:* Maternal heart volume and prematurity. Amer. J. Obstet. Gynec. *105*, 1252, 1969.

Knobloch, H. et al.: A developmental screening inventory for infants. Pediatrics *38*, 1095, 1966.

Kolář, F., Šikýř, M., Popílka, I., and *Kubálková, M.:* Results of prevention and treatment of pregnancies involving health hazards under condition of a small institute (in Czech). Čs. Gynek. *37*, 219, 1972.

Koleta, F.: Justifiability and risk of treatment of the foetal distress in labour by inhalation of concentrated oxygen (in Czech). Čs. Gynek. *33*, 131, 1968.

Koller, Th., and *Leuthardt, F.:* Das quantitative Verhalten der östrogenen Stoffe bei intrauterinem Fruchttod. Zbl. Gynäk. *65*, 1941, 1972.

Kotásek, A.: Late toxaemia (in Czech). 2nd edition, Avicenum, Prague, 1968.

Kotásek, A., Drábková, J., Červenka, J., and *Žák, F.:* Further experiences with analgesia in the management of labour (in Czech). Čs. Gynek. *33*, 215, 1968.

Kotásek, A., Gazárek, F., and *Brutar, V.:* The mortality of mothers in connection with sectio caesarea in the years 1964—1968 in ČSSR (in Czech.) Čs. Gynek. *35*, 513, 1970.

Kouba, K.: On relation of toxoplasmosis to pregnancy (in Czech). Čs. Gynek. *35*, 234, 1970.

Kralert, M., Horská, S., and *Štembera, Z. K.:* The influence of narcosis during sectio caesarea on the metabolic state of foetus (in Czech). Čs. Gynek. *35*, 561, 1970.

Kratochwil, A.: Antenatal diagnosis of the "high-risk" fetus during late pregnancy and labour. In: Perinatal Medicine, edit. Z. Štembera, Avicenum, Prague/G. Thieme, Stuttgart, 32, 1975.

Krátká, L.: Observation of fertility in patients after arteficial interruption of pregnancy (in Czech). Čs. Gynek. *32*, 651, 1976.

Kräubig, H., and *Wolf, H.:* Zur präventiven Behandlung der konnatalen Toxoplasmose. Geburtsh. u. Frauenheilk. *25*, 531, 1965.

Kronus, R., and *Zemanová, M.:* Relation of uterine neck to induction of labour by means of infusion with oxytocine (in Czech). Čs. Gynek. *35*, 106, 1970.

Kubli, F.: Fetale Gefahrenzustände und ihre Diagnose. Thieme, Stuttgart, 1966.

Kubli, F.: The optical evaluation of amniotic fluid. In: Perinatal medicine. 1st Europ. Congr. Berlin. Stuttgart /New York/ London, G. Thieme/Acad. Press, 1969.

Kubli, F. W., Hon, E. H., Khazin, A. F., and *Takemura, H.:* Observations on heart rate and pH in the human fetus during labor. Amer. J. Obstet. Gynec. *104,* 1190, 1969.

Kubli, F.: Measurement of placental function. In: Perinatal Medicine. Edit. P. J. Huntingford, S. Karger London, 23, 1971.

Kubli, F., Rüttgers, H., Haller, U., Bogdan, C., and *Ramzin, M.:* Die antepartale fetale Herzfrequenz. II. Verhalten vom Grundfrequenz, Fluctuation und Dezelerationen bei antepartalem Fruchttod. Z. Guburtsh. Perinat. *176,* 309, 1972.

Larks, S. D., and *Anderson, G. V.:* The abnormal fetal electrocardiogram. Amer. J. Obstet. Gynec. *84,* 1893, 1962.

Larson, S. L., and *Titus, J. L.:* Chromosomes and abortions. Mayo Clin. Proc. *45,* 60, 1970.

Láska, L., and *Kohoutek, M.:* Unsuccessful induction of labour (in Czech). Čs. Gynek. *35,* 110, 1970.

Lauritzen, Ch.: Ausscheidung und Stoffwechsel von DHEA in der normalen und pathologischen Schwangerschaft. In: Das Testosteron − Die Struma. Springer, Berlin, 1968.

Lemberg-Siegfried, S., and *Stamm, O.:* Der Vaginalabstrich am Schwangerschafts-ende und seine diagnostische Verwendung zur Bestimmung des Geburts-termins. Geburtsh. Frauenheilk. *15,* 885, 1955.

Lepage, F., et al.: Insufficiency of the present state of the electronical monitoring of the foetus during labour. Int. J. Gynaec. Obstet. *8,* 172, 1970.

Lesný, I.: Cerebral palsy (in Czech). SZdN Prague, 1959.

Lesný, I.: Cerebral palsy from the neurological point of view (in Czech). Avicenum, Prague 1972.

Liley, A. W.: Liquor amnii analysis in the management of the pregnancy complicated by rhesus sensitization. Amer. J. Obstet. Gynec. *82,* 1359, 1961.

Lindberg, B. B., Nilsson, A., Rooth, G., and *Ylänen, L.:* Estimation of human chorionic somatotropin (HCS) levels during normal pregnancy using a rapid radioimmunoassay. Uppsala J. med. Sci. 77, 129, 1972.

Littlefield, J. W., Milunsky, A., and *Atkins, L.:* Birth defects. Proc. 4th Int. Conf. Vienna, Austria, 2-8 Sept. 1973, p. 221. Exc. med., Int. Congr. Ser. No 310, Amsterdam, 1974.

Loefler, E. E.: Clinical foetal weight prediction. J. Obstet. Gynaec. Brit. Cwlth *74,* 675, 1967.

Loriaux, C.: La thermographie en gynécologie et en obstétrique. Rev. méd. Bruxelles, *28,* 385, 1972.

Ludwig, H.: Mikrocirkulationsstörungen und Diapedeseblutungen im fetalen Gehirn bei Hypoxie. Fortschr. Geburtsh. Gynäk. Bibl. Gynaec. Basel 33, 1968.

Luh, W., and *Brandau, H.:* Enzymologische Studien am normalen menschlichen Endometrium. Z. Geburtsh. Gynäk. *168,* 14, 1967.

Lysgaard, H., and *Lefèvre, H.:* Measurement of uterine circulation whith Xenon[131]. Acta obstet. gynec. scand. *44,* 401, 1965.

Magát, A.: Initial findings in unsuccessful introduction of labours (in Czech). Čs. Gynek. *35,* 109, 1970.

Manzanilla, S. R., Suarez, C. M., Casanova, A. N., and *Maas, E. R.:* Alimentation fetal oral intrauterina. Rev. med. Isste *4,* 625, 1969.

Marx, G. F., and *Greene, N. M.:* Maternal lactate, pyruvate and excess lactate production during labor and delivery. Amer. J. Obstet. Gynec. *90,* 786, 1964.

McDonald, I. A.: Suture of the cervix for inevitable miscarriage. J. Obstet. Gynaec. Brit. Cwlth *64,* 436, 1957.

Messer, R. H.: Heat-stable alkaline phosphatase as an index of placental function. Amer. J. Obstet. Gynec. *98,* 459, 1967.

Méndez-Bauer, C., Arnt, J. C., Gulin, L., Escarcena, L., and *Caldeyro-Barcia, R.:* Relationship between blood pH and heart rate in the human fetus during labor. Amer. J. Obstet. Gynec. *97,* 530, 1967.

Méndez-Bauer, C. et al.: Changes in fetal heart rate associated with acute intrapartum fetal distress. In: Perinatal factors affecting human development. PAHO Scientific Publ. No 185, Washington DC, 178, 1969.

Michalkiewicz, W., Zaremba, Z., Pisarski, T., Volna, M., Konieczny, J., and Kaczmarek, M.: Attempt to assess foetal distress. In: Intra-uterine Dangers to the Foetus, edit. J. Horský and Z. Štembera, Excerpta Medica Foundation, Amsterdam, 283, 1967.

Michel, C. F.: The effect of Dipyridamole on the acid-base status of normal and asphyxiated fetus. Int. J. Gynaec. Obstet. 8, 237, 1970.

Milunsky, A., Littlefield, J. W., Kanfer, J. N.: Prenatal genetic diagnosis. New Engl. J. Med. 24, 1370. 1970.

Millar, D. G., and Neligan, G. A.: The Newcastle maternity survey and survey of child development. J. Obstet. Gynaec. Brit. Cwlth 75, 481, 1968.

Minkowski, M.: Zur Entwicklungsgeschichte, Lokalization und Klinik des Fussohlenreflexes. Schweiz. Arch. Neurol. Psychiat. 13, 475, 1923. cit. sec. Development of normal motor behavior. M. J. Jacobs, Amer. J. phys. Med. 46, 41, 1967.

Minkowski, A., et al.: The assessment of foetal age by examination of the central nervous system. In: Aspects of Prematurity and Dysmaturity. S. Kroese, Leiden, 1968.

Monzon, O. T., Armstrong, D., Pion, R. J., Deigh, R., and Hewitt, W. L.: Bacteriuria during pregnancy. Amer. J. Obstet. Gynec. 85, 511, 1963.

Morris, N., Osborn, S. B., Wright, H. P., and Hart, A.: Effective uterine blood flow during exercise in normal and preeclamptic pregnancies. Lancet II, 481, 1956.

Mosler, K. H.: Klinisch-pharmakologicshe Untersuchungen zur Uterusdynamik. Arzneimittelforsch. 19, 810, 1969.

Mot de E., Muller, G., Irrmann, M., Boog, G., and Gandar, R.: Fetal risk in paracervical block. In: Perinatal Medicine. Edit. P. J. Huntingford; S. Karger, London, 167, 1971.

Moya, F., Morishima, H. O., Shnider, S. M., and James, L. S.: Influence of maternal hyperventilation on the newborn infant. Amer. J. Obstet. Gynaec. 91, 76, 1965.

Nadler, H. L.: Antenatal detection of hereditary disorders. Pediatrics 42, 912, 1968.

Nesbit, R. E. L. Jr., and Aubry, R. H.: High-risk obstetrics. Amer. J. Obstet. Gynec. 103, 972, 1969.

Neumann, H., and Hengst, P.: Behandlung der drohenden Früh- und Fehlgeburt mit Dilatol. Zbl. Gynäk. 93, 849, 1971.

Newman, W., Draid, D., and Wood, C.: Fetal acid-base status I. Relationship between maternal and fetal pCO$_2$. Amer. J. Obstet. Gynec. 97, 43, 1967.

Niswander, K., Friedmann, E. A., and Bayonet-Rivera, N.: Prelabor pelvic score as a predictor of birth weight. Obstet. and Gynec. 29, 256, 1967.

Niswander, K. R., and Berendes, H.: Effect of maternal cardiac disease on the infant. Clin. Obstet. Gynec. 11, 1026, 1968.

Nyirjesy, L.: Relationships between maternal prepregnant weight, low birth weight and perinatal death. J. Gynaec. Obstet. 8, 178, 1790.

Nyklíček, O. et al.: Statistical view on some values in prolonged pregnancies (in Czech). Čs. Gynek. 34, 16, 1969.

Page, E. W.: Pathogenesis and prophylaxis of low birth weights. Clin. Obstet. Gynec. 13, 79, 1970.

Palmer, R. and Laconne, M.: La béance de l'orifice interne, cause d'avortements à réparation? Une observation de déchirure cervico-isthmique réparée chirurgicalement avec gestation à terme consécutive. Gynéc. et Obstét. 47, 905, 1948.

Palmer, R. et al.: L'hystérographie dans l'avortement récidivant. Acta obst. gynec. scand. 44, 126, 1965.

Papiernik-Berkhauer, E., and Kieszkievicz, T.: Prévention de la prématurité. Valeur pronostique du coefficient de risque d'accouchement prématuré (C. R. A. P.) Gynéc. et Obstét. 69, 153, 1970.

Pardi, G., Brambati, B., Dubini, S., Luchetti, D., Polvani, F., and Candiani, G. M.: Analysis of the fetal electrocardiogram by the group averaging technique. In: Perinatal Medicine. Edit. P. J. Huntingford. S. Karger, Longon, 75, 1971.

Parrish, H. M., Rountree, Mary E. L., and Lock, F. R.: Technique and experience with transabdominal amniocentesis in 50 normal patients. Amer. J. Obstet. Gynec. 75, 724, 1958.

295

Pedersen, J., and *Pedersen, L. M.:* Prognosis of the outcome of pregnancies in diabetics. Acta endocr. (Kbh.) *50,* 70, 1965.

Pendleton, H. J.: Fetal heart monitoring. Brit. J. Hosp. Med. *3,* 509, 1970.

Perkin, G. W.: Assessment of reproductive risk in non-pregnant women. Amer. J. Obstet. Gynec. *101,* 709, 1968.

Persianinov, L. S., and *Savelieva, G. M.:* Disturbances in the respiratory functions of foetal blood and their treatment. J. int. Feder. Gynec. Obstet. *6,* 211, 1968.

Pierog, S., Lavery, J. P., and *Faison, J. B.:* Unusual behaviour in the newborn of the out-of-wedlock mother. Int. J. Gynaec. Obstet. *8,* 133, 1970.

Pitkin, R. M., and *Zwirek, S. J.:* Amniotic fluid creatinine. Amer. J. Obstet. Gynec. *98,* 1135, 1967.

Poláček, K.: Unser Verfahren bei der Indikationsstellung zur Austauschtransfusion. Pädiat. Pädol. *1,* 21, 1965.

Poláček, K.: Further experience with the exchange transfusion indication by the bilirubin level (in Czech). Čs. Pediat. *22,* 471, 1967.

Poláček, K., Zwinger, A., and *Vedra, B.:* Antenatal prognosis of haemolytic disease of newborns. Spectro--photometric examination of amniotic fluid (in Czech). Čs. Gynek. *35,* 14, 1970.

Poláček, K.: Tables of birth weights of normal fetuses from the 30th to 42th week of pregnancy (in Czech). Čs. Pediat. *26,* 85, 1971.

Poláček, K., and *Syrovátka, A.:* Wachstum der Kinder mit niedrigem- Geburtsgewicht im Alter von 10 Jahren. Mschr. Kinderheilk. *124,* 1951, 1976.

Pontuch, A., Gazárek, F., and *Dráč, P.:* Perinatal mortality in premature deliveries (in Czech). Čs. Gynek. *29,* 459, 1964.

Poradovský, K., Spišáková, J., Dobayová, I., and *Meszárosová, A.:* Prolonged gestation and endangered foetus (in Czech). Čs. Gynek. *34,* 82, 1969.

Pose, S. V. et al.: Test of foetal tolerance to reduced uterine concentrations for the diagnosis of chronic fetal distress. Int. J. Gynaec. Obstet. *8,* 142, 1970.

Poseiro, J. J., Méndez-Bauer, C., Pose, S. V., and *Caldeyro-Barcia, R.:* Effect of uterine contractions on maternal blood flow through the placenta. In: Perinatal factors affecting human development. Washington, PAHO Scient. Publ. No 185, Washington DC, 161, 1969.

Prát, V., Hatala, M., Beer, O. and *Vágnerová, E.:* Bacteriuria in pregnant women in Prague 4. Analysis of results in 735 women (in Czech). Čs. Gynek. *32,* 727, 1967.

Prechtl, H. F. R., and *Beintema, D.:* The neurological examination of the full-term newborn infant. Clinics in Develop. Med. No 12, Spastics Society & Heinemann, London, 1964.

Prechtl, H. F.: Neurological sequelae of prenatal and perinatal complications. Brit. med. J. *4,* 763, 1967.

Pundel, J. P.: Precis de Colpocytologie Hormonale. Masson, Paris, 1966.

Prindle, R. A., and *Gomez, C. J.:* Identification of maternal risk by the PAHO/WHO system. Official Records of the World Health Organisation, Washington D. C. 1973.

Raboch, J.: Spermiologische Befunde bei wiederholten Schwangerschaftsverlusten. Zbl. Gynäk. *87,* 194, 1965.

Raffaj, J., Tarina, F., Šamšula, M., and *Schmidt, K.:* Oxytocin and disturbed uterine activity (in Czech). Čs. Gynek. *35,* 107, 1970.

Räihä, C. E., Lind, J., and *Johanson, C. E.:* Relation of premature birth to heart volume and Hgb% concentration in women. Ann. paediat. Fenn. *2,* 69, 1956.

Räihä, C. E.: Prevention of perinatal mortality. Intrauterine dangers to the foetus. Exc. med. Found. Amsterdam, 335, 1967.

Renaud, R., Vincendon, G., Boog, G., Brettes, J. P., Schumacher, J. C., Koehl, C., Kirclestetter, L., and *Gandar, R.:* Injections intraamniotiques d'acides aminés dans les cas de malnutrition foetale. J. Gynéc. Obstét. Biol. Reprod. *1,* 231, 1972.

Rendina, G. H., and *Tignanelli, F.*: In: Proceedings of Symposium on Problems of Foetal Distress. Ed. A. Centaro, Picin, Padova, 465, 1967.

Reygaerts, J., Diesche, R.. and *Quevrin, B.*: Epreuves fonctionnelles de la résistance circulatoire du foetus. Bull. Soc. roy. belge Gynéc. Obstét. *30*, 163, 1960.

Rorke, M. J., Davey, D. A., and *Du Toit, H. J.*: Foetal oxygenation during caesarean section. Anesthesia *23*, 585, 1968.

Rooth, G.: Early detection and prevention of foetal acidosis. Lancet *I*, 290, 1964.

Roversi, G. D., and *Canussio, V.*: Neue Aspekte der Diabetes Therapie in der Gravidität. In: Perinatal Medizin, G. Thieme Verlag, Stuttgart, 55, 1972.

Rubowits, F. E. et al.: Habitual abortion: A radiographic technique to demonstrate the incompetent internal os of the cervix. Amer. J. Obstet. Gynec. *66*, 269, 1953.

Russel, J. K., and *Millar, D. G.*: Maternal factors and mental performance in children. In: Perinatal Factors Affecting Human Development. PAHO Scientific Publ. No 185, Washington DC 1969.

Rutter, M., Graham, P., and *Yule, W.*: A neuropsychiatric study in childhood. Clinics in Develop. Med. No 35/36, Spastics Society & Heinemann Med., 1970.

Rüttgers, H., Kubli, F., Haller, V., Bachmann, M., and *Grunder, E.*: Die antepartale fetale Herzfrequenz. I. Verhalten von Grundfrequenz, Fluktuation und Dezelerationen in der ungestörten Schwangerschaft. Z. Geburtsh. Perinat. *176*, 294, 1972.

Šabata, V., Znamenáček, K., Přibylová, H., and *Melichar, V.*: The effect of glucose in the prenatal treatment of small-for-date fetus. Biol. Neonate *22*, 78, 1973.

Saling, E.: Untersuchung des Kindes unter der Geburt durch Blutentnahme am vorangehenden Teil. Zbl. Gynäk. *83*, 1663, 1961.

Saling, E.: Die Amnioskopie, ein neues Verfahren zum Erkennen von Gefahrenzuständen des Feten bei noch stehender Fruchtblase. Geburtsh. u. Frauenheilk. *22*, 830, 1962.

Saling, E.: Die Wirkung einer O_2 – Atmung der Mutter auf die Blutgase und den Säure-Basen-Haushalt des Feten. Geburtsh. u. Frauenheilk. *23*, 528, 1963.

Saling, E.: Das Kind im Bereich der Geburtshilfe. Thieme, Stuttgart, 1966.

Saling, E., and *Schneider, D.*: Biochemical supervision of the foetus during labour. J. Obstet. Gynaec. Brit. Cwlth *74*, 799, 1967.

Saling, E.: Amnioscopy and fetal blood sampling. In: Diagnosis and Treatment of Fetal Disorders. Edit. K. Adamsons, Springer, New York, 141, 1968.

Sapák, K., Sklovská, M., and *Pontuch, A.*: Less known causes of premature labours (in Czech). Čs. Gynek. *29*, 466, 1964.

Schaefer, G., Arditi, L. J., Solomon, H. A., and *Ringland, J. E.*: Congenital heart disease and pregnancy. Clin. Obstet. Gynec. *11*, 1048, 1968.

Schaeffer, A. J., and *Avery, M. E.*: Diseases of the newborn. Saunders W. B., Philadelphia, 1971.

Schmidt-Matthiesen, H.: Histochemische Untersuchungen der Endometrium-Substanz. Acta histochem. (Jena) *13*, 129, 1962.

Schmidt-Matthiesen, H.: Ursachen und therapeutische Ansatzpunkte bei habituelle Aborten. Therapiewoche *18*, 71, 1968.

Schönfeld, V.: The first experiences with spectrophotometric examination of amniotic fluid in Rh-iso--immunized pregnant women (in Czech). Čs. Gynek. *33*, 333, 1968.

Schulte, F. J., Michaelis, R., and *Nolte, R.*: Develop. Med. Child. Neurol. *9*, 511, 1967.

Sciarra, J. J., Kaplan, S. L., and *Grumbach, M. M.*: Localisation of antihuman growth hormone serum within the human placenta: evidence for a human chorionic "growth hormone-prolactin". Nature *199*, 1005, 1963.

Siegel, M., and *Greenberg, M.*: Fetal death, malformation and prematurity after maternal rubella. Results of a prospective study 1949 – 1958. New Engl. J. Med. *262*, 389, 1960.

297

Šikl, O., Mrázek, M., and *Holíková, V.:* Physiologically and pathologically prolonged pregnancy in clinical practice (in Czech). Čs. Gynek. *34,* 8, 1969.

Sinclair, J. C. et al.: Supportive management of the sick neonate. Pediat. Clin. N. A. *17,* 863, 1970.

Sirotný, E. et al.: Contemporary situation of anaesthesia during section caesarea (in Czech). Čs. Gynek. *35,* 557, 1970.

Smyth, C. N.: Der Oxytocin-Empfindlichkeitstest für die Geburtseinleitung. Triangel, 3, 150, 1957/1958.

Soiva, K., and *Salmi, H.:* Phonocardiographic studies of the foetal heart rate. Ann. Chir. gynaec. Fenn *48,* 287, 1959.

Soukup, K., Böswart, J., Bendl, J., Vinšová, N., and *Trnka, V.:* Enzymologic study of prolonged pregnancy (in Czech): Čs. Gynek. *32,* 83, 1967.

Soukup, K., Trnka, V., Hamrová, D., Vinšová, N., and *Bendl, J.:* Evalution of biological readiness for labour (in Czech). Čs. Gynek. *35,* 89, 1970.

Soumar, J. et al.: Die Schilddrüsentätigkeit bei Frauen mit wiederholten Spontangeburten. Z. Geburtsh. Gynäk. *170,* 242, 1969.

Spellacy, W. N., Carlson, K. L., and *Birk, S. A.:* Dynamics of human placental lactogen. Amer. J. Obstet. Gynec. *96,* 1164, 1966.

Spellacy, W. N., Buhi, W. C., Schram, J. D., Birk, S. A., and *McCreary, S. A.:* Control of human chorionic somatomammotrophin levels during pregnancy. Obstet. and Gynaec. 37, 567, 1971.

Srp, B. et al.: Fetal electrocardiography and intrauterine tensometry. International Symposium on Medical Electronics (in Czech). ČVTS, Ostrava, 1970.

Štembera, Z. K.: Einfluss des von der Gebärenden inhalierten Sauerstoffes auf die Frucht- „Sauerstofftest". Arch. Gynäk. *187,* 609, 1956.

Štembera, Z. K., Hodr, J., and *Židovský, J.:* Complex early diagnosis of intrauterine foetal distress. In: Intra-uterine Dangers to the Foetus. Edit. Horský J., Štembera Z. K. Excerpta Medica Foundation, Amsterdam, 373, 1967.

Štembera, Z. K.: Hypoxia of the fetus (in Czech). SZdN Prague, 1967.

Štembera, Z. K.: Fetal tolerance in maternal exercise hypoxia. In: Perinatal factors affecting human development. PAHO Scientific Publ. No 185, Washington DC, 105, 1969.

Štembera, Z. K., and *Horská, S.:* The course of labour and the state of foetus and of newborn infant in prolonged gestation (in Czech). Čs. Gynek. *34,* 91, 1969.

Štembera, Z. K., Horská, S., Hodr, J., and *Janda, J.:* Die Beeinflussung des azidobasischen Gleichgewichtes und der Zirkulation bei der gesunden und hypoxischen Frucht durch Sauerstoffatmung der Mutter. Zbl. Gynäk. 91, 178, 1969.

Štembera, Z. K., and *Znamenáček, K.:* Screening and differentiation of high risk pregnancy (in Czech). Prakt. Lék. (Prague) 50, 874, 1970.

Štembera, Z. K.: The management of fetal distress before and during labour. In: Perinatal Medicine. Edit. P. J. Huntingford. S. Karger, London, 124, 1971.

Štembera, Z. K., Zezuláková, J., and *Znamenáček, K.:* Evaluation of the importance of individual factors of risk pregnancy (in Czech). Čs. Gynek. *37,* 193, 1972.

Štembera, Z. K., and *Horská, S.:* The influence of coiling of the umbilical cord around the neck of the fetus on its gas matabolism and acid-base balance. Biol. neonata *20,* 214, 1972.

Štembera, Z. K.: Timely diagnosis of fetus hypoxia in the first stage of labor defined by auscultation of fetus heart sounds by means of simplified dip II (in Czech). Čs. Gynek. *37,* 150, 1972.

Štembera, Z. K.: Prevention of premature labour by means of Th 1165a (in Czech). Čs. Gynek. *37,* 222, 1972.

Štembera, Z. K., and *Herzmann, J.:* Evaluation of the DHEA − S test as an index of fetoplacental insufficiency. J. perinat. Med. 3, 192, 1973.

Štembera, Z. K.: Temporary improvement of hypoxia of the foetus with Alupent before termination of labour by caesarean section (in Czech). Čs. Gynek. *38,* 666, 1973.

Štembera, Z. K., Zezuláková, J., and *Dittrichová, J.:* Step-test and fetal heart-rate monitoring as a diagnostic means for the prevention of perinatal morbidity. VII. World Congress of Obstetrics and Gynaecology, Moscow, August 12—18, 1973.

Štembera, Z. K., and *Vreclová, S.:* Screening of imminent premature labour by menas of palpation of the cervix uteri (in Czech). Čs. Gynek. *39,* 335, 1974.

Štembera, Z. K.: Actual possibilities considering the decrease of premature labors in ČSSR (in Czech). Čs. Gynek. *39,* 344, 1974.

Štembera, Z. K., Zezuláková, J., Dittrichová, J., and *Znamenáček, K.:* Identification and quantification of high risk factors affecting fetus and newborn. In: Perinatal Medicine, edit. Z. Štembera, Avicenum, Prague/G. Thieme, Stuttgart, 400, 1975.

Stewart, A. M., Webb, J. W., and *Hewitt, D.:* Social medicine studies based on civilian medical board records. Brit. J. prev. soc. Med. *9,* 147, 1955.

Stříbrný, J., Šnaid, V., and *Citterbart, K.:* The problem of protracted pregnancy (in Czech). Čs. Gynek, *34,* 552, 1969.

Šula, F., and *Šilhan, J.:* Haemodynamic changes after oxytocin and methyloxytocin in labour (in Czech). Čs. Gynek. *35,* 74, 1970.

Sureau, C. et al.: L'électrophysiologie utérine. Bull. Féd. Soc. gynéc. obstét. *17,* 79, 1965.

Sweeney, W. J.: Intrauterine synechiae. Obstet. and Gynec. *27,* 284, 1966.

Syrovátka, A. et al.: Dévelopment et morbidité des enfants au cours des trois premières années de la vie en fonction du milieu familial. Courrier CIE, *16,* 517, 1966.

Syrovátka, A., Poláček, K., Melichar, V., and *Zezuláková, J.:* Present condition of children born with a birth-weight of 1000 g or less, today aged over 10 years (in Czech). Čs. Gynek. *37,* 227, 1972.

Takeda, J., Okazaki, T., Shimizu, R., Nakamura, J., Kudo, H., and *Sanfujin, H.:* Prevention and therapy of neonatal asphyxia. Jissal, *18,* 365, 1969.

Teramo, K., and *Widholm, O.:* Studies of the effect of anaesthetics on foetus. Acta obstet. gynec. scand. 46, Supl. 2, 39, 1967.

Teramo, K.: In: Perinatal Medicine. Edit. P. J. Huntingford, G. Thieme, Stuttgart, 13, 1969.

Thomas, A., Chesni, Y., and *Dargassies, Saint-Anne:* The neurological examination of the infant, Spastics Society, London, 1960.

Thorn, I.: Cerebral symptoms in the newborn. Acta paediat. scand. Suppl. *195,* 174, 1969.

Tišer, H., and *Opatrný, E.:* Anamnestic data of perinatally damaged children (in Czech). Prakt. Lék. (Prague) *54,* 449, 1974.

Tosetti, K.: Registrierung pharmakologischer Wirkungen mittels der Herztonkurve am Kinde während der Schwangerschaft. Geburtsh. u. Frauenheilk. *18,* 303, 1958.

Trampuz, V.: Die Rolle der Berufsarbeit der Mutter während der Schwangerschaft in der Pathogenese der Unreife des Neugeborenen. Zbl. Gynäk. *85,* 847, 1963.

Trča, S.: Cigarette smoking in pregnancy and premature delivery. In: Perinatal Medicine, edit. Z. Štembera, Avicenum, Prague/G. Thieme, Stuttgart, 265, 1975.

Turnbull, A. C., and *Anderson, A. B. M.:* Induction of labour. J. Obstet. Gynaec. Brit. Cwlth *75,* 24, 1968.

Ulrich, J., and *Židovský, J.:* The significance of the biological readiness of the organism for the induction of labour in protracted pregnancies (in Czech). Čs. Gynek. *24,* 586, 1959.

Usher, R., Shephard, M., and *Lind, J.:* The blood volume of the newborn infant and placental transfusion. Acta pediat. scand. *52,* 497, 1963.

Vedra, B., and *Pavlíková, E.:* The onset of abnormal weight gain in toxemia of pregnancy. J. Obstet. Gynaec. Brit. Cwlth *76,* 837, 1969.

Vlach, V.: A short outline of neurological examination of the newborn. Čs. Neurol. *27,* 73, 1964.

Vlach, V.: Neurological examination in infancy (in Czech). Čs. Neurol. *31,* 289, 1968.

Vlach, V.: Unconditioned newborn reflexes (in Czech, English summary). SZdN, Prague, 1969.

Vlach, V.: Cerebral palsy (in Czech). Acta Chir. orthop. traum. čech. *33,* 87, 1966.

299

Vlach, V., and *Zezuláková, J.:* Neurological and EEG findings in low birth weight babies at the age of 10 years (in Czech). Čs. Pediat. *26*, 528, 1971.

Vlach, V., and *Čiperová, V.:* Screening test of psychomotoric development of infants (in Czech). Čs. Pediat. *27*, 351, 1972.

Vlach, V., Čiperová, V., and *Zezuláková, J.:* Prospective long-term follow-up study in children at risk. In: Perinatal Medicine, edit. Z. Štembera, Avicenum, Prague/G. Thieme, Stuttgart, 1975.

Vojta, M.: Treatment of toxoplasmosis sequelae with vaccine (in Czech). Čs. Gynek. *34*, 132, 1969.

Wallace, S. J., and *Michie, G. R.:* A follow-up study of infants born to mothers with low oestriol excretion during pregnancy. Lancet, *II*, 560, 1966.

Wallace, H. M.: Factors associated with perinatal mortality and morbidity. Clin. Obstet. Gynec. *13*, 13, 1970.

Watteville, H., Voiet, B., and *Beguin, F.:* Les facteurs médico-sociaux dans l'etiologie de l'accouchement prématuré. Bull Soc. gynéc. obstét. franç. *15*, 174, 1963.

Waxman, S. H. et al.: Cytogenetics of fetal abortions. Pediatrics *39*, 425, 1967.

Weis, Jr. E. H., Bruns, P. D., and *Tylor, E. S.:* A comparative study of the disappearance of radioactive sodium from human uterine muscle in normal and abnormal pregnancy. Amer. J. Obstet. Gynec.*76*, 40, 1958.

Wesselius de Casparis, A., Thiery, M., and *Yo le Sian, A.:* Results of double blind multicentre study with ritodrine in premature labour. Brit. med. J. *3*, 247, 1971.

Whitfield, C. R.: The significance of methods for monitoring the fetal heart rate. In: Perinatal Medicine, edit. P. J. Huntingford, G. Thieme, Stuttgart, 76, 1969.

Wilson, E. W., and *Sill, H. K.:* Identification of the high risk pregnancy by a scoring system, N. Z. med. J. *78*, 437, 1973.

Willerman, L., and *Churchill, J. A.:* Inteligence and birth weight in indentical twins. Child. Develop. *38*, 623, 1969.

Willock, J. et al.: Intrauterine growth assessed by ultrasonic foetal cephalometry. J. Obstet. Gynaec. Brit. Cwlth *74*, 639, 1967.

Winick, M., Velasco, E., and *Rosso, P.:* DNA content of placenta and fetal brain. In: Perinatal factors affecting human development. PAHO Scientific Publ. No 185, Washington DC, 9, 1969.

Wolff, J. A., and *Goodfellow, A. M..* Hematopoesis in premature infants. Pediatrics, *16*, 753, 1955.

Wolff, C. H.: Experimentelle und klinische Untersuchungen zur Therapie der vorzeitigen Wehentätigkeit. Zbl. Gynäk. *90*, 31, 1968.

Wolfik, D.: Minimal brain dysfunction — an approach to treatment. Med. J. Austr. *2*, 601, 1973.

Wood, C.: Use of fetal blood sampling and fetal heart rate monitoring. In: Diagnosis and treatment of fetal disorders, Edit. K. Adamsons, Springer New York, 163, 1968.

Worm, M., and *Jutzi, E.:* Behandlungsergebnisse der von 1952 — 1962 in Karlsburg betreuten diabetischen Schwangeren. IV. Int. Symp. über Diabetesfragen, Karlsburg 1965. Karlsburg, Institut für Diabetes, 45, 1966.

Woyton, J.: Die Beurteilung des Reifegrades der Frucht auf grund der Fruchtwasseruntersuchung. Zbl. Gynäk. *85*, 552, 1963.

Wulf, H., Künzel, W., and *Lehman, V.:* Vergleichende Untersuchungen der aktuellen Blutgase und des Säure-Basen-Status im fetalen und maternen Kapilarblut während der Geburt. Z. Geburtsh. Gynäk. *167*, 113, 1967.

Zander, J.: Die bedrohte Schwangerschaft: Die Behandlung der bedrohten Schwangerschaft. Arch. Gynäk. *204*, 92, 1967.

Židovský, J.: Vaginal cytological changes at the end of normal pregnancy (in Czech). Čs. Gynek. *26*, 280, 1957.

Židovský, J.: Vaginal cytodiagnostics in pregnancy (in Czech). SAV Bratislava 1964.

300

Židovský, J., and *Vedra, B.:* Diagnostic possibilities of colpocytology to prevent the fetal damage in the late gestosis (in Czech). Čs. Gynek. *31,* 718, 1966.

Židovský, J., Vedra, B., Mareš, J., and *Horská, S.:* Cytodiagnostics to the foetus on potential foetal distress from intra-uterine asphyxia. Intrauterine dangers to the foetus. Exc. med. Found. Amsterdam, 291, 1967.

Židovský, J., Hodr, J., Brotánek, V., and *Jungmannová, Č.:* Cytological indices of prognosis of threatening premature labours after therapy with isoxsuprine (in Czech). Čs. Gynek. *35,* 181, 1970.

Židovský, J.: Cytological signs of placental insufficiency in high-risk pregnancies. In: Perinatal Medicine, edit. Z. Štembera, Avicenum, Prague / G. Thieme, Stuttgart, 29, 1975.

Znamenáček, K., and *Jirsová, V.:* Neurological examination of the newborn with CNS trauma (in Czech). Čs. Pediat. *11,* 830, 1956.

Zoltan, J., Kubinyi, J., Fojtha, F., and *Uskerth, J.:* Spätfolgen des Kaiserschnittes für das Kind. Anamnestische Untersuchung geistig zurückgebliebener Kinder. Gynaecologia (Basel) *150,* 280, 1960.

Zuspan, F. P., et al.: Progestational therapy during pregnancy. J. reprod. Med. *3,* 9, 1969.

Zwinger, A., Schönfeld, V., and *Balák, K.:* Der prognostische Wert der Kolpozytologie und des Arborisationsphänomens im Zervikalschleim bei Frauen mit habituellen Fehlgeburten. Gynaecologia (Basel) *166,* 369, 1968.

Zwinger, A., Jirásek, J. E., and *Schönfeld, V.:* Influence of insufficient secretory transformation of endometrium on fertility of women suffering from habitual abortion (in Czech). Čs. Gynek. *34,* 217, 1969.

Zwinger, A., Schönfeld, V., and *Firla, J.:* Preconceptional observation of myometrium factor as a possible cause of habitual abortion in women (in Czech). Čs. Gynek. 34, 405, 1969.

Zwinger, A., Schönfeld, V., Mareš, J., and *Valenta, M.:* Die Applikation eines intrauterinen Antikonzeptionspessars bei der Behandlung der Uterus-Synechien infertiler Frauen. Zbl. Gynäk. *91,* 63, 1969.

Zwinger, A.: Die Bedeutung und pharmakologische Beeinflussung des Myometrium-Faktors bei Frauen mit habituellen Fehlgeburten. Abstr. 2. europ. Sterilitäts-Congr., Dubrovník, 123, 1969.

Zwinger, A., and *Horský, J.:* The importance of metroplasty in treatment of habitual abortion. Com. I. Congr. Ginec., Bucuresti, 97, 1969.

Zwinger, A., Dyková, H., and *Šmeral, P.:* The influence of oxytocin and isoxsuprin on the motility of the nonpregnant uterus in women with habitual abortion. Abstr. Congr. Danub. I., 179, 1970.

Zwinger, A., Šmeral, P., Jirásek, J. E., and *Dyková, H.:* Risk pregnancy in women examined before conception and treated for habitual abortion (in Czech). Čs. Gynek. *37,* 232, 1972.

Zwinger, A., Jirásek, J. E., and *Dyková, H.:* Placental morphology in pregnancies with foetal intrauterine death. Zbornik II, VII. kongr. gin. obst. Jugosl. 313, 1972.

Zwinger, A., Fialová, Z., Jirásek, J. E., and *Dyková, H.:* Preconceptive operative treatment of insufficient uterine neck in women with habitual abortion (in Czech). Čs. Gynek. *38,* 256, 1973.

Zwinger, A., Jirásek, J. E., Dyková, H., and *Šmeral, P.:* Possibilities of hysterography in the diagnosis in women with habitual abortion (in Czech). Čs. Gynek. *39,* 41, 1974.

Zwinger, A., Jirásek, J. E., Michalová, K., Činátl, J., and *Chrz, R.:* Chromosomal aberrations and maldevelopment in habitual spontaneous abortions (in Czech). Čs. Gynek. *41,* 121, 1976.

SUBJECT INDEX